Bionanomaterials

Fundamentals and biomedical applications

Bionanomaterials

Fundamentals and biomedical applications

Edited by
Ravindra Pratap Singh
Department of Biotechnology, Indira Gandhi National Tribal University, Madhya Pradesh, India

Kshitij RB Singh
Department of Chemistry, Govt. V. Y. T. PG. Autonomous College, Chhattisgarh, India

IOP Publishing, Bristol, UK

ISBN 978-0-7503-3767-0 (ebook)
ISBN 978-0-7503-3765-6 (print)
ISBN 978-0-7503-3768-7 (myPrint)
ISBN 978-0-7503-3766-3 (mobi)

DOI 10.1088/978-0-7503-3767-0

Version: 20210601

IOP ebooks

British Library Cataloguing-in-Publication Data: A catalogue record for this book is available from the British Library.

Published by IOP Publishing, wholly owned by The Institute of Physics, London

IOP Publishing, Temple Circus, Temple Way, Bristol, BS1 6HG, UK

US Office: IOP Publishing, Inc., 190 North Independence Mall West, Suite 601, Philadelphia, PA 19106, USA

Dedicated
to those who
care, conserve, protect
but do
not spoil/destroy the beauty
and
unique characteristics
of
Kshit (Earth)
Jal (Water)
Pawak (Fire)
Gagan (Sky)
and
Sameera (Air)

Contents

Preface

Technology is advancing day by day, and the development from applying bulk ointments to the preparation of films and composites to burnt skin is a remarkable example of a journey from microbiology to nanotechnology. The attention and interest towards nanotechnology were mainly derived due to their size, ranging from 1 to 100 nm. The idea of producing nanoscale products is gaining attention due to their capability to mimic the same functions as that of the cell, which is the major driving force in the advancement of nanotechnology in the biomedical fields. The growing demand for science and technology for development in clinical/biomedical, agriculture, and the environment has given rise to nanotechnology, one of the six key enabling technologies (KETs). In 1959, Richard Feynman laid the scientific concept of nanotechnology by quoting 'There is plenty of room at the bottom,' meaning that there is a possibility of material production at the atomic level through direct manipulation. After this, nanotechnology started in the 1970s with the production of materials by reducing their size. The first formal term, 'nanotechnology,' had been introduced by Norio Taniguchi in 1974. The nano-ranged materials show a wide range of specific and peculiar properties, namely optoelectronic, magnetic, mechanical, photoresponsive, catalytic, etc, making them a promising material in various fields.

The potential applications of biological nanomaterials created a new field called bionanotechnology as one of the fundamental and focused sub-disciplines within nanotechnology. Bionanotechnology has also connected the gap among natural sciences and usual remedies by employing nanomaterials' engineering proficiencies. The chemistry of nanostructured material plays an essential role in the multidisciplinary branch of science, including different electronics, biomedical, environmental, and agricultural areas, and they also hold potentiality to play a central role in upcoming research areas. Molecular structures constituting partially/completely constituted biological molecules, namely DNA, RNA, lipids, oligosaccharides, etc at nanoscale dimensions, are known as bionanomaterials. The bionanomaterials show potential applications in various disciplines like physics, mathematics, immunology, biochemistry, chemistry, etc. Owing to their unique properties such as size and biocompatibility, bionanomaterials have found their beneficial role in the field of biology as drug delivery systems, regenerative medicines, biosensors, tissue engineering, etc. To achieve high bio-synergy, the particulate size should be small, and therefore, bionanomaterials are considered the third alternative in the synergistic approach. Due to their unique properties, bionanomaterials have gained a lot of attention in recent years. Further, utilization of bionanomaterials has evolved and is spreading its utility in various fields, affecting humankind directly and indirectly. Moreover, bionanomaterials and their composites can play a key role in uplifting medical complications such as diagnostics and therapeutics; they can also be useful in environmental and agricultural applications. Hence, bionanomaterials and bionanocomposites play a very crucial role in solving problems faced by humanity.

This book, *Bionanomaterials: Fundamentals and biomedical applications*, will be an outstanding collection of reviews based on current research and developments on bionanomaterials' utilization in biomedical applications along with their prospects. Here in this book, we have provided an extensive concept of bionanomaterial classification, properties, and synthesis to help students and professionals better understand bionanomaterials and their biomedical applications. It will also help them understand and address problems faced in the clinical/medical sectors by utilizing bionanomaterials. Moreover, it will serve as a textbook for students and will be of great importance for professionals, scientists, researchers, academicians in this research field.

Aims and scope

This book will help a wide range of readers in the biomedical domain, as it introduces the bionanomaterial concept and will also highlight biomedical applications of bionanomaterials. The major points which this book covers are listed in the facets below.

- Classification, properties, synthesis, and applications of bionanomaterials.
- Biomedical application of bionanomaterials.
- Characterization of bionanomaterials for biosensing applications.
- Bionanocomposite utility in the biomedical domain.
- Bionanomaterials utility in biotechnology and nanobiotechnology.

Ravindra Pratap Singh
Kshitij RB Singh

Acknowledgments

It gives us immense pleasure to acknowledge Professor Shri Prakash Mani Tripathi, Honorable Vice-Chancellor, Indira Gandhi National Tribal University, Amarkantak, India and Professor Ajaya Kumar Singh, Department of Chemistry, Govt. V. Y. T. PG. Autonomous College, Durg, Chhattisgarh, India, for providing constant assistance in all the possible ways. It is also our great pleasure to acknowledge and express our enormous debt to all the contributors who have provided their quality material to prepare this book. We are grateful to our beloved family members (Dr Babita Singh and Aparajita RB Singh), who joyfully supported and stood with us in many hours of our absence to finish this book project. Thanks, are also due to Caroline Mitchell, Robert Trevelyan, and the entire publishing team for their patience and extra care in publishing this book.

Ravindra Pratap Singh
Kshitij RB Singh

Editor biographies

Dr Ravindra Pratap Singh

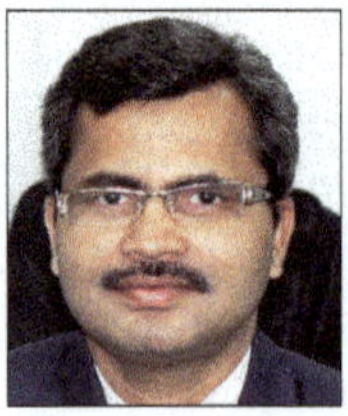

Dr Singh did his BSc from Allahabad University India and his MSc and PhD in Biochemistry from Lucknow University, India. He is currently working as an Assistant Professor in the Department of Biotechnology, Indira Gandhi National Tribal University, Amarkantak M.P. India. He has previously worked as a scientist at various esteemed laboratories globally, namely Sogang University, IGR, Paris, etc. His work and research interests include biochemistry, biosensors, nanobiotechnology, electrochemistry, material sciences, and biosensors applications in biomedical, environmental, agricultural and forensics. He has to his credit several reputed national and international honors/awards. Dr Singh authored over 30 articles in international peer-reviewed journals and more than 20 book chapters of international repute, and he serves as a reviewer of many reputed international journals and is also a member of many international societies. He is currently also involved in editing various books, which will be published in internationally reputed publication houses, namely IOP, CRC Press, Elsevier and Springer Nature. Moreover, he is also appointed as book series editor of "Emerging advances in Bionanotechnology," CRC Press, Taylor and Francis Group and Guest managing editor of Materials Letters, Elsevier, to edit a special issue on "Special Issue on Smart and Intelligent Nanobiosensors: Multidimensional applications".

Mr Kshitij RB Singh

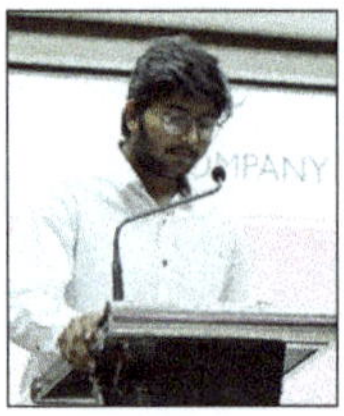

Mr Singh is a Postgraduate in Biotechnology from Indira Gandhi National Tribal University, Amarkantak, Madhya Pradesh, India. He is currently working in the laboratory of Dr Ajaya Singh, Department of Chemistry, Government V.Y.T. PG. Autonomous College Durg, Chhattisgarh, India. He has many publications to his credit and has authored more than ten book chapters published in the internationally reputed press, namely Elsevier, Springer Nature, and CRC Press. He is currently also involved in the editing of books with international publishing houses, including CRC Press, IOP, Elsevier, and Springer Nature. His research interest is in biotechnology, biochemistry, epidemiology, nanotechnology, nanobiotechnology, biosensors, and materials sciences.

Contributors

Isaac Chukwutem Abiodun
Department of Physics, Federal University Otuoke, P.M.B. 126, Yenagoa, Bayelsa State Nigeria

Juliana Bunmi Adetunji
Nutritional and Toxicological Research Laboratory, Department of Biochemistry Sciences, Osun State University, Osogbo, Nigeria

Charles Oluwaseun Adetunji
Applied Microbiology, Biotechnology and Nanotechnology Laboratory, Department of Microbiology, Edo University Iyamho, Nigeria

Uyiosa Osagie Aigbe
Department of Mathematics and Physics, Faculty of Applied Sciences, Cape Peninsula University of Technology, PO Box 1906, Cape Town, South Africa

Semra Akgönüllü
Department of Chemistry, Hacettepe University, Ankara, 06800, Turkey

Osikemekha Anthony Anani
Laboratory of Ecotoxicology and Forensic Biology, Department of Biological Science, Faculty of Science, Edo University, Iyamho, Edo State, Nigeria

Monireh Bakhshpour
Department of Chemistry, Hacettepe University, Ankara, 06800, Turkey

Mamoni Banerjee
Rajendra Mishra school of Engineering and Entrepreneurship, Indian Institute of Technology Kharagpur, Kharagpur, West Bengal, 721302, India

Vinita Bhankar
Department of Biochemistry, Kurukshetra University Kurukshetra, Haryana 136119, India

Ruth Ebunoluwa Bodunrinde
Department of Microbiology, Federal University of Technology Akure, Ondo State, Nigeria

Ayodotun Oluwafemi Bobadoye
Forestry Research Institute of Nigeria (FRIN), P.M.B. 5054, Ibadan, Nigeria

Praveen Kumar Chiruguri
Department of Biotechnology, Vignan's Foundation for Science, Technology & Research, Vadlamudi, Guntur, 522213, India

Adil Denizli
Department of Chemistry, Hacettepe University, Ankara, 06800, Turkey

Santanu dhara
Biomaterials & Tissue Engineering Laboratory, School of Medical Science and Technology, Indian Institute of Technology Kharagpur, Kharagpur, West Bengal, 721302, India

Joseph Onyeka Emegha
Department of Physics, Faculty of Physical Sciences, University of Benin, P.M.B. 1154, Ugbowo, 300283, Benin City, Edo State, Nigeria

Abel Inobeme
Department of Chemistry, Edo University Iyamho, Nigeria

Shikha Kapil
University Institute of Biotechnology, Chandigarh University, Gharuan Mohali, Punjab 140413, India

Vijay Kiran
Department of Chemistry, C.R.A. College, Sonipat, Haryana 131001, India

Krishan Kumar
Physical Chemistry Research Laboratory, Department of Chemistry, D. C. R. University of Science and Technology, Murthal, Sonipat, Haryana 131039, India

Sandeep Kumar
Department of Electrical Engineering, Indian Institute of Technology, Bombay 400076, India

Kalpana Madgula
SAS Nanotechnologies LLC, 550 S College Avenue, Newark, DE 19716, USA

Sadhucharan Mallick
Department of Chemistry, Indira Gandhi National Tribal University, Amarkantak, Madhya Pradesh 484887, India

Padmavati Manchikanti
Plant Metabolic Pathway Laboratory, Rajiv Gandhi school of Intellectual Property and Law, Indian Institute of Technology Kharagpur, Kharagpur, West Bengal, 721302, India

Brij Mohan
School of Science, Harbin Institute of Technology (Shenzhen), Shenzhen 518055, China

Vanya Nayak
Department of Biotechnology, Indira Gandhi National Tribal University, Amarkantak, M.P., India

Godstime Obiajulu Okocha
Department of Science Laboratory Technology, Federal Polytechnic, Auchi, P.B. M. 13, Auchi, 312101, Edo State, Nigeria

Olugbemi T Olaniyan
Laboratory for Reproductive Biology and Developmental Programming, Department of Physiology, Edo University Iyamho, Nigeria

Robert Birundu Onyancha
Department of Physics and Space Science, School of Physical Sciences and Technology, Technical University of Kenya, PO Box 52428—00200, Nairobi, Kenya

Nirmalya Pal
University Institute of Biotechnology, Chandigarh University, Gharuan Mohali, Punjab 140413, India

Jhansi Lakshmi Parimi
Biomaterials & Tissue Engineering Laboratory, School of Medical Science and Technology, Indian Institute of Technology Kharagpur, Kharagpur, West Bengal, 721302, India, and Plant Metabolic Pathway Laboratory, Rajiv Gandhi school of Intellectual Property and Law, Indian Institute of Technology Kharagpur, Kharagpur, West Bengal, 721302, India

Wadzani Dauda Palnam
Crop Science Unit, Department of Agronomy, Federal University, Gashua, Yobe State, Nigeria

Ekta Poonia
Physical Chemistry Research Laboratory, Department of Chemistry, D. C. R. University of Science and Technology, Murthal, Sonipat, Haryana 131039, India

Venkata Sreenivas Puli
Smart Nanomaterials Solutions LLC, Casselberry, Orlando, FL 32707, USA, and Department of Chemistry, Federal University of São Carlos, São Carlos, São Paulo 13565-905, Brazil

Bhavabhuti Prasad
Department of Chemistry, Indira Gandhi National Tribal University, Amarkantak, Madhya Pradesh 484887, India

Narender Ranga
Department of Materials Science and Nanotechnology, D. C. R. University of Science and Technology, Murthal, Sonipat, Haryana 131039, India

Ragavi Rajasekaran
Biomaterials & Tissue Engineering Laboratory, School of Medical Science and Technology, Indian Institute of Technology Kharagpur, Kharagpur, West Bengal, 721302, India and Rajendra Mishra school of Engineering and Entrepreneurship, Indian Institute of Technology Kharagpur, Kharagpur, West Bengal, 721302, India

Jasbir Sangwan
Department of Chemistry, T. D. L. Govt. College for Women, Murthal, Haryana 131027, India

Venkata Sundeep Seesala
Biomaterials & Tissue Engineering Laboratory, School of Medical Science and Technology, Indian Institute of Technology Kharagpur, Kharagpur, West Bengal, 721302, India

Ajay Shankar
Department of Chemistry, Indira Gandhi National Tribal University, Amarkantak, Madhya Pradesh 484887, India

Anand Sharma
Solid State structural Chemistry Unit, Indian Institute of Science, Bangalore 560012, India

Vipasha Sharma
University Institute of Biotechnology, Chandigarh University, Gharuan Mohali, Punjab 140413, India

Ravindra Pratap Singh
Department of Biotechnology, Indira Gandhi National Tribal University, Amarkantak, M.P., India

Kshitij RB Singh
Department of Chemistry, Govt. V. Y. T. PG. Autonomous College, Durg, Chhattisgarh, India

Satya Veer Singh
School of Materials Science and Technology, Indian Institute of Technology (BHU), Varanasi, UP 221005, India

Israel Uzuazor Siloko
Mathematical Statistics/Modelling Unit, Department of Computer Science and Mathematics, Edo University Iyamho, P.B.M. 04, Auchi, 312101, Edo State, Nigeria

Jay Singh
Department of Chemistry, Institute of Science, Banaras Hindu University-Varanasi, UP 221005, India

Jagadish Kumar Suluvoy
Department of Biotechnology, Vignan's Foundation for Science, Technology & Research, Vadlamudi, Guntur, 522213, India

Ankita Vinayak
University Institute of Biotechnology, Chandigarh University, Gharuan Mohali, Punjab 140413, India

Kingsley Eghonghon Ukhurebor
Climatic/Environmental/Telecommunication Unit, Department of Physics, Edo University Iyamho, P.B.M. 04, Auchi, 312101, Edo State, Nigeria

Chapter 1

Introduction to bionanomaterials: an overview

Kshitij RB Singh, Vanya Nayak and Ravindra Pratap Singh

Bionanomaterials are promising materials produced from various biological elements, namely plants, bacteria, fungi, peptides, nucleic acids, etc. Bionanomaterials' utility in the biomedical field has gained them much attention as they are biologically synthesized and biocompatible. Owing to their miniature size, bionanomaterials exhibit extraordinary properties which help them gain potentialities in different domains like aerospace engineering, material science, pharmacology, biosensors, etc. Moreover, to study the properties of the synthesized bionanomaterials, various characterization techniques have been utilized. Hence, this chapter briefly describes the fundamentals of bionanomaterials along with their biomedical applications.

1.1 Introduction

Material at a nanoscale level exhibits unique properties and functions. Nanotechnology is a multidisciplinary subject dealing with nanosized materials (1–100 nm), which has experienced enormous development in the last few decades and has found its profound use in many science domains like biology, robotics, physics, chemistry, materials science, biotechnology, microbiology, etc. The word nanotechnology originates from the Greek word 'nano,' which means one-billionth of a meter and was first used by Norio Taniguchi in 1974. Nanotechnology has efficiently revolutionized the medical field by introducing nanosized particles and materials, which show excellent biocompatibility and low toxicity. The nanosized materials which are synthesized by biological means are known as bionanomaterials. Their extraordinary small size helps them exhibit unique structural, chemical, physical, optical, biological, mechanical, and electrical properties that differentiate them from the bulk matter. These unique properties help them find their diverse roles in the biomedical domain, such as tissue engineering, drug and gene delivery, cancer treatment, neurodegenerative diseases, inflammation, etc. Apart from therapeutics, bionanomaterials are also used in the diagnosis and imaging of various

doi:10.1088/978-0-7503-3767-0ch1

biological compounds that help detect various diseases. Although bionanomaterials are biocompatible, their safety, toxicity, and regulation are still a major concern in both research and market aspects. However, the ongoing research has now become more organized and broadened their research [1].

Bionanomaterial is defined as molecular material composed of partial or non-partial biological molecules like proteins, antibodies, enzymes, nucleic acids, lipids, poly- and oligosaccharides, viruses, secondary metabolites, etc. These can also be utilized to fabricate complex devices through self-assembling in eco-friendly and mild conditions. The objective is to produce one of its kind materials by combining human-made or non-biological material with the natural compound for non-biological use [2]. Therefore, many biodegradable polymers and naturally derived nanomaterials have been extensively used in various biomedical, pharmaceuticals, industrial, packaging, and agriculture fields.

This chapter of this book entitled *Bionanomaterials: Fundamentals and biomedical applications* will highlight bionanomaterial's basic utility in the biomedical domains along with the current trends and prospects. Further, this book will elaborate on bionanomaterial classification, synthesis, properties, and characterization in chapter 2 and chapter 3, followed by chapter 4 about bionanocomposites and their various biomedical domain applications. Furthermore, the fabrication of various biosensors for biomedical utility-based on bionanomaterials is discussed in chapter 5. Chapter 6 will deal with bionanomaterials' emerging role as nanomedicine, followed by chapter 7, which deals with the current bionanomaterials scenario in the biomedical domains for therapeutic utility. Chapter 8 of this book deals with bionanomaterials for tissue implant and regeneration; chapter 9 deals with the molecularly imprinted bionanomaterials for biomedical utility. Finally, chapter 10 deals with the role of bionanomaterials in green bionanotechnology.

1.2 Properties

The properties of a material highly define its applications, and the same is also applied for green synthesized bionanomaterials. Bionanomaterial properties are classified into physical, chemical, biological, mechanical, optical, electric, catalytic properties, etc. These properties are detected using different sophisticated characterization techniques like spectroscopy, microscopy, etc. It has been observed that as the size of the material decreases, the properties of the material are enhanced, and therefore, bionanomaterials are now preferred in every domain these days. The pharmacokinetics and unique properties like shape, size, surface chemistry and properties, and agglomeration state of bionanomaterials make them a suitable candidate for the biomedical domain. These properties decide the role of bionanomaterials like binding with proteins and receptors, drug delivery to the target, transport across epithelial cells, etc [3]. The surface area-by-volume ratio and particle size distribution are the two major relational parameters that are required to study the morphology of synthesized bionanomaterials [4, 5].

The size of the bionanomaterials highly defines their role in the biomedical domain as a smaller-sized particle can easily interact with the body's molecules and help decide the final fate of nanomaterials. Similarly, the mechanical properties of the bionanomaterials help with deciding their role in biomedical applications. The volume, size, and quantum effects of bionanomaterials help them to exhibit commendable mechanical properties. When these bionanoparticles are mixed into a common material, they start refining the grain and form either an intergranular or an intragranular structure, enhancing the grain boundary and increasing the common materials' mechanical properties. For example, when 3% nano palm oil was added to epoxycomposites, it increased their impact strength and tensile strength [6]. Bionanomaterials exhibit potential properties that allow the researcher to explore more about them and explore the their potentialities in the biomedical domain.

1.3 Classification of bionanomaterials

The entry of organic bionanomaterial in the biomedical domain has made them gain much focus, and therefore a sudden increase in their applications in bone or tissue regeneration, the formation of scaffolds, etc. Bionanomaterials should fulfill certain criteria like biodegradability, biocompatibility, and non-toxicity for use of these organic bionanomaterials in the biomedical field [7]. Some organic bionanomaterials include silk fibroin, chitosan, and other biodegradable polymers such as poly(lactic-co-glycolic) acid (PLGA). PLGA is considered as one of the synthetic polymers but, as it shows biocompatible nature, it is now counted under organic bionanomaterial. Silk fibroin is a natural polymer with a large molecular weight obtained from various spider species and silkworms. It shows various biomedical applications like regenerative medicines to control the drug's delivery in the cell efficiently. Moreover, to enhance the applications of bionanomaterials, it can be functionalized by adding different functional groups, as this functionalized silk fibroin helps in drug and gene delivery to the cancer cells, but it also regulates the drug-releasing kinetics [8]. It was observed that silk fibroin acted as nanocarriers loaded with cisplatin, and prevented cytotoxicity and side effects of the drug on normal tissues [9]. Another organic bionanomaterial is chitosan, a linear polysaccharide made up of a deacetylated unit D-glucosamine and acetylated unit β-(1–4)-linked *N*-acetyl-D-glucosamine. Recently, chitosan has found its potentialities in bone formation therapies like developing chitosan nanomaterials-based scaffolds for tissue regeneration, and with the help of collagen, it increased the growth of bone regeneration [10, 11]. PLGA is a copolymer made up of different monomers of lactic and glycolic acid. PLGA nanomaterials could be easily fabricated with various natural and synthetic materials to produce nanofibers or nanoscaffolds, which can be used in tissue engineering and drug delivery applications. It was observed that when PLGA was combined with chitosan, it produced nanostructures that could be used in dentistry and healing of wounds [12–14]. Various cancer-treating drugs such as cisplatin, paclitaxel, doxorubicin, triptorelin, xanthone, 9-nitrocamptothecin, dexamethasone, and 5-fluoracil, have been successfully incorporated in PLGA, PLA and PCL nanoparticles (NPs) [15]. Polymer-based bionanomaterials have also become a new vehicle for the regulated release of drugs. Similarly, silica is considered the most multifaceted compound in the materials family, easily existing with other minerals, and is found abundantly in nature. Organic silica-based bionanomaterials possess special properties like small size, chemical nature, high surface area, high absorption capacity, tunable pore volume and size, hydrophilic nature, and high biocompatibility, which have made them capable of being utilized in the biomedical domain. Organically modified silica-based NPs have been used for the *in vivo* delivery of genes. Unlike other silica NPs, mesoporous silica NPs (MSNs) have gained much utility in the biomedical domain such as for loading large amounts of drugs and producing biosensing molecules. The unique honeycomb-like porous structure, low cytotoxicity, and structural stability have made MSN gain an efficient role in drug delivery applications [16]. Figure 1.1 describes brief classification of bionanomaterials.

Ceramic bionanomaterials predominantly include zirconia, alumina, nitride, hydroxyapatite tricalcium phosphate, etc, as they exhibit many important properties like high resistance, good chemical stability, high biocompatibility, and low density. It has been observed that nanocrystalline hydroxyapatite shows numerous applications in tissue engineering by enhancing the biocompatibility of titanium alloy, and acts as delivery agents of antibody in different bone infections and also works as injectable pastes that can be used as a substitute in producing bone structure as they exhibit great osteoconductive properties [17–20]. Currently, bionanocomposites have gained much interest from researchers as they exhibit a strong platform between nanotechnology, material sciences, biology, and nanobiotechnology. However, nowadays bionanocomposites are gaining utility in the biomedical domain as well. Bionanocomposites are considered precursors of various biopolymers like polysaccharides, polypeptides, poly-nucleic acids, and aliphatic polyesters [21]. The size of biopolymer lies in the range of 1–100 nm, and the method of synthesis and the unique structure of bionanocomposite mainly decide their properties.

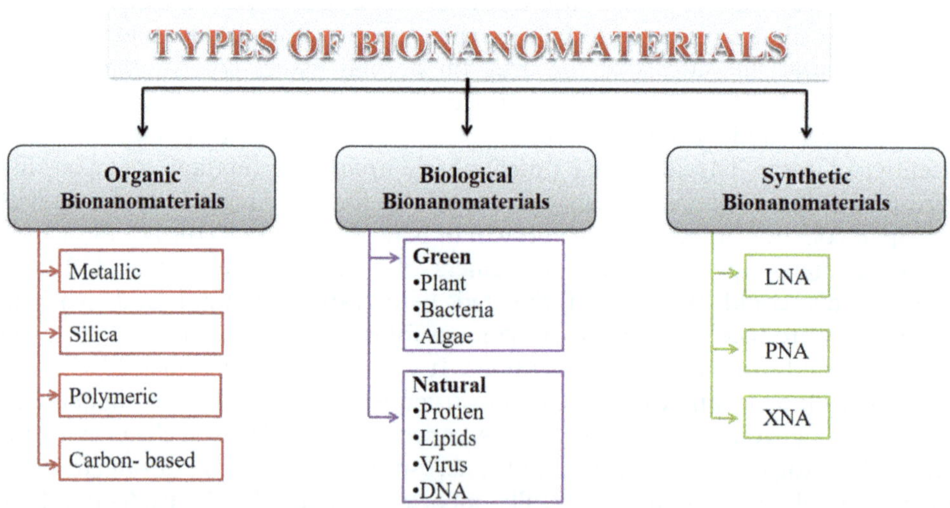

Figure 1.1. Classification of bionanomaterials.

Generally, the biopolymers present in bionanocomposites are soluble in water, although petroleum-derived polymers show non-solubility in the water but are soluble in organic matter. The various properties of bionanocomposites like solubility in water, biodegradability, biocompatibility, and thermal stability help in determining the preparation methods, and applications. Bionanocomposites have found their potentialities in biomedical applications like antimicrobial activity against *Staphylococcus aureus* by tourmaline/cellulose nano-crystal composite films. Moreover, due to the starch's commendable properties like reduced toxicity, high biodegradability, biocompatibility, and tunable mechanical properties, researchers started focusing on starch-based bionanocomposites for the biomedical domain [22–26]. Some starch-based bionanocomposites in biomedical applications include bone regenerating treatments, drug-delivery systems, bone and tissue engineering, and hydrogels production. Similarly, carbon nanotubes (CNTs) have also found their uses in medical applications, like reinforcement, to help initiate formation [27]. An experiment was performed by combining multi-walled carbon nanotubes (MWCNTs) with starch-based nanocomposites to study their biomedical applications; the results showed that they successfully regenerated bone and can be used for regenerating or treating bones or tissue scaffolds [28]. Another nanocomposite material was produced through the self-assembly of oleyl phosphate (OPh) which was stabilized with the help of iron oxide (Fe_3O_4) NPs [29].

Currently, biologically derived bionanomaterials have also gained much attention from researchers in the biomedical domain field. Biologically derived bionanomaterials can be further divided into two types: natural and green-based. The natural bionanomaterials involve certain lipoproteins, DNA or RNA, peptides, etc, whereas green-based bionanomaterials include plant-based, bacteria-based, fungi based and viral-based bionanomaterials. Some naturally derived bionanomaterials are further discussed. Lipoproteins are hydrophobic biomolecules consisting of lipids and proteins, which show spherical shape in nanodimensioned form. Lipoprotein-based nanomaterials are biocompatible, biodegradable, and stable in blood circulation, making them more suitable for biomedical applications. Lipoprotein-based nanomaterials have found their potential role in both therapeutics and imaging. Lipoproteins are widely used in drug delivery and cancer diagnosis [30]. Similarly, peptide bionanomaterials can be structurally modified either through self-assembly of their molecules or by binding with other nanomaterials, leading to variation in their structure such as icosahedron [31, 32]. The small size (6–10 nm) of peptide NPs' central core has found profound use in fluorescence imaging and gene delivery by attaching certain oligonucleotide sequences. It has been found that peptide-based NPs exhibit efficient antimicrobial properties, drug delivery and gene therapy [33]. Also, deoxyribonucleic acid (DNA) is a biomolecule made up of base pairs that store up the genetic information of a living body, and it is considered the most versatile biomolecule in nanotechnology. Its unique physical and chemical properties have been utilized in various biomedical applications; various forms of DNA have been utilized in the biomedical domain, such as in the production of sensors, molecules for imaging, and therapeutics. DNA-based biosensors are under the spotlight as they have been applied in all domains like biological, environmental, industrial, and pharmaceuticals, because DNA plays various roles in biosensors such as target, linking strand recognition motif, probe, etc [34]. Cancer is considered as one of the leading causes of death worldwide and various cures like radiotherapy or chemotherapy cause a lot of side effects on the human body. Therefore, it has became a necessity to develop some alternative agents for the curing of cancer. DNA nanostructures exhibit unique features [35, 36] and are now widely utilized to create various heterogeneous anticancer agents for targeted cancer treatments [37–39]. Also, a variety of DNA nanostructures have been developed for chemotherapeutic drug-loading platforms along with the aptamer-based delivery system, which will specifically decide the uptake of drugs in *in vivo* conditions [40]. Doxorubicin (DOX) is a well-known anticancer drug that is widely used in chemotherapy to treat cancer, as it works by stopping macromolecular biosynthesis by communicating with DNA [41]. Furthermore, it is important to control the release of DOX by modifying DNA's twisting degree. Another approach was developed to overcome multi-drug resistance using targeted drug delivery. In this a combination of an aptamer along with GC-rich dsDNA was prepared which showed great stability, reduced side effects and with good payload capacity. [42]. Similarly, a novel self-assembled DNA nanostructure showed the capacity to particlularly recognize cancer cells and to also control the release of the loaded anticancer drug maintained at pH 5.0 [43, 44].

With the increase in the development of nanotechnology, attention towards green-based bionanomaterials has increased. Certain plants, bacteria, fungi, yeasts, and viruses are used to derive bionanomaterials as they provide great cytocompatibility, less toxicity, eco-friendly techniques and are cost-friendly; therefore, these green-based bionanomaterials have found potentialities in the biomedical domain. Nowadays, it has been proved that viruses can also be utilized in the field of nanobiotechnology as they have found their potential role in various fields like bionanomaterials and bioimaging and the field of science. Some of the viruses that have been used for these applications are cowpea chlorotic mottle virus (CCMV), hepatitis B cores, cowpea mosaic virus (CPMV), vault nanocapsules, MS2 bacteriophages, and M13 bacteriophages. It was observed that the paramagnetic Gd^{3+}-bound NPs exhibited higher relaxivity as compared to the protein-bound Gd^{3+} chelates [45], and therefore they are now used for *in vivo* small animal MRI. Canine parvovirus (CPV), is a natural pathogen of dogs that carries a gene delivery vehicle known as adeno-associated virus (AAV), which has been utilized for targeting tumors [46].

Various bionanomaterials, which are analogs of natural material, can be defined as inorganic bionanomaterials like peptide nucleic acid (PNA), aptamers, xeno nucleic acids (XNAs), etc. PNA is a synthetic analog of DNA/RNA consisting of 2-([2-Aminoethyl] amino) acetic acid backbone that results in the formation of achiral and uncharged mimic. It is generally considered as DNA, but it consists of a neutral peptide backbone instead of a negatively charged sugar-phosphate backbone. This change in the PNA's backbone makes it possess unique physical and chemical properties like resistance to enzymatic degradation inside living cells, which helps it gain consideration in various fields for application [47, 48]. It has also shown potential applications as a biomolecular tool, biosensors, antisense and antigene agent, and molecular probes. The lack of sugar-phosphate backbone in PNA makes it neutral, and therefore it lacks electrostatic repulsion, which helps it to exhibit great affinity towards the target. PNA is polyamide-based synthetic molecules which helps it gain more chemical and pH stability as compared to the DNA or RNA. This property of PNA helps it to bind with more specific sequences. PNA generally consists of uracil, adenine, guanine, and cytosine-N-acetic acids, making it a precursor of RNA. Moreover, PNA's ability to easily recognize specific RNA or DNA sequences using the Watson–Crick hydrogen bonding arrangement helps it show distinctive ionic strength and thermal stability [49]. Therefore, it exhibits a broad range of applications in the biomedical domain as nucleic acid biosensors is one of the tested applications in genetics and biomedicine using PNA specifically. It can be utilized in the development of high-performance affinity biosensors for applicability in DNA genotyping, although studies about specificity and sensitivity are yet to be explored [48]. XNAs are considered as artificial genetic systems which constitute only synthetic nucleotide monomers, with the change in the chemical composition of the sugar moiety. Examples include 3 acyclic L-threoninol (L-aTNA), cyclohexene (CeNA), 2′-O,4′-C-methylene linked ribose (LNA), threose (TNA), acyclic L-threoninol (L-aTNA), or a glycol (GNA) instead of the natural (2′-deoxy) ribose. The formation of homoduplexes by XNAs gives them more stability than heteroduplexes formed with complementary DNA and RNA counterparts [50].

Various bionanomaterial-based metals and their oxides used in the biomedical domain are the most widely studied elements in nanotechnology, and plenty of nanomaterials have found their significant use in different domains. The metal and metal oxide nanomaterials are easy to synthesize and characterize, as they show excellent properties, making them unique and different from the bulk material. They can be easily synthesized using chemical, physical or biological routes, but generally, biologically synthesized bionanomaterials grab the attention as biological synthesis is cost-effective, they are free of chemical toxins and do not produce any side effects in both the environment and in living cells. Various reviews and book chapters have focused on the metal NP and its applications in various domains [51–53]. The commonly used metallic bionanomaterials are gold, silver, iron, copper, zinc and nickel, but researchers have now started to focus on different metals like cerium, selenium, magnesium, etc. The unique properties exhibited by metallic bionanomaterials like size, shape, conductivity, etc have made them the most common bionanomaterials to be used in biomedical applications as they are utilized in both diagnosis and therapeutics. When these metal NPs are fabricated with other compounds their properties are enhanced, which in turn increases their utility [54].

1.4 Synthesis of bionanomaterials

Nanotechnology comprises synthesizing, designing, characterizing and potentiality at a nano-level; therefore, it is also known as 'engineering at a molecular level'. These nano-scaled biomaterials have provided great benefits in the biotechnology and biomedical domain and have connected various domains. There are many approaches like chemical, physical, and biological to synthesize bionanomaterials, but nowadays, biological approaches are preferred more than other approaches as they are easy, convenient, eco-friendly, reduce the use of excess toxic chemicals and are cost-effective. Due to these reasons, green synthesized bionanomaterials are more preferred in the biomedical domain, as these bionanomaterials are biocompatible and non-toxic. Biological approaches include the utilization of various living organisms like bacteria, fungi, yeast, plants, animals, etc, but they also include the use of various natural components like honey, pectin, glucose, starch, etc. The utilization of plant extracts is known as the green synthesis of bionanomaterials and is considered more than other green-based synthesis because plants show immunity to accumulation of heavy metal ions, so there is no need to maintain the culture media of microorganisms, and rate synthesis of the plant is fast as compared to the microorganisms. Another advantage of the green approach for the synthesis of bionanomaterials is that they exhibit slow reaction kinetics so that both stabilization and growth of bionanomaterials can be controlled. Many books, book chapters, and reviews are available, focusing on bionanomaterials' green synthesis [54].

The selection of the correct plant and its part is one of the important criteria in the plant-based synthesis of bionanomaterials, as different plants differ in enzyme activity, phytochemical constituents, biochemical processing, etc. Plant-based synthesis can be either *in vivo* or *in vitro*, where *in vivo* means the synthesis of NPs inside the plant, whereas *in vitro* is the synthesis of NPs using the plant. These plant extracts naturally act as stabilizers and reductants; therefore, they play a vital role in synthesizing nanomaterials [55]. The plant-based synthesis of bionanomaterial follows a common protocol in which plant extract is first washed, squeezed and filtered, followed by salt (metal or non-metal), which causes a visible color change. This color change is considered as the formation of NPs, and they are further characterized.

Nanomaterials' unique properties have increased their role in various research fields and have also developed markets of products containing nano-objects. To understand the physicochemical properties of green synthesized bionanomaterials, various characterization techniques are used. Some of the factors like solvent medium and the stabilizing and reducing agent need to be considered while green synthesizing the bionanomaterials. The characterization techniques are mainly used to study and improve various properties like distinct size, shape, molecular weight, purity, solubility, chemical composition, and stability of the green synthesized bionanomaterials, as these properties help in determining their applications in various domains like biomedical, sensing, agriculture, environment, etc [56–58]. The characterization techniques are divided into two types: structural characterization and chemical characterization. Structural characterization is used to detect the structural morphology of a bionanomaterial like size, shape and crystallinity, whereas chemical characterization is used to detect various surface and chemical atoms and spatial conjugation of the bionanomaterial. The characterization techniques use highly sophisticated instruments. Some structural characterization instruments are x-ray photoelectron spectroscopy (XPS) which is also known as electron spectroscopy used generally for chemical analysis (ESCA) and is required to study the physical and chemical properties of the nanomaterials. XPS works on the principle of photoionization principle and is widely utilized to study surface properties of the bionanomaterials which helps in studying chemical state and energy distribution. XPS was utilized to study the interaction effects of proteins extracted from *Capsicum annuum* in the formation of silver NPs [59]. Scanning electron microscopy (SEM) and transmission electron microscopy (TEM) are among the most highly utilized tools in analyzing green synthesized bionanomaterials because they are simply effortless and convenient to use. They are used to study the morphological characters like size and shape and size distribution of green synthesized bionanomaterials. SEM analysis was used to study the ultra-thin coating of electrically conductive material and various other green synthesized bionanomaterials, but in contrast to SEM, TEM has been considered a more sophisticated technique as it gives details about the chemical composition of the material and it also produces a direct image of high spatial resolution within atomic range. There is not much difference between SEM and TEM except for the sample thickness and the means of data collection from the material. To study detailed information about the chemical composition of bionanomaterials, x-ray spectroscopy can be combined with TEM and SEM [60]. TEM has been utilized for the morphological study of various green synthesized bionanomaterials like silver, copper, nickel, etc [61]. Another technique used for structural detection is atomic force microscopy (AFM), which is considered the most modern, promising and advanced technology as it produces nano and atomic scaled images of the surface, and it can be performed in different surroundings like air, vacuum, liquid, etc. AFM is used to detect and analyze the characteristic properties of many green synthesized bionanomaterials [62]. Energy dispersive x-ray (EDX) is one of the most sophisticated techniques used to study bionanomaterials' composition. SEM and TEM combined with EDX can efficiently detect the elemental composition, microstructure, and spectra [63]. EDX can give qualitative, quantitative or semiquantitative analysis by mapping the spatial distribution of components. EDX is considered as one of the most powerful tools for studying various physical, compositional, and chemical properties of green synthesized bionanomaterials like gold and silver nanomaterials [64], and similarly, the x-ray diffraction (XRD) method is one of the important techniques used in the nanotechnology domain, as it determines the crystal structure, crystallinity, crystal defects, and atomic spacing of the crystalline material. XRD is used to characterize many green synthesized bionanoparticles like silver NPs [65].

To study the chemical composition of the green synthesized bionanomaterials, various techniques are utilized like UV–visible spectroscopy, a basic technique utilized for both quantitative and qualitative characterization of all biochemical compounds. It is generally used to analyze physical and chemical properties such as size, aggregation, and molecules' concentration. It is used to study the optoelectronic properties and the structural conformation of the bionanomaterials. UV–visible spectroscopy works on the principle of Beer–Lambert Law by applying linear relations between absorbance and concentrations. Many green synthesized bionanomaterials like silver, gold, copper, cerium, selenium, etc which have been characterized and used to study the structural properties of the green bionanomaterials. Similarly, Fourier transform infrared spectroscopy (FT-IR) is considered the most sensitive and rapid analysis technique to characterize bionanomaterials. It works by analyzing specific vibration patterns of individual molecules that help determine the functional groups like aldehydes, ketones, alcohols, carboxylic acid, and terpenoids present in the bionanomaterial. Therefore, it is used for both quantitative and qualitative analysis of solid and aqueous samples. Additionally, it is also used to detect the structural composition, dynamics, stability, aggregation, etc. Several green synthesized bionanomaterials like silver NPs, gold NPs, nickel NPs, iron oxide NPs, etc have been analyzed with FT-IR help [66, 67]. Moreover, nuclear magnetic resonance (NMR) spectroscopy is also a non-invasive method used for analyzing various constituents present in the sample. NMR is considered as an efficient analyzing method as it provides high output, high reproducibility, and easy to modify data. NMR is used to analyze properties of various polymers, amorphous materials, biomolecules, and bionanomaterials. Figure 1.2 shows a various characterization technique of bionanomaterials.

1.5 Applications of bionanomaterials

Bionanomaterials are utilized in biomedical applications, including tissue engineering, drug delivery, nanomedicines, and diagnosis of various diseases, as shown in figure 1.3, by nanobiosensors and bioimaging, and various applications have been described below.

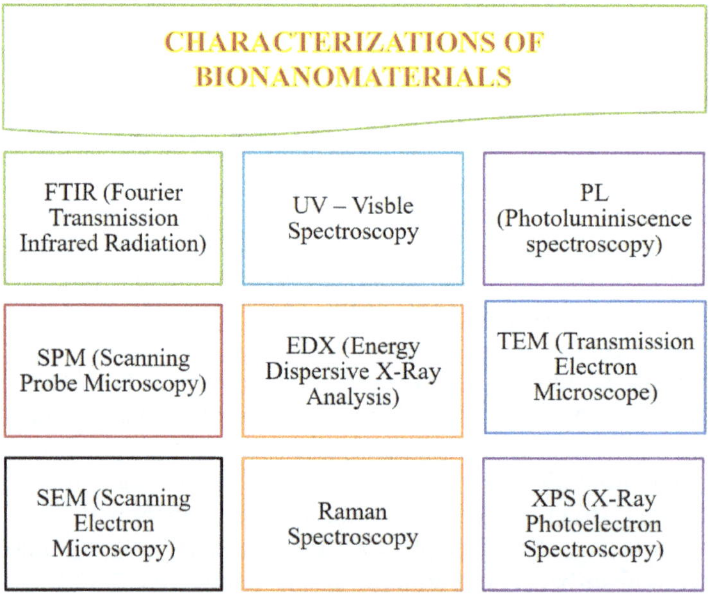

Figure 1.2. Characterization techniques of bionanomaterials.

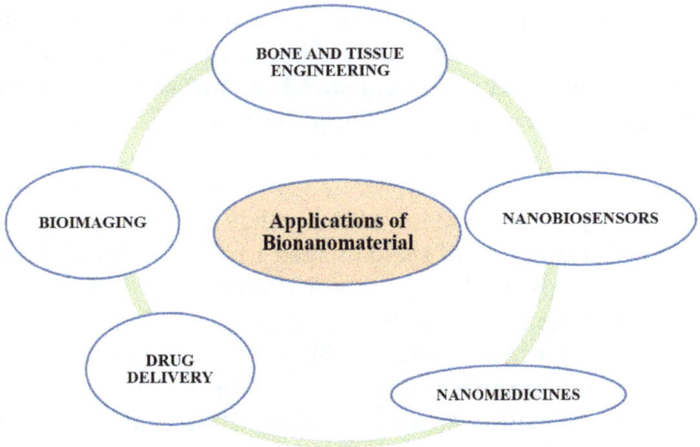

Figure 1.3. Biomedical applications of bionanomaterials.

1.5.1 Tissue engineering

Tissue engineering has occurred as a boon in surgical and therapeutic techniques as it helps develop and identify the desired cell or tissue behavior, functions and structure. It is considered a promising technology that helps to build on defected or damaged tissues and aims to restore partial or full functionality [68]. Tissue engineering utilizes various combinations of scaffolds, biologically active molecules, and cells to construct, maintain, or improve on the damaged tissue or organ functions. In order to produce an ideal scaffold, it should be able to carry active biomolecules, initiate physiological signals and mechanical properties similar to the original tissue [69, 70]. With the introduction of bionanomaterial, tissue engineering's potentialities have enhanced and developed, making it more efficient and more often considered in therapeutic applications. Bionanomaterials possess a superfine structure, which helps them directly interact with the cell or tissue surface receptors, creating a microenvironment to form tissue regeneration [71]. Further, bionanomaterials produce a wide range of basic structural units like NPs, nanofibers, nanofilms, and nanotubes essential in replacing damaged or defected tissue or organs in the body.

Vascular tissue engineering is one of the leading applications in tissue engineering, which replaces or repairs the damaged vessels. Several *in vivo* studies have shown that vascular tissue can efficiently interact with NPs when there is a dire need to create an appropriate method to repair or replace the damaged vessel. In recent times, the formation of allografts or autografts for repairing damaged vascular tissues has not gained much attention because of the formation of compliance incongruity and thrombus. Therefore, several bionanomaterials have been targeted, assembled, and toned to overcome these problems and improve the function of vascular endothelial cells. Comparative studies have concluded that the nanostructured titanium surface provides great adhesion and expansion of vascular endothelial cells as compared to bulk titanium; therefore, this can be used to enhance the vascular endothelial cells [72]. It was observed that nanometer PLGA vascular grafts helped in triggering the proliferation of both smooth muscle cells (SMCs) and vascular endothelial cells, and it also enhanced the absorption of both fibronectin and vitronectin from the serum [73]. Similarly, the repair and restoration of damage in the nervous system are dangerous to life and more complicated and challenging than vascular tissue engineering. However, many biomaterials have been considered a promising technology to date and have been widely explored; complete recovery is not possible, but a full function of the damaged nerve is restored. Unlike vascular tissue damage, nervous tissue damage is considered fatal and dangerous for life because the nervous system is a sophisticated network that works by receiving, analyzing, and responding to information. Slight damage in nervous system could lead to serious illness and in some cases death, and for this reason, reconstruction of nervous system injuries is still a challenge. Autograft and allograft are considered golden approaches in fixing nervous system repairs, but complete recovery of tissue is still not possible, and the allograft causes inflammation reactions, tumor formation, and generation of infections in the body. Another common problem that allograft and autograft possess is the regular uptake of immunosuppressors to prevent graft rejection. [74, 75]. Several bionanomaterials have been studied and explored to overcome these problems, as they exhibit excellent electrical conductivity, phase separation, electrospinning, self-assembly, and cytocompatibility, which help them promote neural regeneration and enhance regeneration of axons [76]. It has been found that several piezoelectric bionanomaterials like Poled PVDF, GO nanosheets, Electrospun PVDF and P(VDF-TrFE), etc, can be used in the regeneration of nervous tissue grafts [77, 78]. Bionanomaterials possess a great future and potential applications in tissue implantation and need more research in this field. A detailed analysis is presented in the further chapters, giving plenty of room to the reader to explore the potentialities of bionanomaterials in tissue engineering.

1.5.2 Nanomedicine

Nanomedicine promises a revolution in traditional clinical practices, as the introduction of novel medicines in both diagnosis and treatment have made it possible to meet some impossible medical needs, like the integration of highly toxic but effective molecules like Mepact, increasing efficacy, bioavailability and decreasing dose toxicity and side effects, increasing targeting of the drug, controlled and site-specific release of the drug. It also enhanced transport across biological barriers [79, 80]. This is possible due to bionanomaterials' unique properties, which have brought many pharmaceutical and biomedical development benefits. The extremely small size and high surface area-to-volume helps them in adsorbing biomolecules, like proteins, lipids, etc, when they contact the biological fluids. This has gained them a potential position in the biomedical field. One of the most important interactions within living matter is the plasma/serum biomolecule adsorption layer, also known as 'corona,' which is formed on the surface of colloidal NPs [81]. Its composition depends on the point of entry inside the body and the particular fluid that the NPs come across like blood, lung fluid, and saliva. Additional dynamic changes can influence the 'corona' constitution as the NPe crosses from one biological compartment to another one [82, 83].

Furthermore, other properties like electrical, optical, and magnetic properties can be modified through electron confinement in nanomaterials. Various polymeric bionanomaterials are considered excellent carriers of the required drugs in the treatment of cancer treatment. Synthetic polymeric bionanomateials include poly (lactic acid), PLGA, and polyethyleneimine, while the natural ones are albumin and collagen chitosan and gelatin. Various anticancer drugs like cisplatin, doxorubicin, paclitaxel, 5-fluorouracil, triptorelin, 9-nitrocamptothecin, xanthone, dexamethasone, etc, have been effectively conjugated with PLGA and have shown effective drug delivery to cancer cells [84].

1.5.3 Bionanomaterials for drug delivery

Bionanomaterials have been found to enhance the pharmacological effects along with minimizing the negative side effects, and giving plenty of room to researchers to explore their potentialities in drug delivery [85, 86]. Various criteria should be kept in mind while preparing an efficient drug delivery material, like, it should be able to enhance water solubility of hydrophobic drugs, control the drug release and also enhance the rate of drug delivery. Carbon-based, silicon based and polymeric based bionanomaterials have gained a lot of attention in the past few decades, in which CNTs have attracted a lot of exploration, because they exhibit unique enclosed nanochannels making them a potential material for drug-delivery applications. It was observed that single-walled carbon nanotubes (SWCNTs) when functionalized with different phospholipids along with a folic acid (FA) terminal group and polyethylene glycol (PEG) chain segment (SWCNTs-(PL-PEG-FA)), selectively killed the cancer cells without causing any harm to the normal cells. This experimemt proved that CNTs can be used as an efficient transport material for carrying drug [87]. Similarly, CNTs covalently bonded with amphotericin B (AmB) were easily taken up by mammalian cells [88]. Apart from various types of CNTs, graphene-based bionanomaterals have also gained a lot of success in drug delivery applications [89]. It was observed that when graphene nanosheets (GNS) were attached to the anticancer drug, it showed high loading capacity which was also found to be useful in cellular imaging [90].

Mesoporous silica NPs (MSNs) exhibiting unique properties like adjustable and uniform pore size makes them suitable for the drug delivery material and an excellent pharmacological agent [91, 92]. It was observed that MSNs when coated with lipid bi-layer (LMSNs) showed excellent biocompatibility and also exhibited great cellular uptake in cancer cells as compared to other cancer treating drugs, therefore making LMSNs effective in cancer treatment [93]. Besides carbon and silica nanomaterials, polymer-based nanomaterials have also proved their potentiality in drug delivery applications by protecting drugs from premature degradation, controlling the release of drug and reducing the drug's side-effects [94]. Natural polymer-based bionanomaterials can easily be loaded with the drug and show a great adsorption pattern which can be used in the development of various devices [95]. On the other hand, synthetic polymer based bionanomaterials show continuous drug release *in vitro* along with high loading efficiency [96]. Recently, the drug delivery system has been enhanced and is now shifting towards three-dimensional (3D) technology as it efficiently controlled the drug release for more than four months [96]. The introduction of bionanomaterials in the biomedicine domain efficiently revolutionized drug delivery applications and has also decreased the toxic effects of many harmful drugs to living cells.

1.5.4 Bionanomaterials for nanobiosensing

In the past decades, biosensors have experienced remarkable growth and have revolutionized the biomedical domain by enhancing diagnostic and therapeutic applications. A biosensor is an analytical device which is used to detect an analyte or to measure physiological signals by combining various biological elements and transducers for converting electrical, optical, and thermal signals [2]. A biosensor is primarily made up of two components: firstly, a probe which is used to detect various biomolecules like DNA, RNA, antibody, aptamer, enzyme, protein, etc, and secondly a transducer which is used to transform physiochemical information into detectable magnetic, electrical, optical, thermal and electrochemical signals. Various types of bionanomaterials have been utilized in the development of different nanobiosensors as they possess unique properties like greater surface area, tunable size, etc. Based on different types of bionanomaterials like, zero-dimensioned, one-dimensioned, two-dimensioned and three-dimensioned biosensors, optical and electrical biosensors have been produced, as different types of material exhibit different configurations helping them to enable enhanced integration of biosensors on the human body. Bionanomaterials have made the production of ultrasensitive biosensors possible, as they provide high surface area, excellent biocompatibility, electrocatalytic activity, and electronic properties. They have made it possible to directly wire the enzymes with the electrode surface, to promote an electrochemical reaction, and to amplify a signal produced by biorecognition reactions. It was observed that CNT-modified electrodes can easily detect NADH at low potential. Similarly, gold NPs were used in electrochemical immunosensors, carbon nanotube-based sensors [97, 98] and NPs-based biosensing [99, 100].

Bionanomaterials have not just shown their potential applications in therapeutics, but they have also exhibited great potentiality in diagnosis. Various bionanomaterials are utilized in sensor-based applications, computed tomography (CT) imaging, magnetic resonance imaging (MRI), and photothermal therapy (PTT). Nanotechnology is considered an emerging technology in diagnostic applications as it is enhancing and simplifying the detection of various biomolecules like DNA, RNA, proteins, enzymes, antibodies, etc, by functionalizing NPs to monitor these molecules at the molecular level. Among many bionanomaterials, quantum dots have gained much popularity due to their semiconductive nature and high resistance against chemical degradation. Quantum dots are also stable, specific, and sensitive, which helps them be considered more diagnostic than other bionanomaterials. Quantum dots have provided a strong base for utilizing FRET-based nanobiosensors (fluorescence resonance energy transfer) to monitor and detect various biological responses, for example, it was observed in FRET-based biosensors that when quantum dots were linked with DNA probes to catch DNA targets, they efficiently monitored the low concentration of DNA in a free-separation format. It was also observed that quantum dots in nano-range efficiently amplified the target signals [101]. This book explains the detailed diagnostic applications of bionanomaterials in the upcoming chapters.

1.5.5 Bio-imaging

The diagnostic branch also includes molecular imaging that uses both nuclear medicines and radiology to check the changes in molecules during the living body's disease process [102]. During any disease condition, the body's tissue or organ starts undergoing certain biochemical changes, and these changes are detected using molecular imaging. To enhance molecular imaging functioning, bionanomaterials are now widely explored as they provide high surface area per volume, biocompatibility, and selective binding with the surface receptor of the biological molecules. This selective binding of bionanomaterials with the biological molecule generates specific signals, resulting in detecting the slightest change at the molecular level. Every bionanomaterial exhibits unique physical and chemical properties that help them detect or report the molecules' changes. Therefore, molecular imaging can be differentiated on the basis of imaging modality, which includes MRI, CT, ultrasound, etc. There are mainly two factors that play an important role in molecular imaging: first, the payload, which means the smaller the NP, the larger the payload, and secondly, the suitable distribution of nanomaterials in the living system and targeting by bionanomaterials can occur by both passive targeting and active means.

1.6 Conclusion

Biotechnology has emerged as a revolutionary field in science over the last decade, and the rise in nanotechnology has increased its popularity. Nanobiotechnology is the combination of biotechnology and nanotechnology, which is utilized for the welfare of human needs. Bionanomaterials are nanosized materials made up of biological products like peptides, plants, bacteria, nucleic acids, etc. These bionanomaterials exhibit great biocompatibility, which helps them find their biomedical domain potentialities like therapeutics, diagnosis and imaging. The therapeutic applications involve bone and tissue engineering, drug delivery, and nanomedicines. The bionanomaterials' size highly defines their properties, which help them find their suitable applications and these properties are studied using various sophisticated analytical techniques. Hence, this chapter is just an overview of bionanomaterials in the biomedical domain; moreover, it will also highlight in brief what this book is all about.

Acknowledgments

KRBS is thankful to Dr Ajaya Singh and Principal of Govt. V. Y. T. PG. Autonomous College, Durg, India, for providing a working platform for completing this work diligently and smoothly. Miss Vanya Nayak extends her gratitude of thanks to MSc Biotechnology thesis supervisor Dr Ravindra Pratap Singh for providing this opportunity to write this chapter. RPS is thankful to Hon'ble Vice-chancellor, Indira Gandhi National Tribal University, Amarkantak, M.P., India for providing financial assistance to work smoothly and diligently.

References

[1] Wang X, Ramalingam M, Kong X-d and Zhao L (ed) 2018 *Nanobiomaterials: Classification, Fabrication and Biomedical Applications* (New York: Wiley-VCH Verlag GmbH Co KGaA) p 512

[2] Singh R P 2011 Prospects of nanobiomaterials for biosensing *Int. J. Electrochem.* **2011** 1–30

[3] Theranostic Bionanomaterials [Internet] 2019 (https://linkinghub.elsevier.com/retrieve/pii/C20170010315)

[4] Bleeker E A J, de Jong W H, Geertsma R E, Groenewold M, Heugens E H W and Koers-Jacquemijns M *et al* 2013 Considerations on the EU definition of a nanomaterial: science to support policy making *Regul. Toxicol. Pharmacol.* **65** 119–25

[5] Boverhof D R, Bramante C M, Butala J H, Clancy S F, Lafranconi M and West J *et al* 2015 Comparative assessment of nanomaterial definitions and safety evaluation considerations *Regul. Toxicol. Pharmacol.* **73** 137–50

[6] Abdul Khalil H P S, Fizree H M, Bhat A H, Jawaid M and Abdullah C K 2013 Development and characterization of epoxy nanocomposites based on nano-structured oil palm ash *Compos. Part B: Eng.* **53** 324–33

[7] Tautzenberger A and Kovtun I 2012 Nanoparticles and their potential for application in bone *Int. J. Nanomed.* **2012** 4545

[8] Virlan M, Miricescu D, Radulescu R, Sabliov C, Totan A and Calenic B *et al* 2016 Organic nanomaterials and their applications in the treatment of oral diseases *Molecules* **21** 207

[9] Qu J, Liu Y, Yu Y, Li J, Luo J and Li M 2014 Silk fibroin nanoparticles prepared by electrospray as controlled release carriers of cisplatin *Mater. Sci. Eng.* C **44** 166–74

[10] Poth N, Seiffart V, Gross G, Menzel H and Dempwolf W 2015 Biodegradable chitosan nanoparticle coatings on titanium for the delivery of BMP-2 *Biomolecules* **5** 3–19

[11] Eap S, Ferrand A, Schiavi J, Keller L, Kokten T and Fioretti F *et al* 2014 Collagen implants equipped with 'fish scale'-like nanoreservoirs of growth factors for bone regeneration *Nanomedicine* **9** 1253–61

[12] Chronopoulou L, Nocca G, Castagnola M, Paludetti G, Ortaggi G and Sciubba F *et al* 2016 Chitosan based nanoparticles functionalized with peptidomimetic derivatives for oral drug delivery *Nat. Biotechnol.* **33** 23–31

[13] Li Y, Chen F, Nie J and Yang D 2012 Electrospun poly(lactic acid)/chitosan core–shell structure nanofibers from homogeneous solution *Carbohydr. Polym.* **90** 1445–51

[14] Ajalloueian F, Tavanai H, Hilborn J, Donzel-Gargand O, Leifer K and Wickham A *et al* 2014 Emulsion electrospinning as an approach to fabricate PLGA/chitosan nanofibers for biomedical applications *Biomed. Res. Int.* **2014** 1–13

[15] Pumera M, Sánchez S, Ichinose I and Tang J 2007 Electrochemical nanobiosensors *Sens. Actuators B Chem.* **123** 1195–205

[16] Slowing I I, Vivero-Escoto J L, Trewyn B G and Lin V S-Y 2010 Mesoporous silica nanoparticles: structural design and applications *J. Mater. Chem.* **20** 7924

[17] Bigi A, Nicoli-Aldini N, Bracci B, Zavan B, Boanini E and Sbaiz F *et al* 2007 *In vitro* culture of mesenchymal cells onto nanocrystalline hydroxyapatite-coated $Ti_{13}Nb_{13}Zr$ alloy *J. Biomed. Mater. Res. Part A* **82A** 213–21

[18] Sato M, Aslani A, Sambito M A, Kalkhoran N M, Slamovich E B and Webster T J 2008 Nanocrystalline hydroxyapatite/titania coatings on titanium improves osteoblast adhesion *J. Biomed. Mater. Res. Part A* **84A** 265–72

[19] Rauschmann M A, Wichelhaus T A, Stirnal V, Dingeldein E, Zichner L and Schnettler R *et al* 2005 Nanocrystalline hydroxyapatite and calcium sulphate as biodegradable composite carrier material for local delivery of antibiotics in bone infections *Biomaterials* **26** 2677–84

[20] Laschke M W, Witt K, Pohlemann T and Menger M D 2007 Injectable nanocrystalline hydroxyapatite paste for bone substitution: *in vivo* analysis of biocompatibility and vascularization *J. Biomed. Mater. Res. Part B Appl. Biomater.* **82B** 494–505

[21] Ruiz-Hitzky E, Darder M and Aranda P 2005 Functional biopolymer nanocomposites based on layered solids *J. Mater. Chem.* **15** 3650

[22] Lane M E 2011 Nanoparticles and the skin—applications and limitations *J. Microencapsul.* **28** 709–16

[23] Eid M 2011 Gamma radiation synthesis and characterization of starch based polyelectrolyte hydrogels loaded silver nanoparticles *J. Inorg. Organomet. Polym. Mater.* **21** 297–305

[24] Gao X, Wei L, Yan H and Xu B 2011 Green synthesis and characteristic of core–shell structure silver/starch nanoparticles *Mater. Lett.* **65** 2963–5

[25] Schmitt H, Prashantha K, Soulestin J, Lacrampe M F and Krawczak P 2012 Preparation and properties of novel melt-blended halloysite nanotubes/wheat starch nanocomposites *Carbohydr. Polym.* **89** 920–7

[26] Valodkar M, Sharma P, Kanchan D K and Thakore S 2010 Conducting and antimicrobial properties of silver nanowire–waxy starch nanocomposites *Int. J. Green Nanotechnol. Phys. Chem.* **2** P10–9

[27] Harrison B S and Atala A 2007 Carbon nanotube applications for tissue engineering *Biomaterials* **28** 344–53

[28] Famá L M, Pettarin V, Goyanes S N and Bernal C R 2011 Starch/multi-walled carbon nanotubes composites with improved mechanical properties *Carbohydr. Polym.* **83** 1226–31

[29] Domènech B, Kampferbeck M, Larsson E, Krekeler T, Bor B and Giuntini D *et al* 2019 Hierarchical supercrystalline nanocomposites through the self-assembly of organically-modified ceramic nanoparticles *Sci. Rep.* **9** 3435

[30] Ng K K, Lovell J F and Zheng G 2011 Lipoprotein-inspired nanoparticles for cancer theranostics *Acc. Chem. Res.* **44** 1105–13

[31] Fraysse-Ailhas C, Graff-Meyer A, Per Rigler C, Mittelhozer S, Raman U and Aebi P B 2007 Peptide nanoparticles for drug delivery applications *Eur. Cells Mater.* **14** 115 (https://researchgate.net/publication/242110858_Peptide_nanoparticles_for_drug_delivery_applications)

[32] Raman S, Machaidze G, Lustig A, Aebi U and Burkhard P 2006 Structure-based design of peptides that self-assemble into regular polyhedral nanoparticles *Nanomed. Nanotechnol. Biol. Med.* **2** 95–102

[33] Patel P C, Giljohann D A, Seferos D S and Mirkin C A 2008 Peptide antisense nanoparticles *Proc. Natl. Acad. Sci.* **105** 17222–6

[34] Rasheed P A and Sandhyarani N 2017 Electrochemical DNA sensors based on the use of gold nanoparticles: a review on recent developments *Microchim. Acta* **184** 981–1000

[35] Rothemund P W K and Folding D N A 2006 To create nanoscale shapes and patterns *Nature* **440** 297–302
[36] Shen X, Jiang Q, Wang J, Dai L, Zou G and Wang Z-G *et al* 2012 Visualization of the intracellular location and stability of DNA origami with a label-free fluorescent probe *Chem. Commun.* **48** 11301
[37] Pal S, Deng Z, Wang H, Zou S, Liu Y and Yan H 2011 DNA directed self-assembly of anisotropic plasmonic nanostructures *J. Am. Chem. Soc.* **133** 17606–9
[38] Jia R, Wang T, Jiang Q, Wang Z, Song C and Ding B 2016 Self-assembled DNA nanostructures for drug delivery *Chinese J. Chem.* **34** 265–72
[39] Saccà B and Niemeyer C M 2011 Functionalization of DNA nanostructures with proteins *Chem. Soc. Rev.* **40** 5910
[40] Soininen S K, Repo J K, Karttunen V, Auriola S, Vähäkangas K H and Ruponen M 2015 Human placental cell and tissue uptake of doxorubicin and its liposomal formulations *Toxicol. Lett.* **239** 108–14
[41] Chang M, Yang C-S and Huang D-M 2011 Aptamer-conjugated DNA icosahedral nanoparticles as a carrier of doxorubicin for cancer therapy *ACS Nano* **5** 6156–63
[42] Suo Z, Chen J, Hou X, Hu Z, Xing F and Feng L 2019 Growing prospects of DNA nanomaterials in novel biomedical applications *RSC Adv.* **9** 16479–91
[43] Liu J, Ma X, Lei C, Xue X, Wei T and Zhao J *et al* 2016 A self-assembled DNA nanostructure for targeted and pH-triggered drug delivery to combat doxorubicin resistance *J. Mater. Chem.* B **4** 3854–8
[44] Zhang Q, Jiang Q, Li N, Dai L, Liu Q and Song L *et al* 2014 DNA origami as an *in vivo* drug delivery vehicle for cancer therapy *ACS Nano* **8** 6633–43
[45] Allen M, Bulte J W M, Liepold L, Basu G, Zywicke H A and Frank J A *et al* 2005 Paramagnetic viral nanoparticles as potential high-relaxivity magnetic resonance contrast agents *Magn. Reson. Med.* **54** 807–12
[46] Tsao J, Chapman M, Agbandje M, Keller W, Smith K and Wu H *et al* 1991 The three-dimensional structure of canine parvovirus and its functional implications *Science* **251** 1456–64
[47] Shakeel S, Karim S and Ali A 2006 Peptide nucleic acid (PNA)—a review *J. Chem. Technol. Biotechnol.* **81** 892–9
[48] Singh K R, Sridevi P and Singh R P 2020 Potential applications of peptide nucleic acid in biomedical domain *Eng. Rep.* **2** e12238
[49] Singh R P, Oh B-K and Choi J-W 2010 Application of peptide nucleic acid towards development of nanobiosensor arrays *Bioelectrochemistry* **79** 153–61
[50] Morihiro K, Kasahara Y and Obika S 2017 Biological applications of xeno nucleic acids *Mol. Biosyst.* **13** 235–45
[51] Singh K R, Nayak V, Sarkar T and Singh R P 2020 Cerium oxide nanoparticles: properties, biosynthesis and biomedical application *RSC Adv.* **10** 27194–214
[52] Nayak V, Singh K R, Singh A K and Singh R P 2021 Potentialities of selenium nanoparticles in biomedical science *New. J. Chem.* **45** 2849–78
[53] Fernandes M 2020 Recent applications of magnesium oxide (MgO) nanoparticles in various domains *Adv. Mater. Lett.* **11** 20081543
[54] Mittal A K, Chisti Y and Banerjee U C 2013 Synthesis of metallic nanoparticles using plant extracts *Biotechnol. Adv.* **31** 346–56

[55] Annu A A and Ahmed S 2018 Green synthesis of metal, metal oxide nanoparticles, and their various applications *Handbook of Ecomaterials* (Cham: Springer International Publishing) 1–45
[56] Biao L, Tan S, Meng Q, Gao J, Zhang X and Liu Z *et al* 2018 Green synthesis, characterization and application of proanthocyanidins-functionalized gold nanoparticles *Nanomaterials* **8** 53
[57] Jain A, Ranjan S, Dasgupta N and Ramalingam C 2018 Nanomaterials in food and agriculture: an overview on their safety concerns and regulatory issues *Crit. Rev. Food Sci. Nutr.* **58** 297–317
[58] Kale R D and Jagtap P 2018 Biogenic synthesis of silver nanoparticles using citrus limon leaves and its structural investigation *Advances in Health and Environment Safety* (Berlin: Springer) pp 11–20
[59] Li X and Zhang W 2007 Sequestration of metal cations with zerovalent iron nanoparticlesa study with high resolution x-ray photoelectron spectroscopy (HR-XPS) *J. Phys. Chem.* C **111** 6939–46
[60] Tripathi D K, Ahmad P, Sharma S, Chauhan D K and Dubey N K 2018 *Nanomaterials in Plants, Algae, and Microorganisms* (New York: Elsevier)
[61] Kouvaris P, Delimitis A, Zaspalis V, Papadopoulos D, Tsipas S A and Michailidis N 2012 Green synthesis and characterization of silver nanoparticles produced using Arbutus Unedo leaf extract *Mater. Lett.* **76** 18–20
[62] Bhattacherjee A, Ghosh T and Datta A 2018 Green synthesis and characterisation of antioxidant-tagged gold nanoparticle (X-GNP) and studies on its potent antimicrobial activity *J. Exp. Nanosci.* **13** 50–61
[63] Anake W U, Ana G R and Benson N Study of surface morphology, elemental composition and sources of airborne fine particulate matter in Agbara industrial estate, Nigeria *Int. J. Appl. Env. Sci.* **11** 881–90
[64] Gangadoo S, Taylor-Robinson A and Chapman J 2015 Nanoparticle and biomaterial characterisation techniques *Mater. Technol.* **30** B44–56
[65] Li S, Shen Y, Xie A, Yu X, Qiu L and Zhang L *et al* 2007 Green synthesis of silver nanoparticles using *Capsicum annuum L.* extract *Green Chem.* **9** 852
[66] Arunachalam K D and Annamalai S K H S 2013 One-step green synthesis and characterization of leaf extract-mediated biocompatible silver and gold nanoparticles from *Memecylon umbellatum Int. J. Nanomed.* **8** 1307–15
[67] Davar F, Fereshteh Z and Salavati-Niasari M 2009 Nanoparticles Ni and NiO: synthesis, characterization and magnetic properties *J. Alloys Compd* **476** 797–801
[68] Langer R and Vacanti J 1993 Tissue engineering *Science* **260** 920–6
[69] Greim H, Borm P, Schins R and Do K 2001 Toxicity of fibers and particles? Report of the workshop held in Munich, Germany, 26–27 October 2000 *Inhal. Toxicol.* **13** 737–54
[70] Wang J, Li H, Tian L and Ramakrishna S 2018 *Nanobiomaterials: State of the Art* (New York: Wiley-VCH Verlag GmbH Co KGaA)
[71] An J, Chua C K, Yu T, Li H and Tan L P 2013 Advanced nanobiomaterial strategies for the development of organized tissue engineering constructs *Nanomedicine* **8** 591–602
[72] Choudhary S, Haberstroh K M and Webster T J 2007 Enhanced functions of vascular cells on nanostructured Ti for improved stent applications *Tissue Eng.* **7** 1421–30

[73] Miller D C, Thapa A, Haberstroh K M and Webster T J 2004 Endothelial and vascular smooth muscle cell function on poly(lactic-co-glycolic acid) with nano-structured surface features *Biomaterials* **25** 53–61
[74] Zalewski A A and Gulati A K 1981 Rejection of nerve allografts after cessation of immunosuppression with cyclosporin A *Transplantation* **1** 88
[75] Pan D, Mackinnon S E and Wood M D 2020 Advances in the repair of segmental nerve injuries and trends in reconstruction *Muscle Nerve.* **61** 726–39
[76] Zimmermann R, Vieira Alves Y, Sperling L E and Pranke P 2021 Nanotechnology for the Treatment of Spinal Cord Injury *Tissue Eng. Part B: Rev.*
[77] Kapat K, Shubhra Q T H, Zhou M and Leeuwenburgh S 2020 Piezoelectric nano-biomaterials for biomedicine and tissue regeneration *Adv. Funct. Mater.* **30** 1909045
[78] Valentini R, Vargo T, Gardellajr J and Aebischer P 1992 Electrically charged polymeric substrates enhance nerve fibre outgrowth *in vitro Biomaterials* **13** 183–90
[79] Chan V S W 2006 Nanomedicine: an unresolved regulatory issue *Regul. Toxicol. Pharmacol.* **46** 218–24
[80] Nano on reflection 2016 *Nat. Nanotechnol.* **11** 828–34
[81] Pino P, del, Pelaz B, Zhang Q, Maffre P, Nienhaus G U and Parak W J 2014 Protein corona formation around nanoparticles—from the past to the future *Mater. Horiz.* **1** 301–13
[82] Pearson R M, Juettner V V and Hong S 2014 Biomolecular corona on nanoparticles: a survey of recent literature and its implications in targeted drug delivery *Front. Chem.* **2** 108
[83] Louro H 2018 Relevance of physicochemical characterization of nanomaterials for understanding nano-cellular interactions *Adv. Exp. Med. Biol.* **1048** 123–42
[84] Ali I, Alsehli M, Scotti L, Tullius Scotti M, Tsai S-T and Yu R-S *et al* 2020 Progress in polymeric nano-medicines for theranostic cancer treatment *Polymers* **12** 598
[85] Ling Y, Wei K, Luo Y, Gao X and Zhong S 2011 Dual docetaxel/superparamagnetic iron oxide loaded nanoparticles for both targeting magnetic resonance imaging and cancer therapy *Biomaterials* **32** 7139–50
[86] Yang X, Hong H, Grailer J J, Rowland I J, Javadi A and Hurley S A *et al* 2011 cRGD-functionalized, DOX-conjugated, and 64Cu-labeled superparamagnetic iron oxide nanoparticles for targeted anticancer drug delivery and PET/MR imaging *Biomaterials* **32** 4151–60
[87] Chen J, Shi M, Liu P, Ko A, Zhong W and Liao W *et al* 2014 Reducible polyamidoamine-magnetic iron oxide self-assembled nanoparticles for doxorubicin delivery *Biomaterials* **35** 1240–8
[88] Xu H-L, Mao K-L, Huang Y-P, Yang J-J, Xu J and Chen P-P *et al* 2016 Glioma-targeted superparamagnetic iron oxide nanoparticles as drug-carrying vehicles for theranostic effects *Nanoscale* **8** 14222–36
[89] Muddineti O S, Ghosh B and Biswas S 2015 Current trends in using polymer coated gold nanoparticles for cancer therapy *Int. J. Pharm.* **484** 252–67
[90] Yang J, Shen D, Zhou L, Li W, Li X and Yao C *et al* 2013 Spatially confined fabrication of core–shell gold nanocages@mesoporous silica for near-infrared controlled photothermal drug release *Chem. Mater* **25** 3030–7
[91] Li X, Takashima M, Yuba E, Harada A and Kono K 2014 PEGylated PAMAM dendrimer–doxorubicin conjugate-hybridized gold nanorod for combined photothermal-chemotherapy *Biomaterials* **35** 6576–84

[92] Larson N, Gormley A, Frazier N and Ghandehari H 2013 Synergistic enhancement of cancer therapy using a combination of heat shock protein targeted HPMA copolymer–drug conjugates and gold nanorod induced hyperthermia *J. Control. Release* **170** 41–50

[93] Topete A, Alatorre-Meda M, Iglesias P, Villar-Alvarez E M, Barbosa S and Costoya J A *et al* 2014 Fluorescent drug-loaded, polymeric-based, branched gold nanoshells for localized multimodal therapy and imaging of tumoral cells *ACS Nano* **8** 2725–38

[94] Jang H, Ryoo S-R, Kostarelos K, Han S W and Min D-H 2013 The effective nuclear delivery of doxorubicin from dextran-coated gold nanoparticles larger than nuclear pores *Biomaterials* **34** 3503–10

[95] de Oliveira R, Zhao P, Li N, de Santa Maria L C, Vergnaud J and Ruiz J *et al* 2013 Synthesis and *in vitro* studies of gold nanoparticles loaded with docetaxel *Int. J. Pharm.* **454** 703–11

[96] Kudgus R A, Bhattacharya R and Mukherjee P 2011 Cancer nanotechnology: emerging role of gold nanoconjugates *Anticancer Agents Med. Chem.* **11** 965–73

[97] Agui L, Yanez-Sedeno P and Pingarrón J M 2008 Role of carbon nanotubes in electroanalytical chemistry. A review *Anal. Chim. Acta* **622** 11–47

[98] Umasankar Y and Chen S M 2008 Recent trends in the application of carbon nanotubes-polymer composite modified electrodes for biosensors: a review *Anal. Lett.* **41** 210–43

[99] Mokhtarzadeh A, Eivazzadeh-Keihan R, Pashazadeh P, Hejazi M, Gharaatifar N and Hasanzadeh M *et al* 2017 Nanomaterial-based biosensors for detection of pathogenic virus *TrAC Trends Anal. Chem.* **97** 445–57

[100] Pingarrón J M, Yáñez-Sedeño P and González-Cortés A 2008 Gold nanoparticle-based electrochemical biosensors. *Electrochim. Acta* **53** 5848–66

[101] Singh R D, Shandilya R, Bhargava A, Kumar R, Tiwari R and Chaudhury K *et al* 2018 Quantum dot based nano-biosensors for detection of circulating cell free miRNAs in lung carcinogenesis: from biology to clinical translation *Front. Genet.* **9** 616

[102] Wu M and Shu J 2018 Multimodal molecular imaging: current status and future directions *Contrast Media Mol. Imag.* **2018** 1–12

IOP Publishing

Bionanomaterials
Fundamentals and biomedical applications
Ravindra Pratap Singh and Kshitij RB Singh

Chapter 2

Properties and classification of bionanomaterials

Ekta Poonia, Jasbir Sangwan, Vinita Bhankar, Brij Mohan, Narender Ranga, Vijay Kiran and Krishan Kumar

Nanomaterials because of their various characteristics like chemical stability, non-toxicity, bio-compatibility and other excellent performance characteristics are known as bionanomaterials. In this chapter we will discuss the classification and properties of bionanomaterials. It covers various types of bionanomaterials like; ceramic, polymeric, metallic, silica-based, semiconductor-based, organic–inorganic and biological bionanomaterials. Different types of bionanomaterials are explained with their high resolution transmission electron micrographs (HRTEMs). Properties of bionanomaterials such as bioactivity, antimicrobial, cytotoxicity and drug delivery etc, are explained in detail in this chapter.

2.1 Introduction

Nanotechnology is also called merged innovation, in which the limits isolating various orders are obscure. Organic chemists, material researchers, electrical designers and atomic scholars can be viewed as specialists in the field when they are associated with the advancement of nano-sized structures [1]. Bones are natural and nanostructure materials with nanostructures, i.e. smaller than 100 nanometers in size, which have received bioengineering attention. The advantage of nanostructures is that they mimic the properties of the treatment site and promote cell adhesion processes and angiogenesis by altering their mechanical, electrical wiring, optics, and magnetic properties [2].

When bio-bionic materials are used for osteopathy, a framework must be provided to enable osteoblasts to adhere to, migrate and multiply, allowing bone substrates to be deposited. Thus, bone-forming properties do not have the physical and chemical properties of scales, for example, topology, harshness, crystallization, mechanical strength, and creating sufficient space for angiogenesis [3]. Expanded surface region of exposure (collagen, fibrin and fiberglass amines) provides more cellular movement during integrator and bone marrow membrane ligands [4].

Bionanomaterials are used in the manufacture of gadgets to supplant a section or capacity of the human body in a protected, reliable and physiologically acceptable mode. A biological material is an implanted material used as a structure or device or material to repair tissue or as a desired application. Biological materials may be natural or artificial. Depending on the source of the material, they are divided into different types. They vary by physical, chemical, mechanical and major biological characteristics. Today, developments are under way because biological materials from natural sources are essentially eco-friendly and biodegradable. These biological materials are currently available for the treatment of diseases or injuries and due to their biological compatibility and biodegradable nature, they are suitable for medical applications. Biomaterials are used on the host body, and have no different effects. The different materials or devices used include sutures, needles, catheters, artificial tissues, etc. Biomaterials have been developed in recent decades as an organ of the life system or as a functioning organism with living tissue [5]. The main biological materials are metals, ceramics, polymers and composite biomaterials. Each material has its own characteristics that help them survive in specific applications.

Biological materials might be characterized as 'materials expected to interface with biological systems to appraise, treat or reinstate any tissue, organ or function of the body' or 'any synthetic material used to supplant part of a life system or to approach into close contact among living tissue' [6]. Bionanomaterials save millions of lives, and the quality of life of millions is further enhanced each year. This field is still a rich field of examination and creation, because a single material is not reasonable for all biomaterial applications, and new applications are being created as medication progresses. In addition, there are still many unsolved mysteries about the optimal role of biomaterial bioreactive and biomaterial in tissue regeneration, which continues to inspire research and new product development in biomaterials. Previously, there was much less knowledge about the biological mechanisms of tissues, which meant that biomedical engineering was the complete replacement of functioning tissues with a simple biological material. As our understanding of tissue, disease, and trauma has improved, the concept of trying to repair damaged tissue has emerged. Recently, with the emergence of stem cell research, medicine believes that cell-based tissue engineering will make it possible to regenerate damaged or diseased tissue. The concept of biological materials has evolved over time and the concept of medicine has changed. Williams defined biomaterials in 1987 as 'non-biological materials employed in medicinal devices designed to interrelate with biological systems' [7]. This definition still applies today, including the earliest use of biological materials to replace configurations (e.g. wooden legs, glass eyes) and the current use of biomaterials in regenerative medical devices, such as biodegradable stents for tissue engineering to transport cells. However, the definition remains the same but the understanding of the level of interaction between biological materials and biological systems (in this case, the human body) has changed dramatically. Expectations for biomaterial function have evolved from being relatively inert in the body to being 'biologically active' and assisting in regeneration. Bioactive materials can start natural responses after implantation, for example, cell attachment, multiplication, or, all the more enthusiastically, stem cell differentiation, prompting the recovery of harmed tissue or whole organs [8].

One of the exciting advances in biomaterials nanoscience and engineering is the capability to design novel materials for a wide range of biological applications at the nanoscale level [9]. Present technical advances in the improvement of electron and scanning probe microscopes and sophisticated experimental methods such as x-rays, neutrinos and optical spectroscopy have prompted the investigation of nanoscale materials. Contrasted with other microscopic or macrostructures, materials of nanoscale show exceptional properties such as mechanical, optical and electrical. Nanotechnology-supported methodologies are being investigated for an assortment of biomedical relevancies e.g., biosensors, drug delivery, tissue designing and bioimaging. Critical extents of these strategies use nanoscale or nanobiomaterials to build up the novel capacities needed for these biomedical frameworks [10]. In this chapter we give an expansive viewpoint on the field of nanobiomaterials. This chapter likewise furnishes researchers with a superior perspective on all parts of nanobiomaterials and their medical benefits. We present different classification of bionanomaterials, discuss their properties, and lastly introduce their future possibilities.

2.2 Properties of bionanomaterials

There is a wide range of properties depending upon the physical chemical behavior, structural arrangements and different mechanical reactions of bionanomaterials.

2.2.1 Mechanical properties of bionanomaterials

Bionanomaterials display various mechanical properties, for example, stress protecting, which can be forestalled by coordinating the versatile modulation of the bionanomaterials with the flexible modulation of the bone, which changes somewhere in the range of 4 and 30 GPa [11]. In addition, the material should be characterized by a combination of low shape and high solidarity to expand the service life of embeds and forestalls detachment, forestalling the requirement for correction medical procedure.

Mechanical properties portray their capacity to withstand outer burdens and removals. Firmness is identified with versatile modulation, which characterizes the power needed to deliver flexible misshapening, and consequently, E the Young's modulus is characterized via underlying incline of linearaxial bend of stress–strain, wherever strain is retrievable (flexible). Strength, characterized through the most extreme strength on yield stress hour or peak load before fracture toward the start of perpetual twisting, is a proportion of the unit area power so that a material can hold out. Hardness is another proportion of solidarity—assessed dependent on infiltration of the head on the outside of the material under an outer burden. Malleability is a proportion of the most extreme strain before a break and is generally assessed as a rate lengthening of the test or an overall change in its cross-section area. Durability is a proportion of the capacity to oppose breakage; it may be surveyed very well by the region under the load dislodging bend yet is better assessed utilizing the systems of fracture mechanics [12].

By and large, the properties of mechanical strength controlled via elastic stress against strain examinations include demonstrated outcomes to facilitate the inside reach for typical gadget plans for medical purposes. Exhaustion potency estimations, while decided, have demonstrated estimations of 25%–90% of those of nonporous materials utilized for comparative applications [13]. This information is restricted, and apprehensions have been communicated regarding the roles of: microstructural and synthetic modifications of the mass and surface attributes; presence of chosen stages along the permeable interfaces that may cause adjusted mechanical properties, particularly consumption weariness; and the impact of unpredictable surface geologies and indents that could actuate mechanical weakness breaks. Large numbers of these inquiries have not been responded to in due order regarding the entirety of the permeable frameworks being proposed for prostheses. Until this point, at around nine years into restricted medical preliminaries, these sorts of issues have not been represented to be colossal. Notwithstanding the accessible and latest plans, the materials should be assessed cautiously in a research center climate to avoid likely issues here.

2.2.2 Biological properties of bionanomaterials

Physical, chemical and organic properties of another recyclable composite platform comprising of nanohydroxyapatite (HA) and normally inferred chitosan (CS) polymers and polymer of carboxymethylcellulose (CMC), for example [n-HA/CS/CMC], were contemplated [14]. CS is a biological-degradable, bio-compatible cationic natural polymer and a deacetyl derivative of chitin, because CS-based materials are similar in structure to glycosaminoglycans, and can accelerate bone formation [15]. Hence, in bone tissue designing [n-HA/CS] a composite framework has been generally concentrated. Carboxymethyl cellulose is an innate biological-degradable, bio-compatible anionic polymer acquired by chemically modified innate cellulose, which has a very similar structure to CS, so there is a strong interlinking effect between carboxymethyl cellulose and CS [16].

2.2.2.1 Calcium phosphate biological properties

Biomaterial of calcium phosphate has attracted much consideration in the field of bone recovery, particularly because of its fantastic biological properties [17]. As referenced before, the profoundly intricate climate of the human body necessitates that calcium phosphate bionanomaterials should have the option to mortify at a suitable rate to accomplish an offset with the recovery of new bone tissue, while simultaneously giving an ideal spot to cell development. As a rule, calcium phosphate material has three characteristics that have been broadly concentrated on by scientists. These are as follows.

2.2.2.1.1 Osteoinductivity

Bone induction means recruiting immature cells and stimulating them to develop into pre-bone cells. On account of bone healing, for example fractures, most bone recuperating is subject to bone enlistment [18] strangely, a number of bone-forming specialists, counting bone morphological proteins (BMPs), TGB-b, Wnt and further development aspects through the related flagging pathways, are essentially significant all through the bone acceptance measure. They show a flexible regulatory function in managing gene articulation, signal transduction, and osteoblast separation in different cells.

Unlike most metal materials that lack bone-forming capacity, several calcium phosphate ceramics are accounted to stimulate bone creation at allions devoid of amassing some bone-forming agents to the materials. This process is known as 'bone induction' or 'bone induction potential'. Normally, regardless of whether a material is bone-initiated relies upon whether it works well, even on account of offside embeds, for example under-skin infusion and intramuscular implantation.

Amongst many biological materials, calcium phosphate bionanomaterials, for example; TCP, BCP, and HA because of their good bone induction, are considered to be prominent candidates for bone reconstruction, which is for interstitial cell adsorption and differentiation into osteoblasts and osteoblasts, step by step to improve the development of blood vessels and bone-tissue regeneration is important [19]. By virtue of bone induction ability, these CaP ceramics can accomplish better bone recovery in the body even in basic size defects, lacking the need to add cells or development factors. Bone acceptance is known to rely intensely upon a few material boundaries, including molecule size, porosity, phase composition and in any event, sintering temperature. With respect to natural variables, calcium phosphate is known to have distinctive bone-prompting impacts on various creatures, including canines, mice, hares and pigs. Curiously, a similar material may show contrasts in various creatures. Cheng *et al* contrasted calcium phosphate ceramics with types of creature bone induction, and level of bone-forming is as per the following: dogs > rabbits > rats [20].

2.2.2.1.2 Osteoconductibility

One phenomenon is that when bioactive nanomaterials are embedded into the bone climate, bone tissue develops along surface or interior pores of embed, which is bone conduction. The additional tissue and bone cells that develop on substitution embed the improved bone conductivity. Bone conductivity is influenced by material dependence factors and defect site conditions. For example, bone conductivity is considered to be a feature of biological materials that, from a biological compatible point of view, are not ideal materials, such as stainless steel and titanium [18], but biological materials that have the ability to obtain special forms, have appropriate internal structures and toughness, and provide the ideal location for cellular activity.

2.2.2.1.3 Biodegradability

When biodegradable materials are implanted into the human body, they dissolve over time, along with a decrease in the mechanical properties of the implanted materials, and the load slowly moves from implants to human bones and delicate tissues, evading stress shielding [21]. There are two clarifications for the biodegradation of calcium phosphate, specifically, 'scattering the material into particles' and 'dissolving the material into ions'. The previous idea depends on the possibility that the embedded material is initially scattered into small particles or sections until the fragments are devoured or the bone-breaking cells are moved; it was later discovered that the two mechanisms appeared to exist together in the bone development measure and could be applied to various conditions as indicated by various conditions and materials. Sheik *et al* sum up the debasement cycle of the embedded material into three responses (biological, physical, chemical) and two stages (first stage: early disintegration; second stage: cell-intervened assimilation) [21]. The actual response is the procedure of deprivation through the disintegration of the material; the surface of the biological material is changed into bone-like apatite through a progression of responses, for example, disintegration, deposition, particle trade, lastly crumbling into small particles [22].

2.2.2.2 Nanohydroxyapatite (HA) properties

In the human body, the fundamental parts of bone are mineralized tissue, enamel and dental essence, which are made out of calcium phosphate mineral stage (45%–70% weight), water (10% weight) collagen (20–45 weight) and a modest quantity of non-collagen speaking to stage organic stuff [23].

Bone minerals are fundamentally made out of hydroxyapatite definitions ($Ca_{10}(PO_4)_6(OH)_2$) which assume a significant job in bone digestion and chemical responses [24]. The actual qualities of calcium phosphate biomaterials are associated with the shape and the surface region can be made into microspheres, powder, plates, films, screens, wipes and hydrogels [25]. Table 2.1 shows the bone compositions of adults.

Calcium phosphate ceramics, for example, hydroxyapatite and tricalcium phosphate are chemically similar to minerals in natural bone and also used as bone filler and bone cement [26]. Thus, their response to physiological liquids structures solid bonds to hard and delicate tissues, expanding bone osteointegration. The nanoscale highlight of n-HA instigates beneficial cell reactions when contrasted with m-HA [25]. Both nanotopography and microtopography direct cell conduct, for example, cell

Table 2.1. Bone composition (%) of adults.

Bone composition	(%) in adults
Sodium	0.9
Phosphorus	15.2
Chlorine	0.13
Potassium	0.03
Calcium	34.8
Magnesium	0.72
Fluorine	0.03
Carbonates	7.4
Other elements	0.04

grip, separation, and expansion. Studies have indicated that nanostructure surfaces advance more noteworthy connections of explicit proteins and invigorate new bone development all the more adequately. This might be one of the essential mechanisms for the noticed development of nanostructure biomaterials with magnificent tissue. This has prompted the plan of different nano-stage ceramics, polymers, metals and composite sections for tissue engineering applications [27].

Webster and others reported that compared to traditional 179 nm HA particles, 67 nm HA particles significantly enhance the adhesion of osteoblasts after 4 h of culture, while strikingly inhibiting the adhesion of competitive fibroblasts [28]. Nano-phase ceramics show the highest adsorption to vitronectin, a protein that promotes bone-breaking cell adhesion. In addition, enhanced bone-breaking cellular function and the formation of absorption pits were monitored on n-HA contrasted to traditional HA. Considering this, n-HA is relied upon to have preferred bioactive activity over coarser crystals and has been utilized in designing tissue inserts, which have enhanced their biostability.

It is reported that higher particle correlations with cells and increased cell intake of n-HA do not essentially direct to an increase in cytotoxicity, representing the task of particle contour in toxicity [29]. Additional investigation and study of in-cell dissolution and cell ingestion mechanisms is essential to understanding the mechanisms of cell detection and response to n-HA.

HA holds just calcium and phosphate ions, so no antagonistic nearby or foundational toxicity has been accounted for in any examination. At the point when embedded, the recently shaped bone ties straightforwardly to HA through the calcium carbonate-phosphorus-deficite film of the bone-implantation interface, and the surface of HA supports the attachment, development and separation of the osteoblasts, and the new bone is supplanted by the peristaltic testimony of adjoining living bones. HA stents can likewise be utilized as conveyance vectors for cytokines, with the capacity to tie and focus BMPs in the body [30].

Bioactive materials dissolve slightly, but they form biophosphate before they interact at atomic levels with tissue; this trend gives great strength to materials that are dependent upon mechanical loads. Biodegradation of HA is typically started by changes in the encompassing biofluids and adsorption of biomolecules. The physicochemical disintegration measure relies upon the surface area-to-volume proportion, acidity, liquid convection, and temperature [31]. The disintegration is normally inversely proportional to the Ca/P proportion, virtue, size of crystal, and surface zone. Normally, HA is steadier than other calcium orthophosphates, for example, TCP.

At first, bioceramics were biologically inert, however, the pattern changed to react to bioceramics. These have been isolated into various ages, which portray the acceptance and properties of HA biomaterials. The bone conduction and bone acceptance qualities of HA scafolds are notable. In the previous few years, broad examination has been directed to comprehend the bone-prompted capability of HA. Bone enlistment has been seen in a few free investigations by different hosts, for example, canines, goats, and primates [32]. Ripamonti *et al* have accomplished broad work on the drawn out utilization of HA inserts in the nonhuman primate *Papio ursinus* [33].

2.2.3 Chemical properties of bionanomaterials

In 2003, Lutolf and Hubbell works on the production of hydrogels by examining the new type of expansion responses among the star polymers and bis-cysteine peptides, whereas star polymer is vinyl-sulfone-ended 4-arm poly(ethylene glycol). This was the early cases where bioclick response was employed for the synthesis of bio-nanomaterials [34]. Furthermore, to introduce the signs to cells in neighbourhood transportation vehicles and to advance injury mending, these peptide-functionalized materials were successfully proposed. For strategies in materials with desirable assets this system and tactic works amazingly in the area of medication transporation. Michael-type formation sciences were applied by Zhong and Feijen for the designing of degradable hydrogels using thiol-functionalized dextran and vinyl-sulfone-formed dextran or acrylate-functionalized 4-arm PEG star polymers [34]. Later on, Wagner and collaborators exposed that this type-of expansion can be used among the thiols and acrylates and maleimides integrating the urea elastomers i.e., biodegradable polyurethane. Various other cycloaddition responses like CuAAC and SPAAC are attracting great attention for the amalgamation of biologically allied polymers [34].

With the occurrence of CuAAC, a large number of interesting options are generated in the zone of water media at normal conditions and even without the usage of a catalyst. Likewise, hyaluronic corrosive hydrogels were organized by Shoichet *et al* by using the furan-adjusted hyaluronic corrosive and PEG dimaleimide with the engagement of Diels–Alder click science [35]. The decomposable shape-memory elastomers with blend reconfigurable was prepared with this science and introduced by Ninh and Bettinger. An additional captivating development scheme is the hetero-Diels–Alder response (HDA) among the approachable dienes and intensely electron-insufficient thiocarbonyl thiol compounds [34]. This procedure is appealing, while polymers that combine such electron-insufficient congregations can be set up by RAFT polymerization operating, for instance, benzyl pyridine-2-yldithioformiate. HAD cycloaddition science has been applied to unite poly(isobornyl acrylate) against cellulose substrates that bear cyclopentadienyl functionalities. The converse electron request Diels–Alder click response was explored by Anseth and associates among the dinorbornene peptide cross-linker to get cell-enlightening hydrogels and tetrazine-functionalized 4-arm PEG prepolymers [36]. Figure 2.1 demonstrates various factors that have influence on the chemical reactivity of bionanomaterials.

2.2.4 Physical properties of bionanomaterials

Physical properties, for example, flexible moduli, are changed with respect to the relative areal divisions of heap-conveying segment. Part moduli are, obviously, reliant on both design qualities and material. Hypothetical calculations and estimations of these sorts of properties are restricted for the majority of the

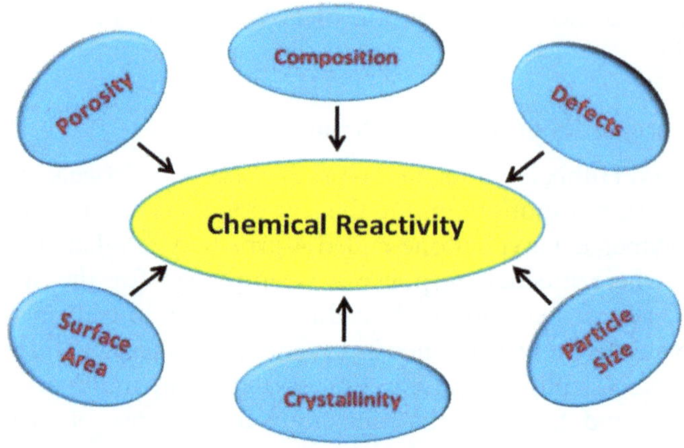

Figure 2.1. Various factors that have influence on the chemical reactivity of bionanomaterials.

accessible permeable frameworks. Additionally, the actual highlights of the porosity, for example, shape, pore size, conveyance, and network, are all perceived from basic to short-term and long-term biological connections. Pore size attributes cover a broad range, with intercept (*l*) estimation esteems covering 10 p.m to 500 p.m ranges, with average qualities (*l*) typically 100 p.m to 250 p.m. Network estimations in some cases show confined pores, however, most frameworks have an interconnected surface porosity. A portion of the splashed plasma frameworks examined in all labs indicated huge measures of confined pores. The mean surface area per unit volume and complete surface area proportions for the different permeable compounds were estimated from 3 to 10 times. These qualities were determined so they could be included for erosion and prosthesis configuration investigations [37]. Porosities states likewise enclosed a broad range, as of ordinary forms created from sintering spheric powders to exceptionally sporadic forms created from coalition or wires of sintering, sintering ranges of powder size portions, sporadically formed powders and splashing of plasma to deliver permeability to surfaces.

2.2.5 Thermal properties of bionanomaterials

Bionanomaterials are efficient in transfer of heat—energy transfer by ideals of a temperature gradient. Regarding a living bionanomaterial, heat transfer capacity of material can be particularly significant on the grounds that the condition of life may rely on the maintenance of a particular temperature. The entirety of the three essential heat transfer mechanisms, radiation, conduction and convection, can happen in actual circumstances including bionanomaterials, yet of these three, conduction is typically most significant in determining the transfer of heat inside the bionanomaterial oneself [38]. The ability of a bionanomaterial to move power via conduction is pre-eminently described in consistent condition through its thermal conductivity (k), and in non-steady state by its thermal diffusivity, α. Due to complex structure of most bionanomaterials, there is no sufficient microscopic hypothesis, for example, that for solids and less significantly for fluids that permits the immediate assurance of k and α of a bionanomaterial from one or a few principal properties. Hence, it is typically important to determine the thermal properties k and α; notwithstanding, a large part of the early work on solids and fluids gave a premise to the investigation and translation of the consequences of these estimations [39].

Any treatment of thermal properties of bionanomaterials, regardless of whether hypothetical or functional, needs a conversation of heat transfer systems for thermal-energy exchange between a living being and its current circumstance [40]. These systems are eventually liable for the condition of thermal support practised by the creature and, in extreme cases, can decide a definitive destiny of the life form. Thermal conductivity and diffusivity of bionanomaterials of which the creature is comprised are significant in such manner on the grounds that these properties decide the degree of the bionanomaterial engaged with the heat transfer interaction as far as time, temperature, and space [41].

Certainly, thermal diffusivity and conductivity are not by any means the single verifiers of the degree of interaction. Thermoregulatory mechanisms include different factors, for example, flow and perspation; a large part of managing heat-transfer components is given to the impact of these physiological variables in thermal cooperations. Due to the complex means by which these physiological elements change that need to be included, it is often important to turn them into a model to assess or clarify their impact [42].

In deciding the idea of thermal communications among human life forms and their current circumstances, especially from the perspective of thermal support, the work of Gagge *et al* has been generally prominent [43]. For almost forty years, we have utilized strategies for fractional calorimetry to recognize and to evaluate different mechanisms for the transfer of heat. Essentially, the method utilizes a calorimeter of copper to determine the different rates of thermal energy transfer for dressed and undressed subjects in exactly inhibited ecological stipulations.

2.2.6 Antimicrobial properties of bionanomaterials

Antimicrobial properties of synthesized bioactive glass nanopowder sample were investigated against four different pathogens/microorganisms, i.e., *Escherichia coli* (*E. coli*), *Staphylococcus aureus* (*S. aureus*), *Bacillus cereus* and *Candida albicans*, as represented in figure 2.2 with the values reported in table 2.2. Undoped bioglass has no significant zone of inhibition while the doped bioactive glass nanopowder has a significant zone of inhibition. The antimicrobial efficiency of the synthesized bioactive glass nanopowder for individual bacteria is also shown in figure 2.2. It can be seen from table 2.2 and figure 2.2 that the synthesized bioactive glass sample is more effective against the growth of *Staphylococcus aureus* and *B. cereus* as compared to the other two bacteria [44].

X-ray diffraction (XRD) results and the presence of the phosphate group in the FTIR-spectra endorse the construction of a calcium phosphate enriched film on the surface of the bioactive glass nanopowder sample. Glass ceramics show good antibacterial results against *B. cereus*, *E. coli*, *Candida albicans*, and *S. aureus* microorganism. This glass matrix would be very useful for distinct biomedical

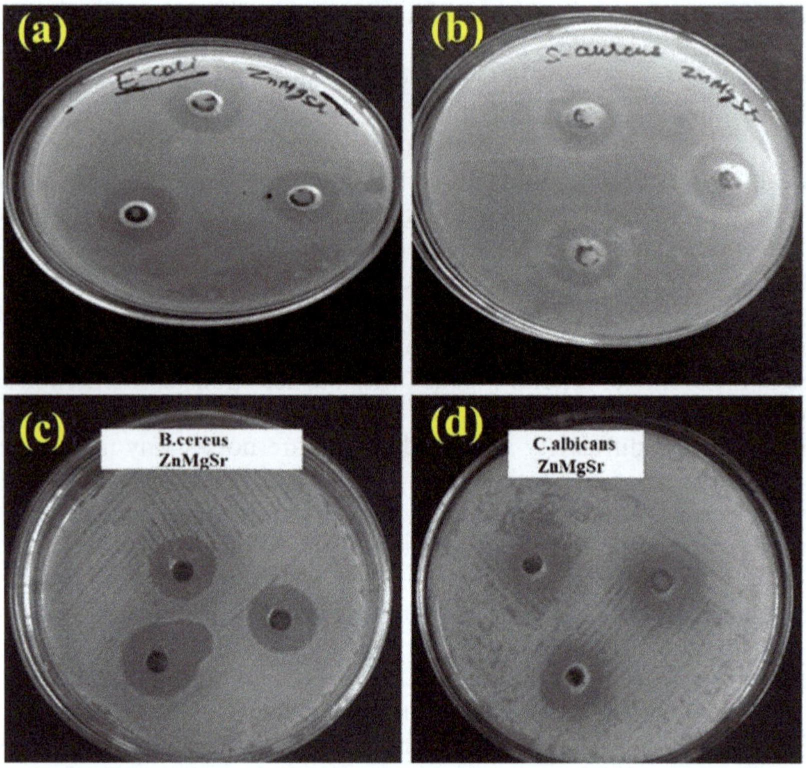

Figure 2.2. Antimicrobial experimental images of the prepared bioactive glass nanopowder against four different pathogen/microorganisms i.e., (a) *Escherichia coli* (*E. coli*), (b) *Staphylococcus aureus* (*S. aureus*), (c) *Bacillus cereus*, (d) *Candida albicans*.

Table 2.2. Zone of inhibition parameters/values of the prepared bioglass sample.

Pathogens/microorganisms	ZOI (mm) after 24h.
S. aureus	15.66
B. cereus	15.0
E. coli	13.0
C. albicans	10.33

applications considering its cost-effectiveness, biocompatibility and its antimicrobial effects. These bioglasses may have a potential application in bone tissue engineering owing to their increased mechanical strength.

2.2.7 Bioactivity

Bioactive testing was carried out using simulated body fluid (SBF), and samples were saturated for 7 and 14 days in SBF in an incubation chamber at 37 °C. Samples were examined by XRD technology and field emission-scanning electron microscope. XRD details following bioactive testing are in figures 2.3(b) and (c). They demonstrate that a hydroxyapatite layer was developed within 7 days of inundation in SBF, and presentation of strontium in a bioglass framework speeded up the development of hydroxyapatite. SBF with ion concentrations approximately equal to those of human blood plasma has been used widely for *in vitro* assessment of the bioactivity of artificial materials and for the formation of bone-like apatite on various substrates. SBF was designed to have a total ion concentration equal to that of blood plasma, except for a few ions like concentration of HCO_3^{-2} , which was set to the saturated level with respect to calcite. Human plasma and SBF (mmol L^{-1}) ion concentration is set out in table 2.3. It is notable that the natural movement of bioglass relies upon the kinetics of the reaction that happens on a superficial level when in contact with SBFs.

Figure 2.3(a) shows an XRD graph of before *in vitro* study of bioglass powder, this unmistakably shows that there are no crystalline pinnacles, for example that the behavior of the sample after calcination at 600 °C is purely amorphous. Compounds AgSr(2) and AgSr(3) demonstrate total amorphous properties of synthesised glass. Figures 2.3 (b) and (c) show an XRD graph of a bioglass sample after *in vitro*

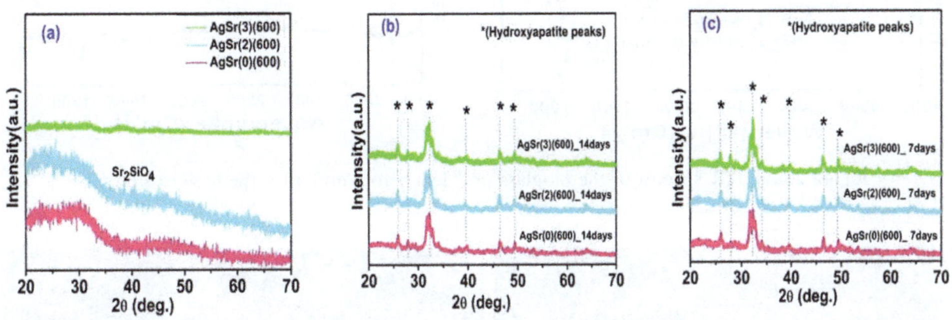

Figure 2.3. (a) XRD prototypes of equipped bioglass powder prior to *in vitro* study calcined at 600 °C, and (b) and (c) XRD prototypes of bioglass following *in vitro* study at diverse soaking times in SBF.

Table 2.3. Human blood plasma and SBF (mmol L^{-1}).

Ion	SBF	Plasma
Na^{+}	142.0	142.0
Mg^{+}	1.5	1.5
K^{+}	5.0	5.0
Ca^{2+}	2.5	2.5
HPO_4^{-2}	1.0	1.0
HCO_3^{-2}	4.2	27.0
SO_4^{-2}	0.5	0.5
Cl^{-}	147.8	103.0

considering, for example a bioglass sample absorbing SBF for 7 and 14 days. It is obvious from the XRD map that when coordinated to the standard hydroxyapatite (JCPDS# 09-0432), there are numerous crystalline peaks relating to hydroxyapatite peaks, as indicated in figure 2.4, which clearly shows the PO bond bending vibration which validates the construction of a hydroxyapatite layer on the surface of bioglass.

Figures 2.5(a)–(d) show FE-SEM images of nanoparticle glass powder soaked in SBF for 7 days and 14 days. It shows irregularly shaped particles of up to 100 nanometers, whose size increases in 7–14 days, which proves hydroxyapatite coating development on the surface of the bioglass template. As the immersion time increased to 14 days, an incessant covering layer considered to be an apatite coating enclosed the outsides of both samples [45].

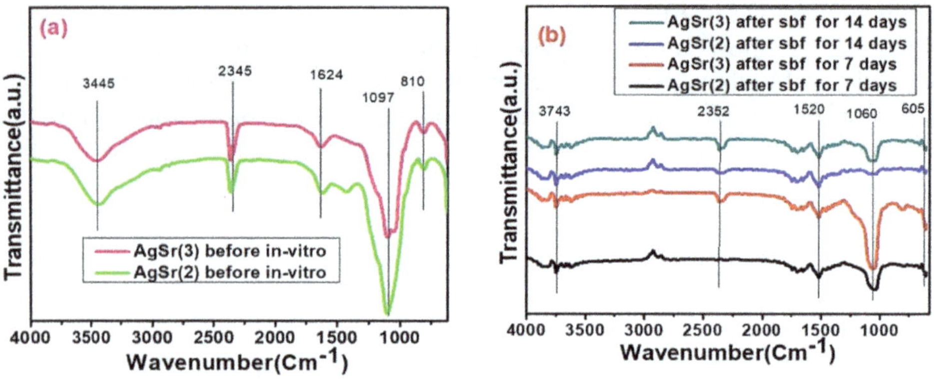

Figure 2.4. FTIR spectra of the bioglass powders before and after the *in vitro* study.

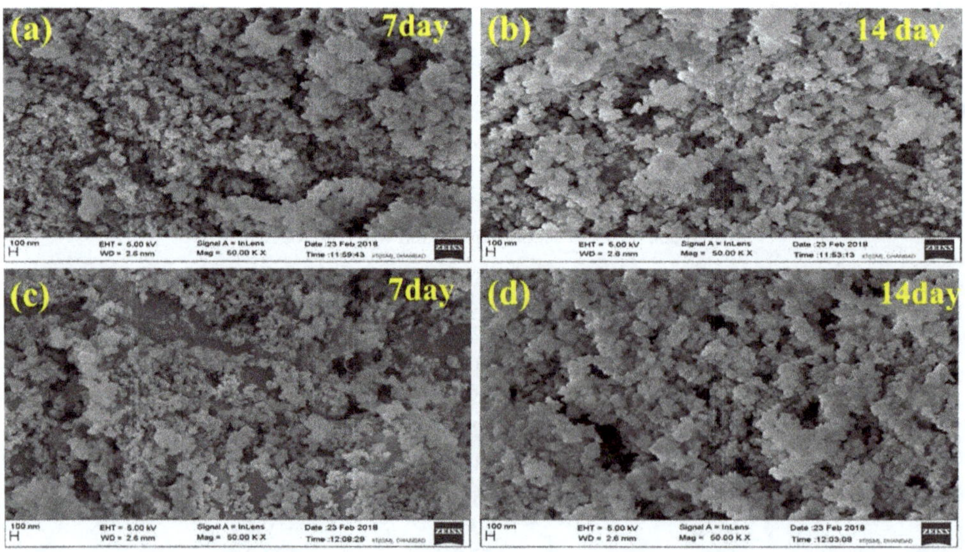

Figure 2.5. FESEM images of (a) and (b) AgSr(2) glass-ceramics and (c) and (d) of AgSr(3) glass-ceramics following *in vitro* study for 7 and 14 days.

2.2.8 Drug delivery

Metal nanoparticle therapy reduces the dose of treatment and improves the efficiency of cancer cells. Chemotherapy drugs inserted into the patient showed toxicity and poor acquiescence. This represents that delivering therapeutic drugs directly to tumor cells is a key objective. It is reported that dox-loaded iron oxide nanoparticles were instantly associated with urinary kinase proton primary activator inhibitors to inhibit the activity of cancer cells. FeO-Dox nanoparticles act in the appreciation phase of improving drug delivery methods. Metal nanoparticles react with biomolecules on the surface (internal and external) of cells. Nanoparticles can also affect the genetic sequence of tumor cells, leading to cell irritation and protein appearance, like cancer necrotic parts [46]. These enlargements of cancer cells rely on exterior and interior signals, for instance cytostebrae function, cell protein, pH, and nucleoprotein and cytoenzyme markers, growth effects, free fundamentals, endogenous stress and oxidation events, and gold-based bimetallic nanoparticles are especially encouraging medication vector competitors because of their small size, great biocompatibility, and basic surface change. For instance, Liu *et al* changed the proton properties of permeable silicon-covered AuAg amalgam nanoparticles to work in problem areas where the electromagnetic field is sufficiently able to enhance the target molecule's Raman dispersing. Different instances of changed gold-based nanoparticles for drug conveyance incorporate the cation BSA implanted in an AuAg bimetallic nanocrystal framework created by Dutta. Notwithstanding investigating the adequacy of medication conveyance, ongoing nanoparticle-constructed examination has centered on building up extra highlights that are useful to treated patients, for example, lessening systemic toxicity. The use of metal nanoparticles for drug delivery is a matter of concern because, although metal particles are inert and biocompatible after administration, some metal particles remain in the body and metal nanoparticles can easily be associated with various preparations such as peptides, antibodies and DNA/RNA binds, specifically targeting different cells, and binding to bio-compatible polymers (polyethyl glycol) to prolong their circulation in the body for drug and gene delivery applications. They can also convert light into heat, which can lead to thermal ablation of targeted cancer cells.

2.3 Classification of bionanomaterials

Bionanomaterials can be classified as described in figure 2.6.

2.3.1 Ceramic bionanomaterials

In recent years, critical advances in ceramics have prompted the improvement of bionanomaterials in dental inserts, tissue designing stents, and hip substitutions [47]. Ceramic bionanomaterials, including zirconium oxide, silicon nitride, hydroxyphosphate tricalcium phoshphate and alumina, have a high wear obstruction, low density, chemical stability, and biocompatible and many other favorable characteristics [48].

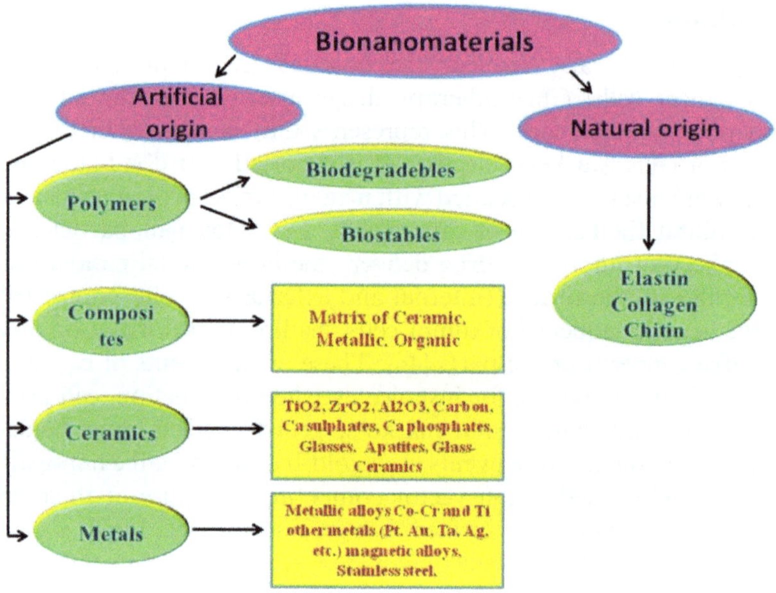

Figure 2.6. Classification of bionanomaterials.

Ceramic materials are generally biocompatible, with very high corrosion and with low conductivity and thermal conductivity. Ceramic biomaterials are mostly suitable for medical implants. Their low toxicity helps to form new bone tissue more efficiently. In ceramics, some examples include calcium phosphate, which mainly contributes to tissue regeneration and is also used for bone repair, and hydroxyapatite, which is mainly used in dental implants due to its excellent hardness properties. The material is structurally made up of metal and non-metallic components. They are highly inert, hard and brittle, with high pressure resistance, but poor pull strength. These materials are mainly used in orthopaedic implants and dental applications where innate inflexible tissues are made up of composites of ceramic polymer such as teeth and bones. Ceramic biomaterials are used in different medical applications based on their biological activity [49]. For example, fully biodegradable materials are used in clinical functions, for example, drug delivery. Today the development of nanostructured ceramics is spectacular. Therefore, the application of ceramic materials depends on the end use.

Tissue transplants and artificial devices have been used to replace the functions of lost or injured hard tissues, like teeth and bones. The entire classes of biological materials, as well as ceramics, metals, composites, and even polymers, have been studied as candidates for rigid tissue alternatives. Metals (Ti-alloys, Co–Cr, etc) and strong static ceramics (zirconia, alumina, etc) have been widely considered for heavy-duty purposes such as hip prosthesis.

Bioactive ceramics, essentially calcium phosphate and bioactive glass, show considerable effect in high biological activity and the development of interface chemical bonds with host tissue, i.e. bone binding [50]. Compared with inert ceramics and metals, the advantages of bioactive ceramics make it possible to develop second-generation hard tissue substitutes with bioactive and equivalent elastic modulations compared to bone [51]. Fascinatingly, bioactive ceramic coverings and permeable brackets show the most capable results in prospect hard tissue substitutes [52].

2.3.1.1 Bioactive glass

Bioactive glass comes under the class of ceramic bionanomaterials. Due to its extraordinary capacity to consolidate with natural bones, bioactive glass has been generally utilized as a bone-filler and bone-grafting material [53]. Ion exchange takes place between the bioglass ceramic materials and simulated bodyfluid whose ionic-concentration is almost identical to human blood plasma, as shown in table 2.3.

This binding capacity provides biological activity and is utilized in a wide scope of biomedical purposes. Numerous analysts are attempting to improve the material biological activity, and created from multiple points of view, for example, its antibacterial properties are additionally identified with their cytotoxicity [54]. The specialists zeroed in on biological glass ceramics shaped by the sol–gel procedure in which CaO, SiO_2, and P_2O_5 are the principle parts. Biological activity of bioglass materials can be improved by presenting an assortment of metal particles into glass frameworks [55]. Scientists have created silver doped bio-glass upgrades biological activity and antimicrobial properties. Similarly, researchers are working on new compositions of bioglass ceramics with the doping of different metal ions such as copper, silver, strontium, magnesium and titanium to enhance their bioacitivity and antimicrobial properties [56]. Ranga *et al*, revealed upgraded antimicrobial properties of bioactive glass utilizing strontium and silver-oxide nano composites. Strontium is additionally extremely valuable in the treatment of osteoporosis. Adding strontium ions to glass matrix can stimulate and improve bone assets. Strontium is also identified as decreasing bone absorption and facilitating injured bone revival procedures. Doped Bioactive glass shows the high quality of Sr-doped glasses and advanced bone mineral development compared to Sr-doped glass. Strontium helps inspire new bone and tissue development and decrease bone absorption [45].

Ranga *et al* have manufactured for the first time a novel system of bioactive bioglass. SiO_2–CaO–SrO–Ag_2O is synthesized through the sol–gel approach and its structural characteristics, biological activity and antibacterial properties are studied using appropriate analytical techniques [45]. Due to the various properties of metal ions in biological glass, the main focus of this study is to add strontium and silver to the glass matrix to improve its biological activity and antibacterial properties.

2.3.1.2 Hydroxyapatite

As discussed above, bone minerals are mainly composed of hydroxyapatite formulations ($Ca_{10}(PO_4)_6(OH)_2$) which assume a significant job in bone digestion and chemical responses. The physical qualities of calcium phosphate biomaterials are associated with the shape and surface zone that can be made into microspheres, layers, screens, sponges, powder, plates, and hydrogels.

2.3.1.2.1 Hydroxyapatite formation in biological fluid

The conceivable mechanism for creation of hydroxyapatite in SBF solution is trading of soluble base and phosphate particles from SBF arrangement through the glass–SBF interface [57]. This phenomenon drives change in the pH of the arrangement. Because of expansion in pH, more OH^- ions hit the silica glass array bringing about arrangement of Si–OH which further goes through polymerization to frame a silica loaded layer.

$$SiOH + SiOH \rightarrow -Si - O - Si - +H_2O \tag{1}$$

Sequential steps involved in formation may be shown as:

Step 1. The PO_4^{2-}, Ca^{2+}, Na^+ and Mg^{2+} ions get unconfined throughout the silica loaded layer.

Step 2. There is a reaction between Ca^{2+} and PO_4^{2-} ions, which results in precipitation of the calcium–phosphate layer.

Step 3. The precipitated calcium-phosphate layer on silica rich layer directs a build-up of the Ca–P layer that nucleates the development of apatite coating.

Step 4. Growth of active interface and apatite–Mg layer results in crystallization of the HA layer that leads to development of a chemical bond between bioactive glass and bone tissues.

2.3.2 Polymeric bionanomaterials

2.3.2.1 Ceramic polymer composites

Ceramics have been successfully used in orthopaedic prosthesis for decades. Ceramic composites are materials made of two or more compositional materials with significantly different physical or chemical properties. At present, composite materials for polymers and ceramics are being developed with the aim of improving the stability of mechanical supports and improving the interaction of tissues [58]. Over the past two decades, various bioactive composites have been studied as alternatives to human lesions or damaged tissue. These ceramic nanobiomaterials are mainly used in bone tissue engineering, dental and hip replacement [5].

Poly lactic acid-glycolic acid (PLGA) and poly lactic acid (PLA) nanoparticles are widely used as compare/drug preparation deliverance schemes in various types of polymer nanoparticles. These two nanoparticles are brilliant artificial biodegradable polymers. Hydrophobic drugs can be summarized in PLA/PLGA nanoparticles and Gd-chelates that can connect or attract terminal active groups or surface charges on the surface of nanoparticles. Table 2.4 clearly shows different types of polymers and their use in the biomedical field.

2.3.2.2 Biodegradable natural polymers

Choosing a biological material for tissue engineering is the most critical step in bracket development. The main requirements should include biocompatibility, non-toxicity, providing beneficial cell interaction and tissue development, in addition to the mechanical strength of synthetic polymers and other properties. According to the chemical structure of a wide variety of polymers synthesized by organisms, they can be

Table 2.4. Different types of polymers used in the biomedical field.

Polymers	Uses
Polyamides	Sutures
Polyethylene	Joint replacement
Polyurethanes	Blood-contacting devices
PVC	Tubing
PET	Vascular prostheses, Sutures
PMMA	Dental restorations, joint Replacement, intraocular lenses
PTFE	Soft-tissue augmentation, vascular prostheses
Polyesters	Drug delivery, vascular prostheses
Silicones	Soft-tissue replacement, ophthalmology

divided into several categories: (i) polysaccharides, (ii) proteins, and (iii) polyester. At the same time, based on the development of biotechnology, natural polymers can be produced by fermentation of microorganisms or *in vitro* production by enzymes. Biomaterials can be classified depending on the material on which they are based; in this case they are classified into four main types of biopolymers: (i) sugar based biopolymers; (ii) starch based biopolymers, (iii) cellulose based biopolymers, (iv) biopolymers based on synthetic materials.

2.3.2.3 Biodegradable synthetic polymers

There are a number of biodegradable synthetic polymers, which are listed in table 2.5.

2.3.3 Metallic bionanomaterials

Metals are used as bionanomaterials due to their tremendous thermal conductivity and mechanical properties. Bionanomaterials are a counterfeit or natural material used to formulate structures or embeds to supplant lost or infected biological structures and re-establish morphology and capacity. As a result, bionanomaterials contribute to improving the quality of life. In various parts of the human body biological materials are used, for instance imitation valves of the heart, shoulder, blood vessel stents, knee, hip, elbow, ear replacement implants and orthopaedic structure, etc [59].

Silver and its composites have been utilized for a wide assortment of purposes, from utensils, gems, and cash to clinical use. During World War I, silver and its composites were discovered to have therapeutic and disease-resistant properties and were utilized to combat contamination. Nano-silver is found to have exceptional chemical, physical, and biological properties contrasted with macroscale measured silver particles. Silver nanoparticles were discovered to have high thermal conductivity, high conductivity, compound stability, catalytic action and improved Raman dispersing. Silver nanoparticles have additionally been found to have antibacterial, antifectal, antiinflammatory, and antiviral properties. Silver

Table 2.5. List of biodegradable synthetic polymers.

S. No.	Name of polymers
1.	Polyglycolide acid (PGA)
2.	Polylactide acid (PLA)
3.	Poly (lactide-co-glycolide)
4.	Polycaprolacton
5.	Poly dioxanone
6.	Polyurethane
7.	Polyhydroxybutyrate (PHB), polyhydroxyvalerate (PHV) and copolymers
8.	Polyanhydried
9.	Poly (ortho esters)
10.	Biopolymers types
11.	Biopolymers made from renewable raw materials (bio-based), and being biodegradable
12.	Biopolymers made from fossil fuels, and being biodegradable

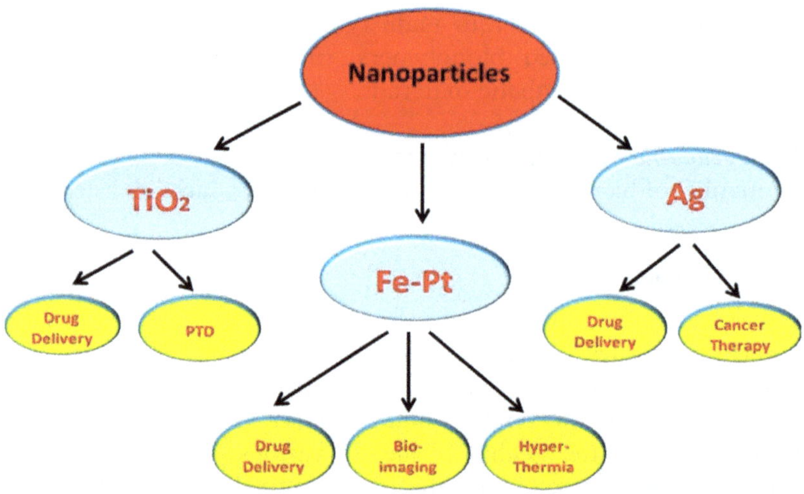

Figure 2.7. Different types of nanoparticles and their biomedical use.

nanoparticles are utilized in biomedical applications, for example, drug conveyance and cancer therapy. Figure 2.7 illustrates the different types of nanoparticles and their biomedical use.

2.3.3.1 Gold nanoparticles

Nanoparticles of gold have been used in biomedical purposes owing to their improved and tunable optical properties, simple amalgamation procedures, and comparatively excellent biocompatibility. They can be adjusted for optical properties, such as surface plasma absorption and scattering or near-infrared (IR) fluorescence by controlling shape, composition, structure and size of nanoparticles [60]. Gold nanoparticles exchange absorbed light into heat through a sequence of non-radiation progressions.

Unique optical and electronic properties of gold make it suitable for exploitation in biosensors and bioimaging, as well as photo-thermal treatment. Gold is easily functional with organic molecules and can be united with antibodies, ligands, or pharmaceutical molecules for active or passive supervision. The chemical inertness of gold gives it good biocompatibility both *in vitro* and *in vivo* and the properties and application of colloidal gold nanoparticles depend on their shape. These resulting gold nanoparticles have unique properties that provides an enlarged surface area-to-volume proportion.

2.3.3.2 Gadolinium nanoparticles

These have favorable magnetic properties and are usually employed as a resonance imaging contrast agent. The advancement of biopolymers to synthesize Gd(III) nanoparticles as therapeutic agents can assume a critical job in nanomedicine [61]. Biocompatible polymers are utilized for complex monovalent biomolecules, yet additionally for the acknowledgment of multivalent dynamic focusing on materials as symptomatic or potentially remedial hybrid nanoparticles. Gd(III) and Au nanoparticles based nanomaterials have as of late indicated essentially expanded esteems in magnetic resonance imaging (MRI) on the grounds that the geometry of Gd(III)-chelating compounds is restricted to permeable structures contrasted with those with openly chelated Gd(III) complexes. Gd_2O_3 has a few alluring attributes in tumor finding and neoadjuvant chemotherapy (NACT), including biocompatibility, colloidal dependability, low cytotoxicity, atomic affinity, and so forth. The Gd chelate has been broadly utilized as an imaging specialist in MRI. Notwithstanding utilizing MRI, they are intriguing, as a radiosensitizer, in neutron catch treatment [62].

2.3.3.3 Iron oxide nanoparticles

Nano-iron oxide particles can be extensively isolated into two classifications as per their size: (i) superparamagnetic iron oxides (SPIOs) with sizes more than 50 nm; (ii) ultrasmall superparamagnetic iron oxides (USPIOs) with sizes less than 50 nm [63]. Contingent upon the size and composition of nano-iron oxide particles, they can be utilized in an assortment of clinical applications, for example, metastatic lymph hubs, location of metastases, provocative infections and degenerative sicknesses.

2.3.4 Silica-based bionanomaterials

2.3.4.1 Mesoporous silica materials

Since the research of mesoporous materials has produced a lot of work in chemical synthesis and brought a lot of exciting practical applications to social welfare, it has attracted much attention. From catalysis to clinical and nanotechnology applications, there are various new materials created with respect to mesoporous silica

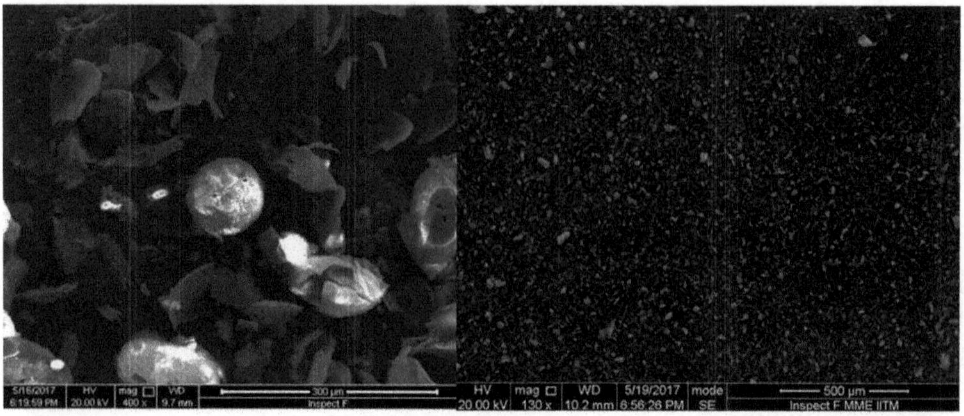

Figure 2.8. Mesoporous silica nanoparticles experiential at diverse scales by electron microscope.

materials [64]. Figure 2.8 shows the mesoporous silica nanoparticles experiential at diverse scales by electron microscope.

In terms of therapeutic capability, silicon-based mesoporous nanomaterials have been demonstrated to be special nano-transporters of an assortment of medications and biomolecules *in vitro* and *in vivo* [65]. For instance, silicon-based mesoporous nanomaterials have been shown to effectively convey little intrusive RNA for gene knockout and numerous anticancer agents [66]. The bio-compatibility and conveyance capacities of silicon-based mesoporous nanomaterials are significant. Finally, silicon dioxide-based mesoporous nanomaterials show incredible possibilities in reasonableness. Advances in sol–gel science and surfactant guideline and amalgamation have made the creation of silicon-based mesoporous nanomaterials moderately simple, with a few straightforward cleaning techniques [67].

2.3.5 Organic–inorganic bionanomaterials

Organic nanoparticles consist of carbon components with a size range of 1–100 nm. These nanoparticles have been generally considered as polymers, liposomes, and dendrimers etc. The polymer structures and beams are utilized in imaging or medication and gene conveyance methods. Simultaneously, inorganic nanoparticles have attracted the consideration of scientists lately because of their remarkable material and dimensional reliance on physico-chemical properties, which are unrivaled by conventional lipid or polymer type nanoparticles [68].

Since organic–inorganic nanomaterials can consolidate intriguing properties of various parts, organic–inorganic hybrid nanomaterials show numerous novel properties, for example, high reactant action, animating optical properties, and different actual properties, which have attracted researchers to develop new intelligent nanocomposites [69]. However, there is still a need to incorporate polymer lattice or an organic segment to additionally improve thermal, chemical, and mechanical properties. The usage of noncovalent connections for the self-assembly and plan of molecules assists with changing the organic nanomaterials into wanted structures, for example, micelles, liposomes, dendrimers, and polymer nanoparticles.

2.3.5.1 Inorganic-based nanomaterials

Metal and metal oxide nanoparticles are found in this type of nanomaterials. Metals like gold, silver, copper, nanoparticles and oxides of metals such as ZnO, WO_3, TiO_2 etc, nanoparticles and ceramics, silicons like semiconductors can be synthesised. There are a number of inorganic nanoparticles in use today which have antimicrobial properties. These materials are being coated onto surfaces or directly incorporated into various substrates, providing a durable long-lasting solution. Nanomaterials can additionally be incorporated onto the surface of implants and devices in an effort to prevent biofilm formation in the body. Furthermore, in some cases, the actual implant is built with metallic or ceramic nanocomposites, making incorporation or coating more facile [70]. Common examples of inorganic nanomaterials used in antimicrobial applications in the healthcare environment and implants and medical device coating include titanium oxide, silver, zinc oxide, and copper.

2.3.6 Biological bionanomaterials

2.3.6.1 Peptide-based nanoparticles

Peptide, as a new material that can not only show protein function but also has a highly modular molecular design, has attracted great interest in the field of biomedical science. Numerous analysts have discovered that combining peptides with non-organic materials, for example, polymers, little sub-atomic compounds, hydrogels, and metal chelates is a promising method to address the natural downsides of peptides [71]. Hence, peptide-nanoparticle forms (PNCs) have been viewed as promising stages for an assortment of biomedical applications. Over recent years, various examinations have exhibited the helpfulness of artificial bioactive peptides, a few of which have been effectively marketed. More than 150 peptide drugs are actively being developed clinically, demonstrating highly promising results for ultimate translation [72]. A few types of peptide are as follows:

1. Dipeptide;
2. Cyclic peptide;
3. Amphiphilic peptide;
4. α-Helical peptide;
5. β-Sheet peptide.

2.3.6.2 Cell biology nanomaterials

Nanoscale range particles in cell science, for example, DNA, proteins, carotenoids, and so forth, have been read top to bottom for quite a while [73]. It is notable that nanomaterials smaller than 100 nm can easily penetrate cells, nanomaterials smaller than 50 nm can enter most cells, and nanomaterials smaller than 20 nm can be transported and penetrated along blood vessels near tissues and jump over the blood–cerebrum barrier [74]. We have arrived at the phase where we can make and strategize nanoparticles for biomedical applications, identified as 'theranostic' techniques, for diagnosis and treatment [75]. Their claim to fame is fundamentally because of two advantageous elements: high surface region-to-volume proportion, which makes it possible to adhere to multi-functional components, for example, fluorophoric groups and targeted on particles; and the chance of pervasive tissue availability [76].

2.4 Conclusion and future perspectives

The interface among biological frameworks and nanomaterials incorporates a progression of dynamic interactions between biological materials and surfaces of nanomaterial. These connections are framed by an enormous strength that decides the colloidal stability, photophysical properties, physical and chemical behavior, and so on of nanomaterials. The advantage of bionanomaterials is their good biomedical performance. Various advances have been made in the development of bio-polymers and in the improvement of the performance of these bionanomaterials in the required applications. Hydroxyapatite has proved to be an important material for biomedical applications due to its biodegradability and bioactive activity. Hydroxyapatite is a biological material beneficial to dental and orthopedic applications. Based on the large surface-to-volume ratio, reaction activity and biological form of hydroxyapatite nanoparticles, HAP nanoparticles are more useful than traditional HAP bulk ceramics and can be used in composite fillings, repair materials for damaged tooth enamel and drug carriers. No single-phase biological material can provide all the basic characteristics of bones and other tissue. Therefore, it is very important that we design multiphase bionanomaterials with mechanical, chemical, structural, and biological properties so that we can mimic native tissues. As the demand for artificial substitutes increases, the biomaterials field needs to innovate. The revelations that natural occurring polymers and BAp ceramics, mostly or altogether created from biological resources, are better acknowledged by living organs and are starting to make these materials more alluring. New elective natural sources, essentially plant sources, present fascinating difficulties for future examination. A lot of exploration has been done on the arrangement of biological nanomaterials and individual components, as well as many studies on its physical chemistry and biological properties. In many cases, however, the outcomes are a long way from business usage, and much remains to be done from lab exploration to clinical practice. This involves viable collaboration between scientific experts, biologists, materials researchers, clinicians, and bioengineers. Although extensive research has been conducted on the use of peptides in nanoparticles to deliver drugs to the brain, there have been no clinical trials of them. The next step, then, will be to use peptides as targeting ligands to develop scalable and repeatable brain-targeted nanoparticle delivery systems. Peptide-based nanoparticles provide an opportunity to make enzyme-reactive or biodegradable delivery systems that may provide less toxicity and immunogenicity and improve efficacy. The development of metal nanoparticles has opened up new innovative applications in the clinical field. The exceptional properties of nanomaterials empower them to profit mankind in numerous areas, counting drugs, catalysis, antimicrobials, biosensors, drug conveyance and gadgets. At present, metal nanomaterials, as a new drug system, are being used in the field of medical science. Nanomaterials in medication conveyance may have a double capacity of determination and treatment. Nanomedicines have discovered better approaches to treat perilous infections. Nonetheless, there are constraints, for example, the way that useful medications conveyed by individual nanoparticles are profoundly confined and hard to evaluate. In order to achieve a targeted dosing system, nanoparticles need to be combined with antibodies or ligand. Nonetheless, the poisonous impacts of metal nanoparticles should be considered before they can be utilized in remedial applications.

References

[1] Avti P K, Patel S C, Uppal P, O'Malley G, Garlow J and Sitharaman B 2012 Nanobiomaterials for tissue engineering *Tissue Eng. Princ. Pract.* **1** 11–24

[2] Chiara G, Letizia F, Lorenzo F, Edoardo S, Diego S, Stefano S, Eriberto B and Barbara Z 2012 Nanostructured biomaterials for tissue engineered bone tissue reconstruction *Int. J. Mol. Sci.* **13** 737–57

[3] Balasundaram G and Webster T J 2006 Nanotechnology and biomaterials for orthopedic medical applications *Nanomedicine (Lond.)* **2** 169–76

[4] Moussy F, Kreutzer D, Burgess D, Koberstein J, Papadimitrakopoulos F and Huang S 2002 inventors; University of Connecticut, assignee Implant coating for control of tissue/implant interactions *United States Patent US* 6,497,729

[5] Chen F M and Liu X 2016 Advancing biomaterials of human origin for tissue engineering *Prog. Polym. Sci.* **53** 86–168

[6] Abdullaeva Z 2017 *Nano-and Biomaterials: Compounds, Properties, Characterization, and Applications* (New York: Wiley)

[7] Williams D F 1987 *Definitions in Biomaterials: Proceedings of a consensus conference of the European Society for Biomaterials, Chester, England* (New York: Elsevier) ch 4 pp 16–30

[8] Gong T *et al* 2016 Current advance and future prospects of tissue engineering approach to dentin/pulp regenerative therapy *Stem Cells Int.* **2016** 9204574

[9] Zhou H and Lee J 2011 Nanoscale hydroxyapatite particles for bone tissue engineering *Acta Biomater.* **7** 2769–81

[10] Saji V S, Choe H C and Yeung K W 2010 Nanotechnology in biomedical applications: a review *Int. J. Nano Biomater.* **3** 119–39

[11] Niinomi M and Boehlert C J 2015 Titanium alloys for biomedical applications *Advances in Metallic Biomaterials* (Berlin: Springer) pp 179–213

[12] Kardomateas G A and Geubelle P H 2010 Fatigue and fracture mechanics in aerospace structures *Encyclopedia Aerosp. Eng.* **1** 1–12

[13] Lemons J E and Lucas L C 1986 Properties of biomaterials *J. Arthroplasty* **1** 143–7

[14] Liuyun J, Yubao L and Chengdong X 2009 Preparation and biological properties of a novel composite scaffold of nano-hydroxyapatite/chitosan/carboxymethyl cellulose for bone tissue engineering *J. Biomed. Sci.* **16** 1–0

[15] Elieh-Ali-Komi D and Hamblin M R 2016 Chitin and chitosan: production and application of versatile biomedical nanomaterials *Int. J. Adv. Res.* **4** 411

[16] Liuyun J, Yubao L and Chengdong X 2009 A novel composite membrane of chitosan-carboxymethyl cellulose polyelectrolyte complex membrane filled with nano-hydroxyapatite I. Preparation and properties *J. Mater. Sci., Mater. Med.* **20** 1645–52

[17] Levingstone T J, Herbaj S and Dunne N J 2019 Calcium phosphate nanoparticles for therapeutic applications in bone regeneration *Nanomaterials.* **9** 1570

[18] Lu J, Yu H and Chen C 2018 Biological properties of calcium phosphate biomaterials for bone repair: a review *RSC Adv.* **8** 2015–33

[19] Barrère F, van Blitterswijk C A and de Groot K 2006 Bone regeneration: molecular and cellular interactions with calcium phosphate ceramics *Int. J. Nanomed.* **1** 317

[20] Cheng L, Wang T, Zhu J and Cai P 2016 Osteoinduction of calcium phosphate ceramics in four kinds of animals for 1 year: dog, rabbit, rat, and mouse *Transplantation Proc.* vol 48 (Amsterdam: Elsevier) 1309–14

[21] Sheikh Z, Najeeb S, Khurshid Z, Verma V, Rashid H and Glogauer M 2015 Biodegradable materials for bone repair and tissue engineering applications *Materials* **8** 5744–94

[22] Nimni M E, Cheung D, Strates B, Kodama M and Sheikh K 1987 Chemically modified collagen: a natural biomaterial for tissue replacement *J. Biomed. Mater. Res.* **21** 741–71

[23] Dey P 2020 Bone mineralisation *Contemporary Topics about Phosphorus in Biology and Materials* (Rijeka: IntechOpen)

[24] Gomes D S, Santos A M, Neves G A and Menezes R R 2019 A brief review on hydroxyapatite production and use in biomedicine *Cerâmica* **65** 282–302

[25] Martín Vilardell A 2017 Functionalized coatings by cold spray for joint prosthesis *Doctoral Dissertation* Universitat de Barcelona

[26] Kenny S M and Buggy M 2003 Bone cements and fillers: a review *J. Mater. Sci., Mater. Med.* **14** 923–38.0

[27] Amini A R, Laurencin C T and Nukavarapu S P 2012 Bone tissue engineering: recent advances and challenges *Crit. Rev. Biomed. Eng.* **40**

[28] Zhang L and Webster T J 2009 Nanotechnology and nanomaterials: promises for improved tissue regeneration *Nano today* **1** 66–80

[29] Miculescu F, Maidaniuc A, Voicu S I, Thakur V K, Stan G E and Ciocan L T 2017 Progress in hydroxyapatite–starch based sustainable biomaterials for biomedical bone substitution applications *ACS Sustain. Chem. Eng.* **5** 8491–512

[30] Kowalczewski C J and Saul J M 2018 Biomaterials for the delivery of growth factors and other therapeutic agents in tissue engineering approaches to bone regeneration *Front. Pharmacol.* **9** 513

[31] Guijt R M, Dodge A, van Dedem G W, de Rooij N F and Verpoorte E 2003 Chemical and physical processes for integrated temperature control in microfluidic devices *Lab Chip* **3** 1–4

[32] Barradas A M, Yuan H, van Blitterswijk C A and Habibovic P 2011 Osteoinductive biomaterials: current knowledge of properties, experimental models and biological mechanisms *Eur. Cell Mater.* **21** 29

[33] Ripamonti U 2007 Recapitulating development: a template for periodontal tissue engineering *Tissue Eng.* **13** 51–71

[34] Jianjun G, Fujimoto K L, Sacks M S and Wagner W R 2005 Preparation and characterization of highly porous, biodegradable polyurethane scaffolds for soft tissue applications *Biomaterials* **18** 3961–71

[35] Yu F, Cao X, Li Y, Zeng L, Yuan B and Chen X 2013 An injectable hyaluronic acid/PEG hydrogel for cartilage tissue engineering formed by integrating enzymatic crosslinking and Diels–Alder ‘click chemistry’ *Polym. Chem.* **5** 1082–90

[36] Cai X Y, Li J Z, Li N N, Chen J C, Kang E T and Xu L Q 2016 PEG-based hydrogels prepared by catalyst-free thiol–yne addition and their post-antibacterial modification *Biomater. Sci.* **4** 1663–72

[37] Hallab N J, Urban R M and Jacobs J J 2004 Corrosion and biocompatibility of orthopedic implants *Biomaterials in Orthopedics* (Boca Raton, FL: CRC Press) pp 63–92

[38] Ray P C, Yu H and Fu P P 2009 Toxicity and environmental risks of nanomaterials: challenges and future needs *J. Environ. Sci. Health Part C.* **27** 1–35

[39] Ali N, Teixeira J A and Addali A 2018 A review on nanofluids: fabrication, stability, and thermophysical properties *J. Nanomater.* **2018** 6978130

[40] Angayarkanni S A and Philip J 2015 Review on thermal properties of nanofluids: recent developments *Adv. Colloid Interface Sci.* **225** 146–76

[41] Ali N, Teixeira J A and Addali A 2018 A review on nanofluids: fabrication, stability, and thermophysical properties *J. Nanomater.* **2018**

[42] Bowman H F, Cravalho E G and Woods M 1975 Theory, measurement, and application of thermal properties of biomaterials *Annu. Rev. Biophys. Bioeng.* **4** 43–80

[43] Gagge A P 1971 An effective temperature scale based on a simple model of human physiological regulatory response *Ashrae Trans* **77** 247–62

[44] Ranga N, Gahlyan S and Duhan S 2020 Antibacterial efficiency of Zn, Mg and Sr doped bioactive glass for bone tissue engineering *J. Nanosci. Nanotechnol.* **20** 2465–72

[45] Ranga N, Poonia E, Jakhar S, Sharma A K, Kumar A, Devi S and Duhan S 2019 Enhanced antimicrobial properties of bioactive glass using strontium and silver oxide nanocomposites *J. Asian Ceram. Soc.* **7** 75–81

[46] AshaRani P V, Sethu S, Lim H K, Balaji G, Valiyaveettil S and Hande M P 2012 Differential regulation of intracellular factors mediating cell cycle, DNA repair and inflammation following exposure to silver nanoparticles in human cells *Genome Integr.* **3** 2

[47] Prasad K *et al* 2017 Metallic biomaterials : current challenges and opportunities *Materials* **10** 884

[48] Velu R, Calais T, Jayakumar A and Raspall F 2020 A comprehensive review on bio-nanomaterials for medical implants and feasibility studies on fabrication of such implants by additive manufacturing technique *Materials* **13** 92

[49] Chevalier J and Gremillard L 2009 Ceramics for medical applications: a picture for the next 20 years *J. Eur. Ceram. Soc.* **29** 1245–55

[50] Ohtsuki C, Kamitakahara M and Miyazaki T 2009 Bioactive ceramic-based materials with designed reactivity for bone tissue regeneration *J. R. Soc. Interface* **6** S349–60

[51] Dhivya S, Ajita J and Selvamurugan N 2015 Metallic nanomaterials for bone tissue engineering *J. Biomed. Nanotechnol.* **11** 1675–700

[52] Baino F, Novajra G and Vitale-Brovarone C 2015 Bioceramics and scaffolds: a winning combination for tissue engineering *Front. Bioeng. Biotechnol.* **3** 202

[53] Gerhardt L C and Boccaccini A R 2010 Bioactive glass and glass-ceramic scaffolds for bone tissue engineering *Materials* **3** 3867–910

[54] Makvandi P, Wang C Y, Zare E N, Borzacchiello A, Niu L N and Tay F R 2020 Metal-based nanomaterials in biomedical applications: antimicrobial activity and cytotoxicity aspects *Adv. Funct. Mater.* **30** 1910021

[55] Nandi S K, Mahato A, Kundu B and Mukherjee P 2016 Doped bioactive glass materials in bone regeneration *Adv. Tech. Bone Regen.* **13** 276–327

[56] Cacciotti I 2017 Bivalent cationic ions doped bioactive glasses: the influence of magnesium, zinc, strontium and copper on the physical and biological properties *J. Mater. Sci.* **52** 8812–31

[57] Kokubo T and Takadama H 2006 How useful is SBF in predicting *in vivo* bone bioactivity? *Biomaterials* **27** 2907–15

[58] Hamdy T M 2018 Polymers and ceramics biomaterials in orthopedics and dentistry: a review article *Egypt. J. Chem.* **61** 723–30

[59] Agrawal C M 1998 Reconstructing the human body using biomaterials *JOM* **50** 31–5

[60] Sumi T, Motono S, Ishida Y, Shirahata N and Yonezawa T 2015 Formation and optical properties of fluorescent gold nanoparticles obtained by matrix sputtering method with volatile mercaptan molecules in the vacuum chamber and consideration of their structures *Langmuir* **31** 4323–9

[61] He C, Liu D and Lin W 2015 Nanomedicine applications of hybrid nanomaterials built from metal–ligand coordination bonds: nanoscale metal–organic frameworks and nanoscale coordination polymers *Chem. Rev.* **115** 11079–108

[62] Cho H K, Cho H J, Lone S, Kim D D, Yeum J H and Cheong I W 2011 Preparation and characterization of MRI-active gadolinium nanocomposite particles for neutron capture therapy *J. Mater. Chem.* **21** 15486–93

[63] Di Marco M, Sadun C, Port M, Guilbert I, Couvreur P and Dubernet C 2007 Physicochemical characterization of ultrasmall superparamagnetic iron oxide particles (USPIO) for biomedical application as MRI contrast agents *Int. J. Nanomed.* **2** 609

[64] ALOthman Z A 2012 A review: fundamental aspects of silicate mesoporous materials *Materials* **5** 2874–902

[65] Jafari S, Derakhshankhah H, Alaei L, Fattahi A, Varnamkhasti B S and Saboury A A 2019 Mesoporous silica nanoparticles for therapeutic/diagnostic applications *Biomed. Pharmacother.* **109** 1100–11

[66] Kesse S *et al* 2019 Mesoporous silica nanomaterials: versatile nanocarriers for cancer theranostics and drug and gene delivery *Pharmaceutics* **11** 77

[67] Mirzaei M, Babaei Zarch M, Darroudi M, Sayyadi K, Keshavarz S T, Sayyadi J, Fallah A and Maleki H 2020 Silica mesoporous structures: effective nanocarriers in drug delivery and nanocatalysts *Appl. Sci.* **10** 7533

[68] Vivero-Escoto J L and Huang Y T 2011 Inorganic-organic hybrid nanomaterials for therapeutic and diagnostic imaging applications *Int. J. Mol. Sci.* **12** 3888–927

[69] Sanchez C, Belleville P, Popall M and Nicole L 2011 Applications of advanced hybrid organic–inorganic nanomaterials: from laboratory to market *Chem. Soc. Rev.* **40** 696–753

[70] Gallo J, Holinka M and Moucha C S 2014 Antibacterial surface treatment for orthopaedic implants *Int. J. Mol. Sci.* **15** 13849–80

[71] Jeong W J, Bu J, Kubiatowicz L J, Chen S S, Kim Y and Hong S 2018 Peptide–nanoparticle conjugates: a next generation of diagnostic and therapeutic platforms? *Nano Converg.* **5** 38

[72] Anselmo A C and Mitragotri S 2014 An overview of clinical and commercial impact of drug delivery systems *J. Control. Release* **190** 15–28

[73] Wong I Y, Bhatia S N and Toner M 2013 Nanotechnology: emerging tools for biology and medicine *Genes Develop.* **27** 2397–408

[74] Buzea C, Pacheco I I and Robbie K 2007 Nanomaterials and nanoparticles: sources and toxicity *Biointerphases* **2** MR17–71

[75] Tao Y, Wang J and Xu X 2020 Emerging and innovative theranostic approaches for mesoporous silica nanoparticles in hepatocellular carcinoma: current status and advances *Front. Bioeng. Biotechnol.* **8** 184

[76] Buzea C, Pacheco I I and Robbie K 2007 Nanomaterials and nanoparticles: sources and toxicity *Biointerphases.* **2** MR17–71

Chapter 3

Synthesis and characterization of bionanomaterials

Shikha Kapil, Nirmalya Pal, Ankita Vinayak and Vipasha Sharma

The prevailing advancements in bio-based nanomaterial composites are gaining attention due to perspective applications around the world. In the past decade, scientific research has opted to synthesize bionanomaterials from natural and synthetic materials which have several advantages such as water solubility, *in vivo* biodegradability, economic values, mechanical stability, and efficient targeting ability, etc which make them more suitable alternatives for the synthesis of bionanomaterials. This chapter presents an overview of the synthesis of bionanomaterials using biopolymers and an update on various imaging, spectroscopic and microscopic techniques to characterize and to determine their chemical composition, molecular weight distribution, and physical properties.

3.1 Introduction

In the present world of advancements and modernization, there is an intense need to look into materials that are green and environment friendly, economical, and sustainable. To replace non-renewable materials with cost-effective, efficient, and usable renewable materials the use of biomaterials is a better substitute. Biomaterials possesses a high sustainability rate due to their overwhelming applications such as reinforcement, biodegradability, and biocompatibility of the resultant product. Biomaterial-derived nanomaterials enable us to conduct new establishments with a wide range of new applications. The nano-structure of biopolymers depends upon two aspects: increased surface area which enhances their reactivity; and the quantum effect offered by the changes in their physio-chemical, mechanical, and optical properties. Bionanomaterials are originally derived from living organisms. These materials are naturally found in nature or can be synthesized artificially using natural resources. In figure 3.1, the classification of bionanomaterials based on their origin and properties is also represented. Moreover, the features of biomaterials at

doi:10.1088/978-0-7503-3767-0ch3

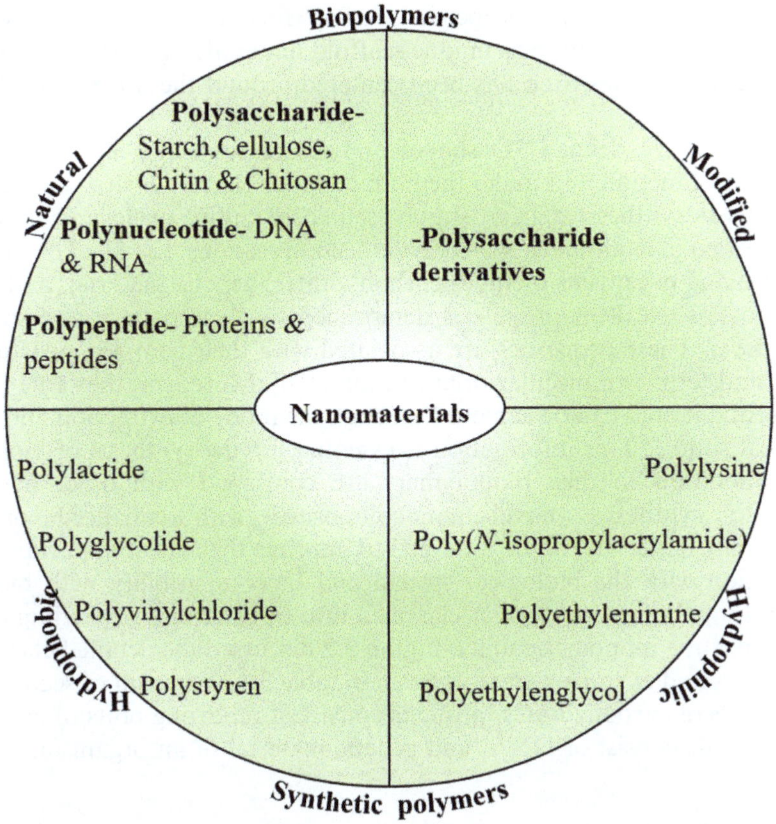

Figure 3.1. Classification of nanobiomaterials based on their origin and property.

the nanoscale level provide us with ultimate properties of low density and strong mechanical strength to enable vast opportunities to develop nanocomposite systems. Therefore, with advanced properties, these nano-biocomposites can be used in medical applications of tissue engineering, drug-delivery carriers, wound healing compounds, and other regenerative medicines. This bio-nano composite is considered to be promising to induce a substantial improvement in cell adhesion and protein absorption at the molecular level and is shown to be biologically desired when compared to its micro-sized proportions. The present chapter gives us in-depth knowledge about the variety of bio-based nanomaterials including polysaccharides (PSs), polynucleotides (PNs), and polypeptides (PPs) that are used for biomedical applications.

3.2 Biopolymers

Biopolymers have polymeric subunits that are covalently bonded with each other to form a complex molecular assembly. Biopolymers are biodegradable and are derived from living sources such as microorganisms, plants, or trees, etc [1]. However, the disadvantage of utilizing natural polymers is that these may quickly degrade with the conceivable loss of organic properties during formulation and storage, often compromising their utilization as unique scaffold materials. Regardless of the minor disadvantage, current research has been centered around the utilization of natural polymers.

Biopolymers have defined 3D shapes and structures which are the important aspects of their function and make them an active molecule *in vivo*. Biodegradable biopolymers are synthesized from starch, cellulose, chitin, nucleic acids, proteins, and other organic components in varying compositions [2, 3]. The molecular makeup of living organisms includes carbohydrates, genetic material, and proteins and they possess excellent properties determined by their pattern and size at the nanoscale level. These properties are associated with their complex structures, i.e., secondary and tertiary molecular organization [4–6]. Moreover, the same polymers with different qualities can be achieved through the mode of extraction and the type of biological source. This information is essential for the synthesis of bionanomaterials. In addition to this, biopolymers are combined with other micro-sized materials to synthesize novel nanocomposites with enhanced properties. Nanocomposite materials can be modified to improve their most important feature, i.e., interaction with the biological system and biocompatibility with biomedical devices [7]. Biopolymers are further classified into three groups depending upon the nature of repeating monomeric units. Figure 3.2 discussed the detailed classification of biopolymers and examples are also given in table 3.1 at the end of section 3.2. PS mainly consists of carbohydrates, proteins consist of repeating units of amino acids and nucleic acids consist of DNA, and genetic material of an organism.

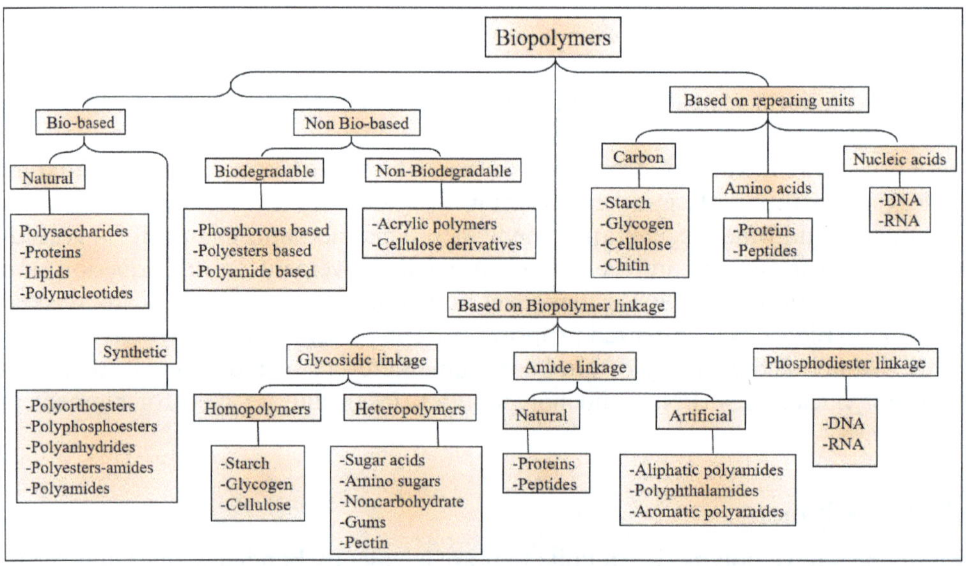

Figure 3.2. Different classes of biopolymers based on their origin, biopolymeric linkage and polymer repeating units.

Table 3.1. Various polymers for nanomaterial fabrication and preparation techniques.

Classification	Polymers	Characteristics	Preparation method	Application	References
Natural polymers	Starch	Mechanical properties, enzymatic degradation, chemical modifications	Dissolution, precipitation, cross-linking, reduction	Biomedical application, drug delivery	[130]
	Chitosan	Biodegradable, no toxic, biocompatible	Precipitation, oxidation, spray drying, freeze-drying	Pharmaceutical application, enhance bioavailability	
	Alginate	Biocompatible, economical, no toxic	Electrostatic interaction, freeze-drying, emulsification, precipitation	Drug delivery	
	Cellulose	Biocompatible, surface properties, colloidal stable	Freeze drying, hydrolysis, solvent evaporation, magnetic decantation	Sustained drug delivery	
	Albumins	Non-toxic, biodegradable, non-immunogenic	Extrusion, precipitation, freeze-drying, desolvation, self-assembly	Drug delivery, tumor-targeting ligand	
	Silk fibroin	Mechanical hard, biocompatible, malleable	Crosslinking, degassing, salting out, degassing	Bioactive molecule delivery	
Synthetic polymers	PLGA—poly (lactic-glycolic acid)	Biodegradable, biocompatible	Solvent evaporation, Precipitation, emulsification	Tissue engineering, biomedical applications	[131]
	Polylactic acid	Biocompatible, non-toxic, mechanical properties	Solvent evaporation	Tissue engineering, drug delivery, bone fixing	[132]
	Polyurethane	Economical, mechanical properties	Polymerization	Medical bandage	[133]
	PMMA—polymethyl methacrylate resin	Biocompatible, easy operation, mechanical stable	Acid hydrolysis, thermal decomposition	Artificial crystal, bone fixation, drug delivery	[134]

3.2.1 Polysaccharide based nanomaterials

PSs including chitin, chitosan, cellulose, and starch are plentiful and are rich in properties such as non-toxic, biodegradability, biocompatibility, the renewable and cheap source that can be used for drug delivery, immobilization, tissue engineering, and regenerative medicines [8]. Properties of these materials are largely governed by their molecular weight and degree of substitution [9]. PSs can be modified by using various modes of physical, chemical, and biochemical reactions. During reaction it involves toxic compounds to initiate the reaction, therefore there is the foremost need to remove these agents by a purification process to ensure the biosafety and biocompatibility of the final products. PSs consist of repeating units of monosaccharides that are joined together employing glycosidic bonds. These are the most abundant biomolecule in nature and are classified according to their origin, including pectin from vegetables, alginate from algae, dextran and xanthan gum from microbes, chitosan, and heparin from animals [10]. Furthermore, PSs are also classified by the charge carriers by their monosaccharides units i.e. cationic includes chitosan, anionic includes hyaluronic acid and heparin, non-ionic includes dextran [11]. Due to these properties, i.e., the presence of a functional group on the PS chain, they are easily modified chemically. PS-nanoparticles (NPs) are fabricated either by top-down or bottom-up processes. In top-down approaches, PS macromolecules are broken down into nanoscale molecules such as cellulose nanocrystals and nanofibrillated cellulose, whereas in the bottom-up process PS macromolecules recombine to generate large-scale NPs [12–16]. In the latter case, PS-NPs are synthesized by using different processes such as chemical crosslinking, ionic crosslinking, self-assembling, supramolecular and hydrophobic interactions. PS-NPs are distinguished according to the methods we use to synthesize them on the nanoscale level.

3.2.1.1 Starch

Starch is generally produced by plants in granular forms which consist of amylose and amylopectin in the majority and lipids, proteins, and minerals as micro-constituents. Starch is used to produce various nanocomposites, NPs, and nano-structured surfaces. Studies have shown that starch granules consist of several nano-sized semi-crystalline blockets [17, 18]. Mild acid or enzyme treatments are sufficient to isolate nano-blockets from starch. The crystalline moieties of the starch granules are more resistant to acids and thus through acid hydrolysis (hydrochloric or sulphuric acids) it is possible to breakdown the starch granules into several hundred nano-meters' sized particles. Acid hydrolysis is a time-consuming approach and also generates a very low yield of the recovery product [19–21]. In addition to this, sonication, high-pressure homogenization, and micro-emulsion-based methodologies are also used to synthesize starch-based NPs [22, 23]. The synthesis techniques are classified into 'top-down' and 'bottom-up' processes [24, 25]. Also, the characteristics of the end product are crucially determined by the type of processing method applied for their synthesis. For instance, NPs obtained after acid hydrolysis and nanoprecipitation are size-dependent and size-independent, respectively, of their source of isolation [26, 27]. Mechanical properties of the starch nanocomposite film also depend upon the starch strength and its source. So both aspects must be considered to tailor the final NPs' features including molecule size, amylose content, and crystalline nature, for the intended application [28]. Besides, starch NPs contain crystalline moiety and have inherent properties of renewability and biodegradability from starch. Various researches have mentioned starch as a potential biomedical material as a safe drug release regulator to generate a sustained drug delivery system [29–32].

3.2.1.2 Cellulose

Cellulose is one of the most pervasive and abundant polysaccharides that has been used and commercially exploited as a resource for many centuries. Cellulose is majorly derived from wood and plant fibers and exists in various forms such as bacterial cellulose, algal cellulose, and tunicate cellulose. Cellulose is a homopolymer chain composed of linear β-1,4-linked anhydrous glucose subunits [33]. The intramolecular H-bonds are required for the stiffness and stability of crystalline cellulose whereas, intermolecular H-bonds are required for the sheet-like characteristic of the native cellulose [34]. The intra-and intermolecular hydrogen bonds (H-bonds) cause the parallel alignment of the polymer chains to give rise to well-defined microfibrils. Microfibrils have a crystalline region (where the polymer chains are highly ordered) and an amorphous region (disordered region) [35]. There are four polymorphs such as cellulose I, II, III, and cellulose IV. Cellulose I is the most important and abundant crystalline form of cellulose which represents the largest biomass on the planet and is found in the major structural component of the plant cell wall [36].

Based on the extraction source and processing approach, cellulose nanomaterials are classified as nanofibrillated cellulose (NFC) (top-down), bacterial nanocellulose (BNC) (bottom-up), and cellulose nanocrystals (CNC) (bottom-up). The processing approaches include acid hydrolysis and mechanical treatments such as high-pressure homogenization and refining [37–39], microfluidization [40, 41], ultrasonication [42, 43], cryocrushing, and grinding [44, 45]. Furthermore, enzyme or chemical pre-treatments are also given in combination with these chemical and physical methods to give rise to sustainable nano-size fibers [46]. In acid hydrolysis, several factors need to be controlled such as the concentration of cellulose and acid to be used for hydrolysis, process temperature, time for agitation, ultrasonication, and hydrolysis [47]. Cellulose nanomaterials have prominent results in the pharmaceutical and biomedical fields due to their excellent cytocompatibility [48]. Applications include wound dressing, bioactive implants, scaffolds in artificial ligaments, or tendon substitutes [12, 49, 50].

3.2.1.3 Chitin

Chitin is present in the exoskeleton and is another abundant polymer in the environment [51]. Moreover, seafood waste such as shrimps, shellfish, and crabs from the food industry is a valuable source of chitin [52, 53]. Chitin is composed of 2-acetamido-2-deoxy-d-glucopyranose units linked together by a β-1,4 glycosidic bond to form a linear biopolymer. Like cellulose, chitin is also arranged in crystalline nanofibrils and considered as a structural biopolymer strengthening the exoskeleton of many insects and arthropods [54, 55]. Based on the alignment of the polymeric chain, chitin is further classified into α- and β-chitin [56]. In α-chitin, the polymer chains are aligned in parallel mode and are found in the exoskeletons of insects, shells of crustaceans, and cell walls of fungi [57–59]. In contrast, in the β-chitin polymer, chains are aligned in an antiparallel mode and it is present in some mollusks and squid pens shell [60–62]. Chitin shares structure similarity and methods used for the synthesis of chitin nanomaterials to that of cellulose. Primarily two types of chitin nanomaterials such as nanowhiskers (NWs) and nanofibrils (NFs) are reported to date. NWs are 100–800 nm long with 6–60 nm diameter, whereas NFs are 1000 nm long with 10–100 nm diameter. Methods reported for chitin nanomaterial synthesis are acid hydrolysis, oxidation, and deacetylation mediated by 2,6,6-tetramethylpiperidinooxy (TEMPO) [63]. Other techniques used are mechanical procedures such as grinding and homogenization in combination with ultra-sonication techniques. Due to its hydrophobic nature chitin is insoluble in water and other organic solvents, which limits its processing and applications. Nevertheless, several studies have shown its biocompatibility and stable immunological responses *in vitro* [64, 65].

3.2.1.4 Chitosan

Chitosan is a cationic biopolyaminosaccharide that consists of repeating units such as *N*-acetyl-D-glucosamine and D-glucosamine joined together by β-1,4-glycosidic linkage [66]. Chitosan is soluble in weak acids (pH < 6.5) such as formic, oxalic, lactic, and acetic acids, is a deacetylated derivative of chitin and is synthesized by alkaline deacetylation process [67]. Generally, chitosan is derived from aquatic fauna such as shrimps and sea crustaceans by using sodium hydroxide during its synthesis. Moreover, chitosan is mucoadhesive, and easy to modify chemically to synthesize derivatives of various characteristics that can be applied in multiple applications [68]. In the medical field, chitosan is used as a potential carrier to successfully deliver drugs/vaccines, growth factors, and anti-inflammatory agents, etc [69, 70]. In addition to low toxicity, biodegradability, biocompatibility, ease of chemical modification, and mucoadhesive properties chitosan has an undesirable drug burst effect which limits its usage in the drug delivery system [71–73]. In this regard, the coating of the chitosan microsphere by using another polymer after loading drugs is a potential approach to overcome its drug-burst effect and to stabilize the drug delivery system. Chitosan is hydrophilic and soluble in a mildly acidic medium, so its surface coating by using acid-resistant polymer is a suitable approach that has been followed by some researchers [74, 75]. Generally, top-down and bottom-up approaches are followed to develop micro-and nanomaterials. Chitosan-derived particles are largely dependent upon their molecular weight [76]. Conventionally, chitosan micro-and nanomaterial synthesis is done by using bottom-up techniques [77]. During synthesis, there are several factors such as particle size, the active compound, and final product stability, residual toxicity, drug release kinetics which should be considered during the selection of synthesis method [78].

3.2.2 Polysaccharide derivatives

PS derivative synthesis by using acetates and methyl ethers has been in use for a long time and is still in trend. Along with this, currently, more attention has been drawn toward newer derivatives with hydrophobic and hydrophilic properties. *De novo* design strategy has been implied to synthesize sustained regioselective [79, 80], block-like [81–87], or another undefined pattern [88] of the substituent. In addition to starch and cellulose, glucans such as dextran are also being utilized for the modification and synthesis of PS derivatives [89]. Although, this field requires more expertise in characterization, treatment, and research to progress in the field of substitution pattern analysis.

3.2.3 Polypeptide based nanomaterials

PPs recently emerged as a remarkable tool for the fabrication of bionanomaterials. They exhibit huge diversity in structure and functionality, making them potent agents for nanomaterials. Peptide-based nanomaterials are comprised of small peptide sequences, having the flexibility to show desired biophysical characteristics through self-assembly or interacting with another nanomaterial. The individual size of the peptide molecule is 2–30 nm, enabling peptides to be formally assigned as nanomaterials. Due to the structural characteristics of peptide groups, the molecules are arranged in spatial ordering ensuring their association with other ordered structures. The desired supramolecular arrangement can be formed by adding more monomer molecules. Nanomaterials such as nanorods, nanotubes, nanofibers, and nanotapes can be generated using peptides and have numerous applications.

In recent years, the development of peptide-based nanomaterials has been of increasing research interest because of biocompatibility, self-assembly, and several other features. Depending upon the usage field and application, PPs offer several advantages viz, easy modifiability, bio functionality, and enhanced biological activity. They are also most stable and can be stored for the long term. The most prominent characteristics of the peptides are self-assembly and substrate recognition for the creation of other nanomaterials by themselves [90]. The unique self-assembly attribute renders them useful biomolecules for the construction of various peptide-based nanomaterials with multivalent effect and high stability. They offer significant medical applications like regenerative medicines, gene therapy, vaccines, and drug delivery [91]. The different types of peptides such as cyclic peptides, dipeptides, alpha-helical peptides, beta-sheet peptides, and cyclic peptides have been used for the generation of peptide-based nanomaterials.

3.2.3.1 Cyclic peptides

Cyclic peptides are attracting special attention for a build-up of nanomaterials. Having rigid and stable conformation in comparison to linear peptides, they have the potential to be used as a soft material for biomaterials. The naturally found cyclic peptides occur in all living forms, exhibiting various biological functions such as being antimicrobial, anti-tumor, antifungal, and anti-inflammatory. Cyclic peptides have alternating L and D type amino acids, forming a flat ring that assembles into cylindrical structures. They self-assemble into a flat conformation structure through the aggregation of cyclic peptides as their building blocks [92]. In the cylindrical configuration, peptide backbone exists on the inner side and carbonyl and amino side chains on the outer side, perpendicular to the ring. The diameter and surface properties of so formed nanomaterials can be controlled by the number and choice of amino acids used for synthesis [93]. The nanomaterials synthesized from cyclic peptides such as nanotubes are formed by self-assembly and are stabilized by hydrogen bonding. Various cyclic peptides including β, δ-amino acids, and alternating α-amino acids (D and L type) are employed for self-assembly and nanomaterials. Cyclic peptides-based nanomaterials possess unique properties such as resistance to enzymatic proteolysis, stable conformation, and diameter control through peptide side-chain modification [94]. The appropriate design and self-assembly conditions optimization allows the tailoring of properties of nanostructures for a specific desired application. In one study, the construction of supramolecular nanotubes from cyclic peptide polymer conjugate was performed and revealed the potential of cyclic peptide-based nanostructures for systematic circulation and renal clearance, thus making them an effective drug carrier [95].

3.2.3.2 Dipeptides

The self-association of small peptides such as dipeptides is being greatly explored and studied for the generation of nanostructures. Short peptides offer several advantages like stability, lowering the cost of the nanomaterial fabrication process, and also minimizing process difficulties [96]. The dipeptide, diphenylalanine (FF, Phe-Phe), core motif of β-amyloid segment was the first studied peptide for the formation of nanomaterial. It was used for the preparation of various nanostructures through self-assembly. Depending on the type of peptide and solvent, they can be ordered into various nanostructures such as nanotubes, nanowires, ribbon, and nanoforests. They exhibit a vast array of applications in material sciences like for the formation of nanobiosensors, nanowires and in the biomedical field also such as in tissue engineering, immune response, and drug delivery [97]. Some other aromatic dipeptides such as KLVFF associate with nanofibrils, nanogels, nanoplates, and nanospheres having clinical application including molecular imaging, bio imaging, etc. Modified dipeptides such as ω amino acids (N terminal) have also joined the race for the formation of functional nanostructures. Carboxyl modified FF analogues also have the potential for the generation of nanoscale materials [98].

3.2.3.3 Amphiphilic peptides

Amphiphilic peptides include linear peptides, peptides phospholipids, ionic complementary polypeptides, peptide-based copolymers, and long-chain alkylated peptides. These peptides are composed of a charged hydrophilic head and a hydrophilic tail. The hydrophobic interactions are attributed to the self-assembly of peptides into nanomaterials like nanomicelles, nanovesicles, and nanotubes [99]. The amino acid residues such as E, D, H, K, and K are used in the hydrophilic head domain of peptides, and A, I, G, F, L, and V are considered as potential candidates for the hydrophobic domain. The self-assembly of peptides is governed by various physical properties like shape, size, and also by chemical properties such as concentration, overall hydrophobicity, peptide charge, and sequence. Unlike the conventional surfactants, amphiphilic peptides involve hydrogen bonding responsible for the aggregation of peptides into nanostructures. In contrast, the hydrophobic interactions in conventional surfactants form vesicles and micelles. The amphiphilic nature of peptides endows them with enhanced solubility in liquid media, favouring their medical applications [100, 101]. Being a short peptide sequence, they facilitate the formation of structure–property relationships, easy design and synthesis, and also large-scale production useful for studies and practical applications. The versatility, simplicity, and biocompatibility enable them to be used in nanotechnology and biomedical applications [102].

3.2.3.4 Alpha-helix peptides

The physical and biological properties of peptides favour their assembly into helical conformation. Alpha-helix peptide is a commonly known secondary structure of proteins and peptides. It is a right-handed helical spiral coil conformation. Each helix occurs with a periodicity of 3.6 amino acid residues per turn. The side chains of residues interact with the helical structure and are responsible for the self-association of peptides into the helix [97]. The chirality of alpha-helix peptides is another predominant factor for the construction of nanomaterials. These peptides are used for the formation of various fibrous bionanomaterials. The so-formed nanostructures from alpha-helix peptides resemble extracellular matrix and cytoskeleton molecules of the biological system, displaying the application in the biomedical field. The alpha-helix peptides can be fabricated into nanofibers and filamentous nanostructures. For example, alpha-helix peptides having 25–30 amino acid residues can assemble into filamentous nanomaterials. The coiled configuration can be manipulated by altering the abiotic factors like ionic strength, pH, and temperature, which enhances biocompatibility as well as potential for application in tissue engineering and drug delivery [103].

3.2.3.5 Beta-sheet peptides

Beta-sheet peptides are another naturally occurring motif employed for the self-assembly of peptides into nanostructures. They are comprised of alternating hydrophobic and hydrophilic amino acid units in their peptide sequence, which imparts amphiphilic nature to them and drives their association into beta-sheets. Various strategies such as enhancing and modulating the interaction of peptides in beta conformation have been used for the fabrication of nanostructures. They are utilized to form nanomaterials like nanoribbons and nanotubes [104].

3.2.4 Polynucleotide based nanomaterials

In the manufacturing and development of nanostructures and devices, molecules of biological substances like nucleic acid have demonstrated excessive potential. Depending on the context, and scope of each application, nano-science, and nanotechnology are distinct contrarily. A nucleic acid is also a suitable molecule for the programming itself due to its propensities that render it as genetic material. The use of nucleic acid has been expanded to create metallic nanowires and functional nanotubes to assemble metals or semiconducting particles [105].

Nanoscience and nanotechnology include atomic, molecular, or macromolecular research and technology advances in the range between 1 and 100 nm. This may contribute to the idea of renaming biological and chemical (molecules) nano-sized structures as small machines [106]. For example, adenosine triphosphate (ATP) synthase catalyzing, the basic currency of free-energy in life systems, can be referred to as a nano-motor; the enzymes also catalyze bonds in other molecules that are formed, disintegrated, or rearranged [107]. The actin-myosin molecular machine is another example that can move fibers past each other. DNA also acts as a 'data storage device' and transmits digital guidance to molecular machines, and the ribosomes which in turn produce protein and enzyme molecules are the major molecular types of machinery in live systems [108]. Nanobiotechnology uses the concepts and techniques of nanoscale for the understanding and transformation of bio-systems (living or non-living) and it uses biological ideologies and materials to construct new nanoscale-integrated devices and systems. Nanotechnologies are estimated to grow exponentially in the coming years in the integration with biotechnologies as well as with cognitive testing. The flexibility of RNA structure and function, bottom-up assembly pricing, its determined dimensions and structure, its favourable *in vivo* attributes, and its great therapeutic potential make this a biomaterial attractive applicant for the delivery of NPs [109].

RNA has the ability to follow several complicated quaternary structures, to stack the foundation, to form as recognized Watson–Crick (G–C, A–T), and to form as non-canonical (A–U reverse hoogsteen, G–U wobble, G–A imino, sheared G–A) [110]. NPs for nanomedicine and bio-nanotechnology use these proprieties for RNA nanotechnology use. Various secondary and tertiary structural RNA patterns are easily scannable by the RNA designer. These motifs are used by engineering factors like the angle of the motif and the arrangement length as building blocks to design varying sizes of NPs [109]. RNA NPS' physicochemical properties can be easily adapted *in vitro* and *in vivo* for the desired applications.

3.2.4.1 Deoxyribonucleic acid (DNA)

DNA is an excellent option to work as a nanotechnological construction material. The extremely precise Watson–Crick hydrogen binding enables the artificial DNA receptor moieties to be programmed conveniently. As a molecular weapon, the strength of DNA lies in the huge mechanical rigidity of small double-helixes, which enables them to act as a hard rod separator on either side of two tied-up functional molecular components. Besides, the physical–chemical stability of DNA is relatively high [110–112]. DNA is rapidly expanding in three major directions for nano-structure manufacturing: (a) the manufacture of native DNA artificial networks; (b) assembly or incorporation of DNA on solid surfaces of state; (c) the development of NPs in metals or semiconductors along with DNA. The missing issue to transform normal DNA into the foundations for stimulating nanomaterial is a branching point on the helix. DNA division points including transient structures, including replication and repair, occur in the cellular metabolism of DNA [110–112]. In the Holliday structure, they are prominent, a four-arm branched intermediate in chromosomes [113]. Arrangements of molecules of DNA can be engineered to create steady synthetic versions of 'Holliday' joints, branched, multi-number molecules, and more complicated motifs [114].

Theories and methods for self-assembled schemes have been established with enormous interest in recent years. Three different methods can mainly be used to assembly metals or semiconducting NPs using DNA: (a) the electrostatic connection to the negative charged DNA of positively charged colloids; (b) the basic binding by chemical bonds of colloids to DNA. DNA and/or colloids, for instance, thiol grouping or biotin–streptavidin complexes, can be changed. Colloids with single sections of DNA containing oligonucleotides are also possible to hybridize; (c) NPs' direct growth in the molecules of DNA. The formation of nucleation on DNA molecules, followed by the chemical deposition of the corresponding salt, will accomplish this [105–109].

There have been several studies to assemble colloidal gold NPs with DNA as binding elements into macroscopic aggregates. In one study, phosphorothioate DNA was used to cross-link the surface of AuNPs in the solution to arrange them in different dimensions [115]. Alivisatos *et al* also documented another approach to successfully arrange gold nano-crystals into a unique structure [116]. Maeda *et al* used the Au-thiol reactors and a technique of hybridization of the DNA to create Au particles inserted on a two-dimensional DNA network template [117]. Besides, when assembling DNA-modified gold NPs, a colour shift of red-to-blue into normal arrays was also observed [118]. Reiss *et al* also described a DNA assembly guided to 'lithographically' well-defined surfaces and to the solution of anisotropic NPs [119].

3.2.4.2 Ribonucleic acid (RNA)

RNA's nanotechnology is the study of RNA architectures of nanometre-scale and its core structure is made up of RNA. The central scaffold, ligand-targeted, regulatory, and modules of therapeutic can all be entirely made up of RNA. The simplified existence of the DNA canonical base combination of NPs reveals RNA comprising the structural stability and functional variety of proteins. Non-canonical baseline simple stacking, pairing, and intricate tertiary networks improve the flexibility of RNA structures and increase thermodynamic stability [109–112].

RNAs are chain-like biopolymers consisting of nucleotide subunits joined with phosphodiester links, close to DNA. Both nucleotides are made up of ribose sugar, a group of phosphates, and a base of nitrogen. Guanine (G), cytosine (C), uracil (U), and adenine (A) are the most common bases. The combination of metal NPs, and particularly gold, with RNA fragments, has been effective, with the cell membrane being crossed. Thiol or electrostatic, non-covalent interactions may be used for the connection of RNA with the surface of metal NPS [120, 121]. However, the stronger bond is formed through the interaction of thiol-metal. A metal NP (e.g., AuNPs), with the thiol group replacing thiolate NA residues originally used for metal nanoparticulate stabilization, is inserted in SNAs (spherical nucleic acids), RNA, or DNA portion with a group of thiol in its 50 termini [122]. These interactions have been typical to date in RNA-metal hybrids [120–123]. In addition to thiol-based interactions, NPs of RNA-metal conjugate are less common. These interactions are typically electrostatic between positive Me-NPs surfaces and RNA [124, 125]. The use of pRNA-3WJ-folate NPs has been aimed at cancer forms such as glioblastoma, gastric cancer, colorectal cancer, head, and neck cancer. The usage of major areas of metastasis containing the liver, lymphatic nodes, and lungs of folic acid as an agent was used by RNA NPs [126]. The flexibility of RNA NPs makes it possible to incorporate immune system motives, such as CpG, in a series of stimulating systems serving as a complement [127]. The RNA polygons with CpG DNA are an exemplification of this, showing a 100-fold increase in the induction of IL-6, and TNF-α (cytokine) [128, 129].

3.3 Synthesis of bionanomaterials

Bionanomaterials are synthesized by using numerous techniques which are further categorized into two groups, i.e., top-down and bottom-up approaches. The performance of bionanomaterials is dependent upon their properties and the technique used for nanofabrication. Nanomaterials are further categorized into NPs, nanofibers, nanotubes, nanorods, nanoplates, and nanoribbons according to their size and dimensions, as represented in figure 3.3. NPs (diameter ranges from 1–100 nm) have equal longest and shortest axes with all three external dimensions (3D), nanofibers (diameter <100 nm) have two dimensions (2D) in the nanoscale, nanotubes are hollow nanofibers, nanorods are solid nanofibers and nanoplates have one dimension (1D). Due to the small size, nanomaterials carry different properties including colloidal properties, optical properties, and chemical properties. The various

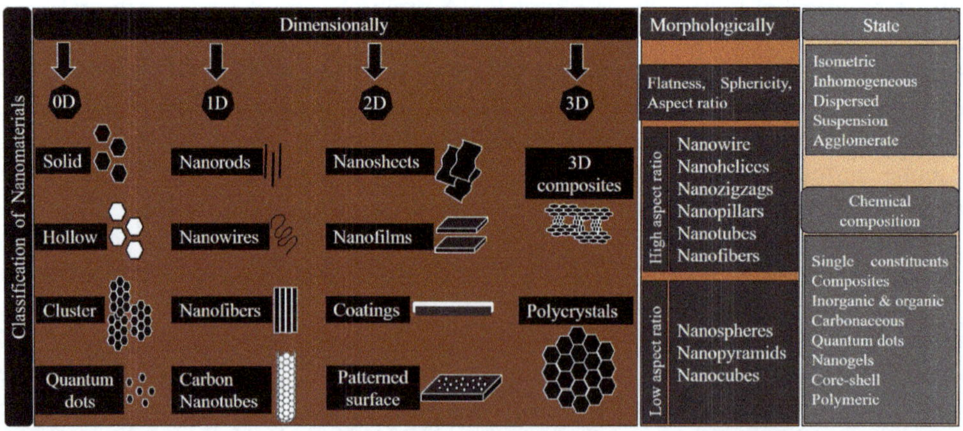

Figure 3.3. Classification of nanomaterials according to their dimensions, morphology, state, and chemical compositions [136].

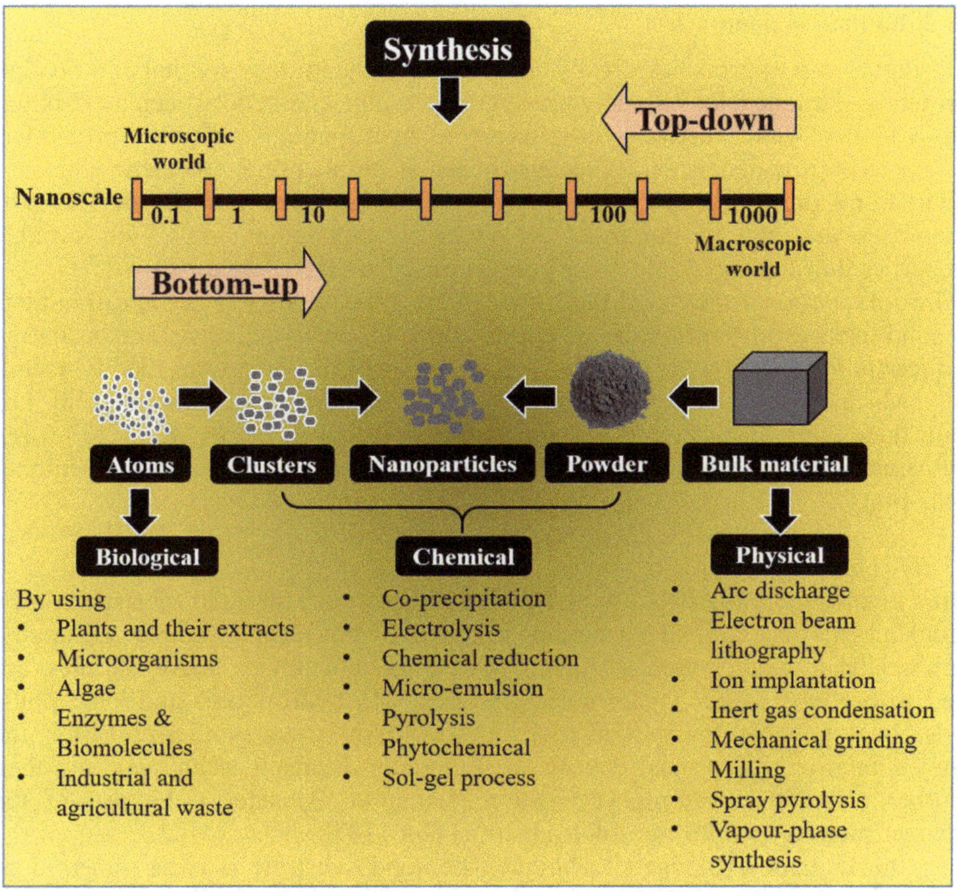

Figure 3.4. An overview of different approaches used for the synthesis of the bionanomaterials is discussed in the given figure.

methods employed to synthesize NPs consist of mechanical, chemical, and biological methods, and are also shown in figure 3.4 [134].

3.3.1 Top-down approach

In the top-down approach during nanofabrication, the complex or bulk material is broken down into the required nanostructures. This approach is inherently simpler and is achieved by Nano-lithographic pattern techniques by using an optical source of a short wavelength [135, 136]. To obtain 10–100 nanometers' size nanomaterials a source of short-wavelength such as extreme UV, x-rays, and electron beam are used. There are certain challenges associated with top-down approaches. Generally, this technique works well at the microscale but is difficult to apply at nanoscale magnitude. Another limitation involves the imperfection of polymer surface structure and difficulty of synthesizing 3D objects as it involves planer techniques [137].

3.3.2 Bottom-up approach

The bottom-up approaches greatly mimics Nature's strategy for nanofabrication through supramolecular interactions. Supramolecular interactions such as H-bonding, Van der Waals forces, hydrophilic- and hydrophobic-interaction, π–π interactions have provided us with a concept of self-assembly of the polymeric units into ordered and functional 3D nanomaterials. There are numerous 2D and 3D self-assemblies that can be employed to synthesize bionanomaterials with variable properties that have multiple applications in the biomedical field.

Two-dimensional thin solid films involve the self-assembly of 2D ultrathin films on solid surfaces with properties such as conducting, semiconducting, and insulating surfaces to synthesize nanoscale films. These nano-films are easy to modify chemically, which consists of a variety of functional groups and applications [68, 138]. The main three types of ultrathin films are Langmuir–Blodgett films (LBFs) [139, 140], self-assembled monolayers (SAMs) [141–143], and 2D supramolecular assemblies [144, 145].

3.3.2.1 Langmuir–Blodgett films

LBFs involve the transfer of a polymeric monolayer onto the solid substrate from a liquid–air interface and this generates an ordered molecular assembly. Generally, amphiphilic molecules such as fatty acids, lipids, and other macromolecules, are used to produce LBFs. These molecules have both hydrophobic and hydrophilic ends. It is possible for two methods to be followed to synthesize LBFs: the conventional one of vertical deposition (Langmuir–Blodgett technique); and then another one with horizontal deposition (Langmuir–Schaefer technique) of the polymer monomers onto the solid substrate. [146, 147].

In the Langmuir–Blodgett technique, the solid substrate is either emersed or dipped/immersed into the LBFs. The deposition of monolayers also depends upon the property of the solid surface, i.e., hydrophobic and hydrophilic. In the hydrophilic substrate, the polymer monolayer is transferred from the liquid–air interface as the substrate is emersed, whereas in the hydrophobic substrate, the polymer monolayer is transferred from the liquid–air interface as the substrate is dipped. The time and speed of immersion and retraction of the substrate also define the quality and the number of LBFs formed in a controlled manner.

In the Langmuir–Schaefer technique, the polymeric monolayer is transferred horizontally onto the substrate. Initially, on the liquid–air interface, a flat solid substrate is placed over the compressed monolayer. Then the substrate is removed horizontally, which separates the monolayer from the water sub-phase. In this horizontal removal, the monolayer is transferred onto the substrate. The method is applicable to transfer viscous films, monolayers of protein, and lipids [139, 148].

3.3.2.2 Self-assembled monolayers

In SAMs, the 2D, quasi-ordered molecule assemblies are synthesized by the adsorption of molecules from the polymer solution. SAMs offer several advantages of stability and flexibility of the synthesized assemblies over LBFs [143, 148, 149].

During SAMs synthesis, one can surpass the barriers of amphiphilic molecules. Moreover, by studying the terminal functionality it is easy to modify the molecules to synthesize SAMs with potential properties such as wettability and adhesion [150, 151]. The surfactant molecule has three main components, backbone, head, and terminal groups. The head group acts as an anchor and enables the surfactant to bind with the substrate. Moreover, the selection is largely affected by the type of substrate used as molecules with varied head groups having different affinity for a particular substrate. The backbone acts as a linker between the head group and terminal group of the molecule and enables control of molecular ordering and stability. In macromolecules, the backbone consists of an aromatic compound and an aliphatic chain. The functionalities of the backbone also influence the interaction of each molecule in SAMs with the neighboring molecules through weaker bonding such as forces of attraction and repulsion. The terminal group is present on the surface of the molecule and its properties such as wettability, flexibility, and corrosion are monitored. The affinity of attraction and repulsive forces (Van der Waals forces and π–π interaction) is further influenced by numerous factors like pH, concentration, temperature, ionic strength (polarity), mechanical factors (pressure, ultra-sonication, shearing, and extension), electrical and magnetic field strength [152, 153].

3.3.3 Hybrid approach

The hybrid approach is a combination of a bottom-up and top-down approach to organizing the self-assembled nanoscale components onto the substrate for nanofabrication. Moreover, for potential properties, it is necessary to control the relative position and orientation of the nanocomponents (NPs, proteins, organic molecules, polymers, and NPs, etc). Usage of both approaches is a potential approach to create a bridge between the macroscopic world and nanoscale entities. For instance, the use of top-down lithography technique to synthesize nanostructures and then its organization into 3D nano-entities by using the bottom-up self-assembling technique [154–156]. Other strategies include the formation of ultrathin films by using SAMs followed by the nanolithography technique to chemically transform the film surface, and finally, immobilization of nano-components on the surface of interest through weak forces of attraction or repulsion, i.e., covalent bonding and supramolecular interactions to synthesize well-defined 3D NPs [154–157].

3.4 Characterization of bionanomaterials

Nanomaterials exhibit a broad range of properties such as their chemical composition, their structures, particle size, and shape, which is the major challenge that needs to be characterized. Characterization of NPs is necessary to identify their characteristics of toxicity, biocompatibility, stability, and flexibility. It is also mandatory to understand the challenges and selection of suitable characterization techniques. Generally, characterization is done to emphasize the NPs' pore size and porosity, size and surface area of the NPs, solubility, aggregation, wettability, adsorption potential, crystallinity, interaction with the substrate, intercalation, and dispersion of NPs, zeta potential, and flexibility, etc [158]. Many techniques are applicable to determine all these parameters appropriately. Techniques used for the formation of NPs include: spectroscopic techniques (UV–visible spectroscopy); studying morphology and particle size of NPs including microscopic techniques (atomic force microscopy (AFM), transmission electron microscopy (TEM), scanning electron microscopy (SEM), and dynamic light scattering (DLS)); studying surface charge of NPs including techniques such as zeta potential, Fourier transform infrared spectroscopy (FT-IR spectroscopy), x-ray photoelectron spectroscopy, and thermal gravimetric analysis, to determine crystallinity x-ray diffraction (XRD); studying magnetic properties techniques given as vibrating sample magnetometry (VSM), superconducting quantum interference device (SQUID), and device magnetometry; other techniques such as matrix-assisted laser desorption time-of-flight mass spectrometry (MALDI-TOF MS), chromatography, filtration, and centrifugation [159–161].

3.4.1 Spectroscopic techniques

3.4.1.1 UV–visible spectroscopy

The formation analysis of bionanomaterials is done by using the UV–visible spectroscopy technique. UV–vis spectroscopy works on the principle of using electromagnetic waves (EM-waves) and measures the plasmon-resonance by collecting oscillations of conduction band electrons against EM-waves [158]. Spectroscopy tends to infer about the optical properties such as size, shape, stability, and conglomeration of the bionanomaterials. Each NP is capable of producing a specific absorbance peak on the nm scale. During spectrum, when light is focused on the sample of NPs, an absorbance pattern appears on the screen of the equipment which varies according to the size and surface plasmon of the particles [162].

3.4.1.2 FT-IR spectroscopy

This technique is used to infer the chemical bonds (covalent bond) and a functional group that presents on the NPs. Moreover, this analysis also interprets the absorption and infrared emission spectrum, photoconductivity of the NPs. Each NP consists of a varying combination of atoms and hence, knowledge about the type of functional group that presents on the NPs is predicted by the FT-IR spectrum [163]. For the analysis, a drop of the liquid sample is placed between two salt plates. These plates are fine and made up of different salts such as potassium bromide (KBr) or sodium chloride (NaCl) which are transparent to IR light. Moreover, the sample preparation is the most crucial step as most of the substances gives IR spectrum at the same wavelength. For a solid sample, a fine powder is prepared by grounding it with KBr or paraffin oil to convert it into a pasty mull. Then the prepared sample is placed between two salt plates and a beam of incident light (IR) is focused on them. Finally, transmission spectra are obtained against the reference (as a blank) sample [161].

3.4.1.3 Dynamic light scattering

DLS is also known as photon correlation spectroscopy. DLS is the fastest and widely used to determine the autocorrelation function of NPs. DLS measures the correlation between the time-dependent fluctuations in the scattered light intensity in a colloidal suspension to enumerate size distribution assuming Brownian motion of NPs [164, 165]. In this method, a monochromatic beam of light is focused on the particles in the solution. After hitting, Doppler shift occurs and fluctuation in the incident light intensity being measured over time to generate autocorrelation function. Then NPs' diffusion coefficient is used to measure the hydrodynamic diameter of NPs by fitting the autocorrelation diffusion coefficient [166].

3.4.2 Microscopic techniques

In microscopic techniques, morphological and particle size determination was done by using TEM, SEM, and AFM [167]. Ranges of applications such as drug delivery, tissue targeting, and *in vivo* distribution of NPs are depended upon the size of nanomaterials. Studies have shown the inefficiency of microparticles due to their large size over NPs to cross and deliver drugs [167–169]. These techniques generate surface images with the help of physical probes which are used for scanning the specimen, which is why these techniques are considered the most useful techniques for characterization. Based on their functionalities, different microscopic techniques used are as follows.

3.4.2.1 Transmission electron microscopy

The characteristics such as shape, size, and morphological identification of the nanomaterials are done by TEM [165, 170]. TEM is a common technique used in morphological identification, although sample preparation is very critical and time cumbersome. For TEM, ultrathin samples 10^{-10} m in size are required. Prepare an NPs mixed solution and sonicate it a few times. Then take a carbon-coated copper grid on a Whatman filter paper and place a small drop (5–10 ul) onto the grid. Let the sample dry naturally or blot dry to remove excess solution. During analysis, a sample must withstand the vacuum pressure for which negative staining is performed after which it is embedded in plastic or exposed to liquid nitrogen. Finally, NPs are allowed to dry under a mercury lamp and are introduced into the TEM [166, 167]. The incident light interacting with the sample undergoes both elastic and inelastic diffraction. The diffracted light then passes through the objective lens and is further introduced to the magnifying lens to generate the final enlarged image.

3.4.2.2 Scanning electron microscopy

In this technique, direct visualization of the NPs is done. Visualization of the biological specimens is not a complicated step as image formation is mostly dependent upon the nature of electrons and the specimen. For SEM, the sample should have a conductive surface and be heavily processed to withstand a high vacuum. Thus, sample preparation is a crucial step during analysis and is divided into six steps. In the very first step, the primary fixation of the sample is done with aldehydes to stabilize the ultrastructure. Then in the next step, secondary fixation of the sample is done with osmium tetroxide to prevent extraction by solvents during dehydration. During this step, black precipitates of osmium tetroxide are formed which enhances image quality (lowers the chances of image deformation due to the presence of charges) and sample conductivity. Then in the next step, the fixed sample is dehydrated by using suitable organic solvents. In the next step, samples are allowed to dry and mounted on a metal stub. For mounting, a carbon disc or silver-containing glue is used which in turn increases sample conductivity. In some cases, the sample surface is coated with conductive material (100 nm thick coating) to avoid charge build-up on the sample surface. The column of SEM contains an electron gun and electromagnetic lenses. Lenses are meant to produce a very fine beam of electrons and to focus the electron beam on the sample surface. A beam is scanned over the sample surface, at a given moment the electron is bombarded and absorbed by the sample to emit low-energy secondary electrons together with x-rays. This phenomenon is used to generate images in SEM. Information is provided about the external morphology, crystallinity, chemical composition, and orientation of the sample. However, SEM is time cumbersome, costly, and requires additional information about the size distribution [171].

3.4.2.3 Atomic force microscopy

AFM is also used to study the morphological features of NPs and generates 3D images which enable one to do quantitative studies of the sample such as volume and height of NPs [172, 173]. AFM is based upon the physical scanning of the NPs and gives ultra-high resolution for particle size at the submicron scale using a probe tip [174]. In this method, a small volume of NPs (liquid or gas medium) is placed and spread evenly on the glass slide mounted on the AFM. Then a stream of liquid nitrogen is introduced to dry the sample at room temperature. Then multiple images are captured by the instrument and generate a topographical map based on the forces between the tip and surface of the NPs which are scanned in a contact mode. AFM has the advantage of its ability to image non-conducting samples without any prior treatment, delicate biological samples, polymer-based micro, and nanostructures [172, 173].

3.4.3 Surface charge analysis

Surface charge analysis is an important parameter that needs to be considered during the characterization of NPs. Surface charge is present on the surface due to the adsorption or desorption of hydrogen ions on hydroxylated sites of the NPs. To measure the surface charge, related zeta potential is generally measured. Zeta potential is a function of the sample of interest and its surrounding medium. It is a calculated property and is used as an indicator of colloidal stability. Zeta potential is measured by using electrophoresis techniques, i.e., laser Doppler electrophoresis or by titration techniques to determine the isoelectric point. The intensity and nature of surface charge enable one to determine the electrostatic interaction of NPs with the surrounding medium.

3.4.4 Crystallinity analysis

In this analysis, XRD is implied to infer the crystallinity of the synthesized NPs. In this method incident light of x-rays is focused on the diffracted powdered sample to analyze NPs' structure and lattice parameter. Further, the angle of diffraction and the width of the peaks are used to determine the particle size.

3.4.5 Magnetic properties

To analyze the magnetic properties of the NPs, VSM and SQUID are used. In SQUID, NPs are cooled and warmed in the presence of the magnetic field. In this technique, magnetization is monitored as a function of temperature and is generally used to estimate the properties of magnetic NPs, whereas VSM is used to monitor the magnetization of magnetic NPs as a function of an externally applied magnetic field (−3 to 3 tesla). VSM is a potential technique to observe the magnetic behavior of NPs on saturation magnetization based on the VSM curve obtained at low or at room temperature [161].

3.4.6 Other techniques

Numerous other techniques are used to characterize NPS, including chromatography techniques to separate NPs based on their affinity toward the organic mobile phase [175, 176], energy dispersive x-ray spectra technique to determine the elemental composition of NPs [158], field flow flotation technique to separate NPs depending upon their magnetic susceptibility [177], filtration and centrifugation technique to fractionate the NPs according to their size [178, 179], hyperspectral imaging technique to determine the surface chemistry and functional groups added to the NPs [180], laser-induced breakdown of NPs' colloids to determine their size and concentration [181], mass-spectrometry to determine the fluorescent-labeled NPs [182], etc.

3.5 Safety aspects of bionanomaterials

In most cases, biomaterials are considered nontoxic due to their natural origin, which is nevertheless contradictory among toxicological studies. Cellulose fibers are reported to have a biopersistence effect among individuals. According to the fiber pathogenicity prototype, long exposure to biopersistence material and other thin high-aspect-ratio fibers are carcinogenic and can lead to lung cancer and mesothelioma [183]. Nanotechnology imparts certain advantages of easy penetration and biocompatibility/properties of nanomaterials over conventional material and methodology. Reduced size enables the increased dosages and easy translocation within the host cell, whereas a large surface area enables nanomaterial to interact well with biological surroundings. Nevertheless, the physicochemical features of nanostructures can alter their toxicity, for example, the length and thickness of nanofibrillated cellulose are responsible for its interaction with dendritic cells [184]. Therefore, the production methodology prominently affects the physicochemical properties of cellulose-based nanomaterials. Moreover, the route of exposure also defines the toxicological behavior of bionanomaterials. The port of passages in the human body includes lungs (through inhalation), gastrointestinal tract, skin, and systemic circulation. Due to the biopersistence property, chronic inhalation exposures of cellulosic material might be a concern [185].

3.6 Factors affecting the synthesis of bionanomaterials

During synthesis, many factors are involved that affect the nature and characterization of bionanomaterials. Various factors such as pH of the solution, the temperature during synthesis, concentration of extract and raw material used, size of the material, and above all the method have affected bionanomaterials synthesis [186]. Methods include physical disruption, chemical hydrolysis using organic/inorganic chemicals, and biological techniques using living organisms. Each method is applicable for the synthesis with both applications and drawbacks but preferably biological methods due to their nontoxic nature and eco-friendly outcomes. Further, pH and pressure are also important and by varying their range the size and shape of bionanomaterials can be modified. Temperature ranges and time of incubation also determine the nature of the end product in different techniques (biological, chemical, and physical).

3.7 Conclusion

The widespread application of nanomaterials in various fields including medicine, food, diagnosis, waste management, and agriculture has gained increased research attention, primarily focussed on the development of green synthesis methods for the fabrication of environmentally friendly, nontoxic bionanomaterials. In a very short period, nanobiomaterials have shown remarkable progress in various applications and have developed with new technologies. No wonder nanotechnology derived biomaterials have entered the 'nanotechnology era' and become the fastest developing and emerging arenas at the intersection of material science and biology, with an extraordinary impact on various fields of science. For example, 'nano-bioengineering' of different enzymes aims to facilitate the conversion of cellulose from wood chips, corn stalks, unfertilized perennial grasses, etc, into ethanol for fuel production. Cellulosic nanomaterials have proven successful applications in a wide group of industrial sectors, electronics, construction, packaging, food, energy, health care, automotive, and defense. The strategy of elegant nano-structures with the exact layout of functional modules in three-dimensional space and self-assembly in a programmable structure of 4D has advanced the arena. Owing to its exclusive structural, physical–chemical properties and capacities, the research into nano-structures using cellulose, starch, chitin, proteins, and DNA/RNA is an attractive field. These biopolymer alternatives offer various advantages such as being cost-effective, renewable, biocompatible, biodegradable, and eco-friendly. The various environmental factors such as source materials, pH, temperature, influence the formation of nanomaterials in terms of quality and quantity. Suitable characterization methods like AFM, SEM, and XRD characterize the synthesized nanomaterial efficiently, thereby paving a way for its enhanced application in drug delivery, biomedical and other fields wherever required. In this chapter, we focused on fundamental aspects of various biopolymers including PSs, peptides, and nucleic acids for the synthesis of green nanomaterials along with structural properties, processing methods, and noteworthy applications in different fields. Moreover, the field of nanomaterials is very young but attractive with extraordinary properties by characterizing novel smart and intelligent biomaterials. In addition to this, various characterization techniques for the exploration of structural and functional properties of bionanomaterials have also been discussed. New computational approaches have added a better vision of how nanostructure serves biological purposes and it is believed that in the future, development of computer-aided tools can help in focusing and facilitating the choice of proper nanomaterials for designing and creating novel nanobiomaterials. Current and advanced research investigation for the formation of bionanomaterials will help to gain complete insight into various factors affecting the development of a promising approach for the fabrication of bionanomaterials. With the development of new nanoproducts, an continuous influx of new knowledge from different areas of science is leading to better biomaterials and is expected to be a very exciting period for nanoscale research and applications in the next decades.

References

[1] Hernández N, Williams R C and Cochran E W 2014 The battle for the 'green' polymer. Different approaches for biopolymer synthesis: bioadvantaged vs. bioreplacement *Org. Biomol. Chem.* **12** 2834–49

[2] Tomalia D A 2009 In quest of a systematic framework for unifying and defining nanoscience *J. Nanopart. Res.* **11** 1251–310

[3] Boles M A, Engel M and Talapin D V 2016 Self-assembly of colloidal nanocrystals: from intricate structures to functional materials *Chem. Rev.* **116** 11220–89

[4] Lefèvre T and Subirade M 2001 Molecular structure and interaction of biopolymers as viewed by Fourier transform infrared spectroscopy: model studies on β-lactoglobulin *Food Hydrocoll.* **15** 365–76

[5] Diener M, Adamcik J, Sánchez-Ferrer A, Jaedig F, Schefer L and Mezzenga R 2019 Primary, secondary, tertiary and quaternary structure levels in linear polysaccharides: from random coil, to single helix to supramolecular assembly *Biomacromolecules.* **20** 1731–9

[6] Gupta P and Nayak K K 2015 Characteristics of protein-based biopolymer and its application *Polym. Eng. Sci.* **55** 485–98

[7] Kulkarni A A and Rao P S 2013 Synthesis of polymeric nanomaterials for biomedical applications *Nanomaterials in Tissue Engineering* (Amsterdam: Elsevier) pp 27–63

[8] Wen Y and Oh J K 2014 Recent strategies to develop polysaccharide-based nanomaterials for biomedical applications *Macromol. Rapid Commun.* **35** 1819–32

[9] Peter M G 2005 Chitin and chitosan from animal sources *Biopolymers: Biology Chemistry Biotechnology Applications* (New York: Wiley) Part 6

[10] Sinha V R and Kumria R 2001 Polysaccharides in colon-specific drug delivery *Int. J. Pharm.* **224** 19–38

[11] Quignard F, Di Renzo F and Guibal E 2010 From natural polysaccharides to materials for catalysis, adsorption, and remediation *Carbohydrates in Sustainable Development I* (Berlin: Springer) pp 165–97

[12] Klemm D, Kramer F, Moritz S, Lindström T, Ankerfors M and Gray D *et al* 2011 Nanocelluloses : a new family of nature-based materials *Angew. Chem. Int. Ed.* **50** 5438–66
[13] Brinchi L, Cotana F, Fortunati E and Kenny J M 2013 Production of nanocrystalline cellulose from lignocellulosic biomass: technology and applications *Carbohydr. Polym.* **94** 154–69
[14] Eyley S and Thielemans W 2014 Surface modification of cellulose nanocrystals *Nanoscale* **6** 7764–79
[15] Khalil H A, Davoudpour Y, Islam M N, Mustapha A, Sudesh K and Dungani R *et al* 2014 Production and modification of nanofibrillated cellulose using various mechanical processes: a review *Carbohydr. Polym.* **99** 649–65
[16] Nechyporchuk O, Belgacem M N and Bras J 2016 Production of cellulose nanofibrils: a review of recent advances *Ind. Crops Prod.* **93** 2–25
[17] Gallant D J, Bouchet B and Baldwin P M 1997 Microscopy of starch: evidence of a new level of granule organization *Carbohydr. Polym.* **32** 177–91
[18] Tang H, Mitsunaga T and Kawamura Y 2006 Molecular arrangement in blocklets and starch granule architecture *Carbohydr. Polym.* **63** 555–60
[19] Dufresne A, Cavaille J-Y and Helbert W 1996 New nanocomposite materials: microcrystalline starch reinforced thermoplastic *Macromolecules* **29** 7624–6
[20] Torres F G, Troncoso O P, Gamucci O, Corvaglia S, Brunetti V and Bardi G 2015 Immunological properties of Andean starch films are independent of their nanometric roughness and stiffness *Int. J. Biol. Macromol.* **75** 460–6
[21] Putaux J-L, Molina-Boisseau S, Momaur T and Dufresne A 2003 Platelet nanocrystals resulting from the disruption of waxy maize starch granules by acid hydrolysis *Biomacromolecules* **4** 1198–202
[22] Liu D, Wu Q, Chen H and Chang P R 2009 Transitional properties of starch colloid with particle size reduction from micro-to nanometer *J. Colloid Interface Sci.* **339** 117–24
[23] Shi A, Li D, Wang L, Li B and Adhikari B 2011 Preparation of starch-based nanoparticles through high-pressure homogenization and miniemulsion cross-linking: influence of various process parameters on particle size and stability *Carbohydr. Polym.* **83** 1604–10
[24] Ma X, Jian R, Chang P R and Yu J 2008 Fabrication and characterization of citric acid-modified starch nanoparticles/plasticized-starch composites *Biomacromolecules* **9** 3314–20
[25] Tan Y, Xu K, Li L, Liu C, Song C and Wang P 2009 Fabrication of size-controlled starch-based nanospheres by nanoprecipitation *ACS Appl. Mater. Interfaces* **1** 956–59
[26] Torres F G, Troncoso O P, Grande C G and Díaz D A 2011 Biocompatibilty of starch-based films from starch of Andean crops for biomedical applications *Mater. Sci. Eng.* C **31** 1737–40
[27] Torres F G, Troncoso O P, Vega J and Wong M 2015 Influence of botanic origin on the morphology and size of starch nanoparticles from andean native starch sources *Polym. Renew. Resour.* **6** 91–103
[28] Martinez S, Rivon C, Troncoso O P and Torres F G 2016 Botanical origin as a determinant for the mechanical properties of starch films with nanoparticle reinforcements *Starch-Stärke* **68** 935–42
[29] Santander-Ortega M J, Stauner T, Loretz B, Ortega-Vinuesa J L, Bastos-González D and Wenz G *et al* 2010 Nanoparticles made from novel starch derivatives for transdermal drug delivery *J. Controll. Release* **141** 85–92

[30] Xiao S, Liu X, Tong C, Zhao L, Liu X and Zhou A *et al* 2012 Dialdehyde starch nanoparticles as antitumor drug delivery system: an *in vitro*, *in vivo*, and immunohistological evaluation *Chin. Sci. Bull.* **57** 3226–32
[31] Kim H-Y, Park S S and Lim S-T 2015 Preparation, characterization and utilization of starch nanoparticles *Colloids Surf.* B **126** 607–20
[32] Zhou G, Luo Z and Fu X 2014 Preparation of starch nanoparticles in a water-in-ionic liquid microemulsion system and their drug loading and releasing properties *J. Agric. Food Chem.* **62** 8214–20
[33] Ciolacu D and Popa V I 2011 Cellulose allomorphs: structure, accessibility and reactivity *Environ. Eng. Manage. J.* **10** 467–8
[34] Ciolacu D E and Darie R N 2016 Nanocomposites based on cellulose, hemicelluloses, and lignin *Nanomaterials and Nanocomposites: Zero-to Three-Dimensional Materials and Their Composites* (New York: Wiley) ch 11
[35] Pérez S and Mazeau K 2005 Conformations, structures, and morphologies of celluloses *Polysaccharides: Structural Diversity and Functional Versatility* ed S Dumitriu (Boca Raton, FL: CRC Press) ch 2
[36] Atalla R H and Vanderhart D L 1984 Native cellulose: a composite of two distinct crystalline forms *Science* **223** 283–5
[37] Malainine M E, Mahrouz M and Dufresne A 2005 Thermoplastic nanocomposites based on cellulose microfibrils from *Opuntia ficus*-indica parenchyma cell *Compos. Sci. Technol.* **65** 1520–6
[38] Siró I and Plackett D 2010 Microfibrillated cellulose and new nanocomposite materials: a review *Cellulose.* **17** 459–94
[39] Lavoine N, Desloges I, Dufresne A and Bras J 2012 Microfibrillated cellulose—its barrier properties and applications in cellulosic materials: a review *Carbohydr. Polym.* **90** 735–64
[40] Lee S-Y, Chun S-J, Kang I-A and Park J-Y 2009 Preparation of cellulose nanofibrils by high-pressure homogenizer and cellulose-based composite films *J. Ind. Eng. Chem.* **15** 50–5
[41] Ferrer A, Filpponen I, Rodríguez A, Laine J and Rojas O J 2012 Valorization of residual empty palm fruit bunch fibers (EPFBF) by microfluidization: production of nanofibrillated cellulose and EPFBF nanopaper *Bioresour. Technol.* **125** 249–55
[42] Johnson R K, Zink-Sharp A, Renneckar S H and Glasser W G 2009 A new bio-based nanocomposite: fibrillated TEMPO-oxidized celluloses in hydroxypropylcellulose matrix *Cellulose.* **16** 227–38
[43] Frone A N, Panaitescu D M, Donescu D, Spataru C I, Radovici C and Trusca R *et al* 2011 Preparation and characterization of PVA composites with cellulose nanofibers obtained by ultrasonication *BioResources.* **6** 487–512
[44] Panthapulakkal S and Sain M 2012 Preparation and characterization of cellulose nanofibril films from wood fibre and their thermoplastic polycarbonate composites *Int. J. Polym. Sci.* **2012**
[45] Chakraborty A, Sain M and Kortschot M 2005 Cellulose microfibrils: a novel method of preparation using high shear refining and cryocrushing *Holzforschung.* **59** 102–7
[46] Hubbe M A, Rojas O J, Lucia L A and Sain M 2008 Cellulosic nanocomposites: a review *BioResources.* **3** 929–80
[47] Azizi Samir M A S, Alloin F and Dufresne A 2005 Review of recent research into cellulosic whiskers, their properties and their application in nanocomposite field *Biomacromolecules.* **6** 612–26

[48] Mathew A P, Oksman K, Pierron D and Harmand M-F 2012 Fibrous cellulose nanocomposite scaffolds prepared by partial dissolution for potential use as ligament or tendon substitutes *Carbohydr. Polym.* **87** 2291–8
[49] Zhang J M and Zhang J 2010 Advanced functional materials based on cellulose *Acta Polym. Sin.* **12** 1376–98
[50] Kalia S, Dufresne A, Cherian B M, Kaith B S, Avérous L and Njuguna J *et al* 2011 Cellulose-based bio-and nanocomposites: a review *Int. J. Polym. Sci.* **2011** 837875
[51] Olatunji O 2016 Classification of natural polymers *Natural Polymers* (Berlin: Springer) pp 1–17
[52] Dhillon G S, Kaur S, Brar S K and Verma M 2013 Green synthesis approach: extraction of chitosan from fungus mycelia *Crit. Rev. Biotechnol.* **33** 379–403
[53] Gabius H-J 2011 *The Sugar Code: Fundamentals of Glycosciences* (New York: Wiley)
[54] Raabe D, Romano P, Sachs C, Fabritius H, Al-Sawalmih A and Yi S-B *et al* 2006 Microstructure and crystallographic texture of the chitin–protein network in the biological composite material of the exoskeleton of the lobster *Homarus americanus Mater. Sci. Eng.* A **421** 143–53
[55] Chen P-Y, Lin A Y-M, McKittrick J and Meyers M A 2008 Structure and mechanical properties of crab exoskeletons *Acta Biomater.* **4** 587–96
[56] Faria R R, Guerra R F, de Sousa Neto L R, Motta L F, de Faria and Franca E 2016 Computational study of polymorphic structures of α-and β-chitin and chitosan in aqueous solution *J. Mol. Graphics Modell.* **63** 78–84
[57] Rinaudo M 2006 Chitin and chitosan: properties and applications *Prog. Polym. Sci.* **31** 603–32
[58] Torres F G, Troncoso O P, Pisani A, Gatto F and Bardi G 2019 Natural polysaccharide nanomaterials: an overview of their immunological properties *Int. J. Mol. Sci.* **20** 5092
[59] Prashanth K H and Tharanathan R N 2007 Chitin/chitosan: modifications and their unlimited application potential—an overview *Trends Food Sci. Technol.* **18** 117–31
[60] Nishiyama Y, Noishiki Y and Wada M 2011 X-ray structure of anhydrous β-chitin at 1 Å resolution *Macromolecules* **44** 950–7
[61] Weiner S and Addadi L 1997 Design strategies in mineralized biological materials *J. Mater. Chem.* **7** 689–702
[62] Zargar V, Asghari M and Dashti A 2015 A review on chitin and chitosan polymers: structure, chemistry, solubility, derivatives, and applications *ChemBioEng Rev.* **2** 204–26
[63] Zeng J-B, He Y-S, Li S-L and Wang Y-Z 2012 Chitin whiskers: an overview *Biomacromolecules.* **13** 1–11
[64] Cuesta A, Esteban M Á and Meseguer J 2003 *In vitro* effect of chitin particles on the innate cellular immune system of gilthead seabream (*Sparus aurata L.*) *Fish Shellfish Immunol.* **15** 1–11
[65] Esteban M A, Mulero V, Cuesta A, Ortuno J and Meseguer J 2000 Effects of injecting chitin particles on the innate immune response of gilthead seabream (*Sparus aurata L.*) *Fish Shellfish Immunol.* **10** 543–54
[66] Prashanth K H, Kittur F S and Tharanathan R N 2002 Solid state structure of chitosan prepared under different N-deacetylating conditions *Carbohydr. Polym.* **50** 27–33
[67] LeHoux J G and Grondin F 1993 Some effects of chitosan on liver function in the rat *Endocrinology* **132** 1078–84

[68] Huo M, Zhang Y, Zhou J, Zou A, Yu D and Wu Y *et al* 2010 Synthesis and characterization of low-toxic amphiphilic chitosan derivatives and their application as micelle carrier for antitumor drug *Int. J. Pharm.* **394** 162–73
[69] Dash M, Chiellini F, Ottenbrite R M and Chiellini E 2011 Chitosan—a versatile semi-synthetic polymer in biomedical applications *Prog. Polym. Sci.* **36** 981–1014
[70] Calderón L, Harris R, Cordoba-Diaz M, Elorza M, Elorza B and Lenoir J *et al* 2013 Nano and microparticulate chitosan-based systems for antiviral topical delivery *Eur. J. Pharm. Sci.* **48** 216–22
[71] Giunchedi P, Juliano C, Gavini E, Cossu M and Sorrenti M 2002 Formulation and *in vivo* evaluation of chlorhexidine buccal tablets prepared using drug-loaded chitosan microspheres *Eur. J. Pharm. Biopharm.* **53** 233–9
[72] Corrigan D O, Healy A M and Corrigan O I 2006 Preparation and release of salbutamol from chitosan and chitosan co-spray dried compacts and multiparticulates *Eur. J. Pharm. Biopharm.* **62** 295–305
[73] Alhalaweh A, Andersson S and Velaga S P 2009 Preparation of zolmitriptan–chitosan microparticles by spray drying for nasal delivery *Eur. J. Pharm. Sci.* **38** 206–14
[74] Li X, Kong X, Shi S, Zheng X, Guo G and Wei Y *et al* 2008 Preparation of alginate coated chitosan microparticles for vaccine delivery *BMC Biotech.* **8** 89
[75] Abreu F O S, Forte M M, Kist T B L and Honaiser L P 2010 Effect of the preparation method on the drug loading of alginate-chitosan microspheres *Exp. Polym. Lett.* **4** 456–64
[76] Luangtana-anan M, Opanasopit P, Ngawhirunpat T, Nunthanid J, Sriamornsak P and Limmatvapirat S *et al* 2005 Effect of chitosan salts and molecular weight on a nanoparticulate carrier for therapeutic protein *Pharm. Dev. Technol.* **10** 189–96
[77] Zhang Y, Chan H F and Leong K W 2013 Advanced materials and processing for drug delivery: the past and the future *Adv. Drug Deliv. Rev.* **65** 104–20
[78] Agnihotri S A, Mallikarjuna N N and Aminabhavi T M 2004 Recent advances on chitosan-based micro-and nanoparticles in drug delivery *J. Controll. Release* **100** 5–28
[79] Kumar P S, Srinivasan S, Lakshmanan V-K, Tamura H, Nair S V and Jayakumar R 2011 β-Chitin hydrogel/nano hydroxyapatite composite scaffolds for tissue engineering applications *Carbohydr. Polym.* **85** 584–91
[80] Kim J, Cai Z and Chen Y 2010 Biocompatible bacterial cellulose composites for biomedical application *J. Nanotechnol. Eng. Med.* **1** 011006
[81] Khan F, Tare R S, Oreffo R O and Bradley M 2009 Versatile biocompatible polymer hydrogels: scaffolds for cell growth *Angew. Chem. Int. Ed.* **48** 978–82
[82] Tvl H B, Vidyavathi M, Kavitha K and Sastry T P 2010 Preparation and evaluation of ciprofloxacin loaded chitosan-gelatin composite films for wound healing activity *Int. J. Drug Deliv.* **2**
[83] Hong H-J, Jin S-E, Park J-S, Ahn W S and Kim C-K 2008 Accelerated wound healing by smad3 antisense oligonucleotides-impregnated chitosan/alginate polyelectrolyte complex *Biomaterials* **29** 4831–37
[84] Hsieh C-Y, Tsai S-P, Wang D-M, Chang Y-N and Hsieh H-J 2005 Preparation of γ-PGA/chitosan composite tissue engineering matrices *Biomaterials* **26** 5617–23
[85] Tanabe T, Okitsu N, Tachibana A and Yamauchi K 2002 Preparation and characterization of keratin–chitosan composite film *Biomaterials* **23** 817–25

[86] Wang T-J, Wang I-J, Chen S, Chen Y-H and Young T-H 2012 The phenotypic response of bovine corneal endothelial cells on chitosan/polycaprolactone blends *Colloids Surf.* B **90** 236–43
[87] Mathews S, Bhonde R, Gupta P K and Totey S 2011 A novel tripolymer coating demonstrating the synergistic effect of chitosan, collagen type 1 and hyaluronic acid on osteogenic differentiation of human bone marrow derived mesenchymal stem cells *Biochem. Biophys. Res. Commun.* **414** 270–76
[88] Cooper A, Bhattarai N and Zhang M 2011 Fabrication and cellular compatibility of aligned chitosan–PCL fibers for nerve tissue regeneration *Carbohydr. Polym.* **85** 149–56
[89] Nirmala R, Navamathavan R, Kang H-S, El-Newehy M H and Kim H Y 2011 Preparation of polyamide-6/chitosan composite nanofibers by a single solvent system via electrospinning for biomedical applications *Colloids Surf.* B **83** 173–78
[90] Zhang C, Wu W, Li R-Q, Qiu W-X, Zhuang Z-N and Cheng S-X *et al* 2018 Peptide-based multifunctional nanomaterials for tumor imaging and therapy *Adv. Funct. Mater.* **28** 1804492
[91] Hamley I W 2017 Small bioactive peptides for biomaterials design and therapeutics *Chem. Rev.* **117** 14015–41
[92] Amorín M, Castedo L and Granja J R 2003 New cyclic peptide assemblies with hydrophobic cavities: the structural and thermodynamic basis of a new class of peptide nanotubes *JACS* **125** 2844–5
[93] Clerici F, Erba E, Gelmi M L and Pellegrino S 2016 Non-standard amino acids and peptides: from self-assembly to nanomaterials *Tetrahedron Lett.* **57** 5540–50
[94] Hu K, Xiong W, Sun C, Wang C, Li J and Yin F *et al* 2020 Self-assembly of constrained cyclic peptides controlled by ring size *CCS Chem.* **2** 42–51
[95] Larnaudie S C, Sanchis J, Nguyen T-H, Peltier R, Catrouillet S and Brendel J C *et al* 2018 Cyclic peptide-poly (HPMA) nanotubes as drug delivery vectors: *in vitro* assessment, pharmacokinetics and biodistribution *Biomaterials* **178** 570–82
[96] Pappas C G, Shafi R, Sasselli I R, Siccardi H, Wang T and Narang V *et al* 2016 Dynamic peptide libraries for the discovery of supramolecular nanomaterials *Nat. Nanotechnol.* **11** 960–67
[97] Katyal P, Meleties M and Montclare J K 2019 Self-assembled protein-and peptide-based nanomaterials *ACS Biomater. Sci. Eng.* **5** 4132–47
[98] Panda J J and Chauhan V S 2014 Short peptide based self-assembled nanostructures: implications in drug delivery and tissue engineering *Polym. Chem.* **5** 4418–36
[99] Mikhalevich V, Craciun I, Kyropoulou M, Palivan C G and Meier W 2017 Amphiphilic peptide self-assembly: expansion to hybrid materials *Biomacromolecules* **18** 3471–80
[100] Qiu F, Chen Y, Tang C and Zhao X 2018 Amphiphilic peptides as novel nanomaterials: design, self-assembly and application *Int. J. Nanomed.* **13** 5003
[101] Cavalli S, Albericio F and Kros A 2010 Amphiphilic peptides and their cross-disciplinary role as building blocks for nanoscience *Chem. Soc. Rev.* **39** 241–63
[102] Zhao Y, Yang W, Chen C, Wang J, Zhang L and Xu H 2018 Rational design and self-assembly of short amphiphilic peptides and applications *Curr. Opin. Coll. Interface Sci.* **35** 112–23
[103] De La Rica R and Matsui H 2010 Applications of peptide and protein-based materials in bionanotechnology *Chem. Soc. Rev.* **39** 3499–509

[104] Wang M, Wang J, Zhou P, Deng J, Zhao Y and Sun Y *et al* 2018 Nanoribbons self-assembled from short peptides demonstrate the formation of polar zippers between β-sheets *Nat. Commun.* **9** 1–11

[105] Abu-Salah K M, Ansari A A and Alrokayan S A 2010 DNA-based applications in nanobiotechnology *J. Biomed. Biotechnol.* **2010** 715295

[106] Roco M C and Bainbridge W S 2002 Converging technologies for improving human performance: integrating from the nanoscale *J. Nanopart. Res.* **4** 281–95

[107] Roco M C and Bainbridge W S 2003 Overview converging technologies for improving human performance *Converging Technologies for Improving Human Performance* (Berlin: Springer) pp 1–27

[108] Daksh D, Rawtani D and Agrawal Y K 2016 Recent developments in bio-nanoelectronics devices: a review *J. Bionanosci.* **10** 81–93

[109] Jasinski D, Haque F, Binzel D W and Guo P 2017 Advancement of the emerging field of RNA nanotechnology *ACS Nano* **11** 1142–64

[110] Guo P 2010 The emerging field of RNA nanotechnology *Nat. Nanotechnol.* **5** 833

[111] Zuo H, Wu S, Li M, Li Y, Jiang W and Mao C 2015 A case study of the likes and dislikes of DNA and RNA in self-assembly *Angew. Chem. Int. Ed.* **54** 15118–21

[112] Guo P, Zhang C, Chen C, Garver K and Trottier M 1998 Inter-RNA interaction of phage φ29 pRNA to form a hexameric complex for viral DNA transportation *Mol. Cell.* **2** 149–55

[113] Lee J B, Hong J, Bonner D K, Poon Z and Hammond P T 2012 Self-assembled RNA interference microsponges for efficient siRNA delivery *Nat. Mater.* **11** 316–22

[114] Guo S, Tschammer N, Mohammed S and Guo P 2005 Specific delivery of therapeutic RNAs to cancer cells via the dimerization mechanism of phi29 motor pRNA *Hum. Gene Ther.* **16** 1097–110

[115] Kumar A, Phadtare S, Pasricha R, Guga P, Ganesh K N and Sastry M 2003 Assembling gold nanoparticles in solution using phosphorothioate DNA as structural interconnects *Curr. Sci.* **84** 71–4

[116] Alivisatos A P *et al* 1996 Organization of 'nanocrystal molecules' using DNA *Nature* **382** 609–11

[117] Maeda Y, Tabata H and Kawai T 2001 Two-dimensional assembly of gold nanoparticles with a DNA network template *Appl. Phys. Lett.* **79** 1181–3

[118] Li Z, Jin R, Mirkin C A and Letsinger R L 2002 Multiple thiol-anchor capped DNA–gold nanoparticle conjugates *Nucleic Acids Res.* **30** 1558–62

[119] Reiss B D, Mbindyo J N, Martin B R, Nicewarner S R and Mallouk T E 2001 *DNA-Directed Assembly of Anisotropic Nanoparticles on Lithographically Defined Surfaces and in Solution* University Park: Department of Chemistry, Pennsylvania State University

[120] Graczyk A, Pawlowska R, Jedrzejczyk D and Chworos A 2020 Gold nanoparticles in conjunction with nucleic acids as a modern molecular system for cellular delivery *Molecules* **25** 204

[121] Giljohann D A, Seferos D S, Prigodich A E, Patel P C and Mirkin C A 2009 Gene regulation with polyvalent siRNA—nanoparticle conjugates *JACS* **131** 2072–3

[122] Patel P C, Hao L, Au Yeung W S and Mirkin C A 2011 Duplex end breathing determines serum stability and intracellular potency of siRNA–Au NPs *Mol. Pharm.* **8** 1285–91

[123] Zheng D, Giljohann D A, Chen D L, Massich M D, Wang X-Q and Iordanov H *et al* 2012 Topical delivery of siRNA-based spherical nucleic acid nanoparticle conjugates for gene regulation *Proc. Natl. Acad. Sci.* **109** 11975–80

[124] Jensen S A, Day E S, Ko C H, Hurley L A, Luciano J P and Kouri F M *et al* 2013 Spherical nucleic acid nanoparticle conjugates as an RNAi-based therapy for glioblastoma *Sci. Transl. Med.* **5** 209ra152

[125] Kim H J, Takemoto H, Yi Y, Zheng M, Maeda Y and Chaya H *et al* 2014 Precise engineering of siRNA delivery vehicles to tumors using polyion complexes and gold nanoparticles *ACS Nano* **8** 8979–91

[126] Barnaby S N, Lee A and Mirkin C A 2014 Probing the inherent stability of siRNA immobilized on nanoparticle constructs *Proc. Natl. Acad. Sci.* **111** 9739–44

[127] Kranz L M, Diken M, Haas H, Kreiter S, Loquai C and Reuter K C *et al* 2016 Systemic RNA delivery to dendritic cells exploits antiviral defence for cancer immunotherapy *Nature* **534** 396–401

[128] Koyfman A Y, Braun G, Magonov S, Chworos A, Reich N O and Jaeger L 2005 Controlled spacing of cationic gold nanoparticles by nanocrown RNA *JACS* **127** 11886–87

[129] Hou W, Wei P, Kong L, Guo R, Wang S and Shi X 2016 Partially PEGylated dendrimer-entrapped gold nanoparticles: a promising nanoplatform for highly efficient DNA and siRNA delivery *J. Mater. Chem.* B **4** 2933–43

[130] Jacob J, Haponiuk J T, Thomas S and Gopi S 2018 Biopolymer based nanomaterials in drug delivery systems: a review *Mater. Today Chem.* **9** 43–55

[131] Lü J-M, Wang X, Marin-Muller C, Wang H, Lin P H and Yao Q *et al* 2009 Current advances in research and clinical applications of PLGA-based nanotechnology *Expert Rev. Mol. Diagn.* **9** 325–41

[132] Gonçalves C, Gonçalves I C, Magalhães F D and Pinto A M 2017 Poly (lactic acid) composites containing carbon-based nanomaterials: a review *Polymers* **9** 269

[133] Karak N 2017 *Biobased Smart Polyurethane Nanocomposites: From Synthesis to Applications* (London: Royal Society of Chemistry)

[134] Jokar M, Pedersen G A and Loeschner K 2017 Six open questions about the migration of engineered nano-objects from polymer-based food-contact materials: a review *Food Addit. Contam. Part A* **34** 434–50

[135] Teo B K and Sun X H 2006 From top-down to bottom-up to hybrid nanotechnologies: road to nanodevices *J. Cluster Sci.* **17** 529–40

[136] Ochekpe N A, Olorunfemi P O and Ngwuluka N C 2009 Nanotechnology and drug delivery part 2: nanostructures for drug delivery *Trop. J. Pharm. Res.* **8** 275–82

[137] Arole V M and Munde S V 2014 Fabrication of nanomaterials by top-down and bottom-up approaches-an overview *J. Mater. Sci.* **1** 89–93

[138] Corres J M, Sanz A, Arregui F J, Matías I R and Roca J 2008 Fiber optic glucose sensor based on bionanofilms *Sens. Actuators* B **131** 633–39

[139] Bashar M M, Ohara H, Zhu H, Yamamoto S, Matsui J and Miyashita T *et al* 2019 Cellulose nanofiber nanosheet multilayers by the Langmuir–Blodgett technique *Langmuir* **35** 8052–59

[140] Scholl F A, Morais P V, Gabriel R C, Schöning M J, Siqueira J R Jr and Caseli L 2017 Carbon nanotubes arranged as smart interfaces in lipid Langmuir–Blodgett films enhancing the enzymatic properties of penicillinase for biosensing applications *ACS Appl. Mater. Interfaces* **9** 31054–66

[141] Arslan B, Egerton K, Zhang X and Abu-Lail N I 2017 Effects of the surface morphology and conformations of lignocellulosic biomass biopolymers on their nanoscale interactions with hydrophobic self-assembled monolayers *Langmuir* **33** 6857–68

[142] Motealleh A, Dorri P and Kehr N S 2019 Self-assembled monolayers of chiral periodic mesoporous organosilica as a stimuli responsive local drug delivery system *J. Mater. Chem.* B **7** 2362–71

[143] Acosta S, Quintanilla L, Alonso M, Aparicio C and Rodríguez-Cabello J C 2019 Recombinant AMP/polypeptide self-assembled monolayers with synergistic antimicrobial properties for bacterial strains of medical relevance *ACS Biomater. Sci. Eng.* **5** 4708–16

[144] Yang D, He H and Xu B 2020 Enzyme-instructed morphological transition of the supramolecular assemblies of branched peptides *Beilstein J. Org. Chem.* **16** 2709–18

[145] Han Q, Tao F, Xu Y, Su H, Yang F and Körstgens V *et al* 2020 Tuning chain relaxation from an amorphous biopolymer film to crystals by removing air/water interface limitations *Angew. Chem. Int. Ed.* **59** 20192–200

[146] De Cuyper M and Bulte J W 2001 *Physics and Chemistry Basis of Biotechnology* vol 7 (Berlin: Springer Science & Business Media)

[147] Drazenovic J 2015 Characterization, exchange dynamics, and supported bilayer formation of phosphatidylcholine vesicles *PhD Thesis* Temple University. Libraries

[148] Ulman A 2013 *An Introduction to Ultrathin Organic Films: From Langmuir–Blodgett to Self–Assembly* (New York: Academic)

[149] Shi S-C and Peng Y-Q 2020 Preparation and tribological studies of stearic acid-modified biopolymer coating *Prog. Org. Coat.* **138** 105304

[150] Rukmanikrishnan B, Ismail F R M, Manoharan R K, Kim S S and Lee J 2020 Blends of gellan gum/xanthan gum/zinc oxide based nanocomposites for packaging application: rheological and antimicrobial properties *Int. J. Biol. Macromol.* **148** 1182–9

[151] Cai S, Wu C, Yang W, Liang W, Yu H and Liu L 2020 Recent advance in surface modification for regulating cell adhesion and behaviors *Nanotechnol. Rev.* **9** 971–89

[152] Roy A, Shrivastava S L and Mandal S M 2016 Self-assembled carbohydrate nanostructures: synthesis strategies to functional application in food *Novel Approaches of Nanotechnology in Food* (Amsterdam: Elsevier) pp 133–64

[153] Battigelli A 2019 Design and preparation of organic nanomaterials using self-assembled peptoids *Biopolymers.* **110** e23265

[154] Mendes P M and Preece J A 2004 Precision chemical engineering: integrating nanolithography and nanoassembly *Curr. Opin. Colloid Interface Sci.* **9** 236–48

[155] Mijatovic D, Eijkel J C and van den Berg A 2005 Technologies for nanofluidic systems: top-down vs. bottom-up—a review *Lab Chip* **5** 492–500

[156] Cheng J Y, Ross C A, Smith H I and Thomas E L 2006 Templated self-assembly of block copolymers: top-down helps bottom-up *Adv. Mater.* **18** 2505–21

[157] Dhawan A, Du Y, Batchelor D, Wang H-N, Leonard D and Misra V *et al* 2011 Hybrid top-down and bottom-up fabrication approach for wafer-scale plasmonic nanoplatforms *Small.* **7** 727–31

[158] Ingale A G and Chaudhari A N 2013 Biogenic synthesis of nanoparticles and potential applications: an eco-friendly approach *J. Nanomed. Nanotechol.* **4** 1–7

[159] Khomutov G B and Gubin S P 2002 Interfacial synthesis of noble metal nanoparticles *Mater. Sci. Eng.* C **22** 141–6

[160] Choi Y, Ho N-H and Tung C-H 2007 Sensing phosphatase activity by using gold nanoparticles *Angew. Chem.* **119** 721–3

[161] Gupta A R and Kant V 2013 Synthesis, characterization and biomedical applications of nanoparticles *Sci. Int.* **1** 167–74

[162] Dong F, Guo S, Wang H, Li X and Wu Z 2011 Enhancement of the visible light photocatalytic activity of C-doped TiO_2 nanomaterials prepared by a green synthetic approach *J. Phys. Chem.* C **115** 13285–92

[163] Faraji M, Yamini Y and Rezaee M 2010 Magnetic nanoparticles: synthesis, stabilization, functionalization, characterization, and applications *J. Iran. Chem. Soc.* **7** 1–37

[164] De Jaeger N, Demeyere H, Finsy R, Sneyers R, Vanderdeelen J and Van der Meeren P *et al* 1991 Particle sizing by photon correlation spectroscopy Part I: monodisperse latices: influence of scattering angle and concentration of dispersed material *Part. Part. Syst. Charact.* **8** 179–86

[165] Chauhan R P S, Gupta C and Prakash D 2012 Methodological advancements in green nanotechnology and their applications in biological synthesis of herbal nanoparticles Int *J. Bioassays* **1** 6–10

[166] Parmar A, Kaur G, Kapil S, Sharma V, Sachar S and Sandhir R *et al* 2019 Green chemistry mediated synthesis of PLGA-silver nanocomposites for antibacterial synergy: introspection of formulation parameters on structural and bactericidal aspects *React. Funct. Polym.* **141** 68–81

[167] Pal S L, Jana U, Manna P K, Mohanta G P and Manavalan R 2011 Nanoparticle: an overview of preparation and characterization *J. Appl. Pharm. Sci.* **1** 228–34

[168] Kreuter J 1991 Peroral administration of nanoparticles *Adv. Drug Deliv. Rev.* **7** 71–86

[169] Panyam J, Dali M M, Sahoo S K, Ma W, Chakravarthi S S and Amidon G L *et al* 2003 Polymer degradation and *in vitro* release of a model protein from poly (D, L-lactide-co-glycolide) nano-and microparticles *J. Control. Release* **92** 173–87

[170] Zargar M, Hamid A A, Bakar F A, Shamsudin M N, Shameli K and Jahanshiri F *et al* 2011 Green synthesis and antibacterial effect of silver nanoparticles using *Vitex negundo L Molecules* **16** 6667–76

[171] Visakh P M and Thomas S 2010 Preparation of bionanomaterials and their polymer nanocomposites from waste and biomass *Waste Biomass Valori.* **1** 121–34

[172] Manea F, Garda V G, Rad B and Ajo-Franklin C M 2020 Programmable assembly of 2D crystalline protein arrays into covalently stacked 3D bionanomaterials *Biotechnol. Bioeng.* **117** 912–23

[173] Mishra R K, Ha S K, Verma K and Tiwari S K 2018 Recent progress in selected bio-nanomaterials and their engineering applications: an overview *J. Sci.: Adv. Mater. Devices* **3** 263–88

[174] Zur Mühlen A, Zur Mühlen E, Niehus H and Mehnert W 1996 Atomic force microscopy studies of solid lipid nanoparticles *Pharm. Res.* **13** 1411–16

[175] Tiede K, Boxall A B, Tear S P, Lewis J, David H and Hassellöv M 2008 Detection and characterization of engineered nanoparticles in food and the environment *Food Addit. Contam.* **25** 795–821

[176] López-Serrano A, Olivas R M, Landaluze J S and Cámara C 2014 Nanoparticles: a global vision. Characterization, separation, and quantification methods. Potential environmental and health impact *Anal. Methods* **6** 38–56

[177] Vickrey T M and Garcia-Ramirez J A 1980 Magnetic field-flow fractionation: theoretical basis *Sep. Sci. Technol.* **15** 1297–304

[178] Bekdemir A and Stellacci F 2016 A centrifugation-based physicochemical characterization method for the interaction between proteins and nanoparticles *Nat. Commun.* **7** 1–8

[179] Faccini M, Borja G, Boerrigter M, Morillo Martín D, Martìnez Crespiera S and Vázquez-Campos S *et al* 2015 Electrospun carbon nanofiber membranes for filtration of nanoparticles from water *J. Nanomater.* **2015**

[180] Dong X, Jakobi M, Wang S, Köhler M H, Zhang X and Koch A W 2019 A review of hyperspectral imaging for nanoscale materials research *Appl. Spectrosc. Rev.* **54** 285–305

[181] Barreda F-A, Nicolas C, Sirven J-B, Ouf F-X, Lacour J-L and Robert E *et al* 2015 In-situ characterization of nanoparticle beams focused with an aerodynamic lens by laser-induced breakdown detection *Sci. Rep.* **5** 1–7

[182] Snijder J, van de Waterbeemd M, Damoc E, Denisov E, Grinfeld D and Bennett A *et al* 2014 Defining the stoichiometry and cargo load of viral and bacterial nanoparticles by Orbitrap mass spectrometry *JACS* **136** 7295–9

[183] Donaldson K and Poland C A 2009 New insights into nanotubes *Nat. Nanotechnol.* **4** 708–10

[184] Tomić S, Kokol V, Mihajlović D, Mirčić A and Čolić M 2016 Native cellulose nanofibrills induce immune tolerance *in vitro* by acting on dendritic cells *Sci. Rep.* **6** 1–14

[185] Endes C, Camarero-Espinosa S, Mueller S, Foster E J, Petri-Fink A and Rothen-Rutishauser B *et al* 2016 A critical review of the current knowledge regarding the biological impact of nanocellulose *J. Nanobiotechnol.* **14** 1–14

[186] Baker S, Rakshith D, Kavitha K S, Santosh P, Kavitha H U and Rao Y *et al* 2013 Plants: emerging as nanofactories towards facile route in synthesis of nanoparticles *BioImpacts: BI* **3** 111

Chapter 4

Bionanocomposites and their multifunctional applications

Satya Veer Singh, Sandeep Kumar, Anand Sharma and Jay Singh

This chapter focuses on bionanocomposite materials and their multifunctional applications such as nanomedicine, tissue engineering, cardiovascular stent, etc. Bionanocomposites are the emerging class of nanostructured materials as they constitute particles and biological entities with at least one dimension less than 100 nm. They are very similar to nanocomposites, but they have fundamental differences in synthesis method, functionalities, properties, biocompatibility, biodegradability and their applications. Bionanocomposite science is a tremendous and interesting field because it merges materials science with nanotechnology, physics, and biology. This chapter in four sections elaborates on the definition and classifications of bionanocomposites, preparation methods, properties, and applications.

4.1 Introduction

In the recent past, biocompatible-based bionanocomposites with different nanostructures have been developed for a range of promising applications encompassing wider areas of materials science, medicine and nanotechnology etc [1–3]. Many groups of researchers are consistently working towards developing multifunctional bionanocomposites and more advanced science will be seen in upcoming years. In practice, there exist two key components of bionanocomposites, i.e., biopolymer matrix and nanosized reinforcement or filler constituent. Nanosized fillers or reinforcements exhibit at least one of the nanometer range dimensions, typically below 100 nm [4, 5]. The chemical bonding and strength of the interaction between the biopolymers and fillers decide the functionality and actual properties of synthesized bionanocomposites. Such bionanocomposites hold tremendous potential because of their excellent multi-functionality, and they are known renewable and abundant resources present in Nature. To develop an efficient bionanocomposite, both the sources of biopolymer and reinforcement/filler should be highly

doi:10.1088/978-0-7503-3767-0ch4

biocompatible and offer better biodegradable character along with facile processability. Any new bionanocomposite is believed to be the most proficient and beneficial when it has good competence in association with the existing industrial process and methodology. These factors ensure its maximum reach and advantage to our society. Bionanocomposites show improved and interesting properties which the biopolymer alone cannot possess. One realizes the enhanced physical and chemical behaviors of specific nanosized fillers' related properties and the very high surface-to-volume ratio. The research focus is on obtaining bionanocomposites with better mechanical behavior, improved thermal stability, good solubility and gas-barrier characteristics [6, 7]. Owing to the high biocompatibility of multifunctional bionanocomposites, they deliver prospective applications in various fields, including agriculture, bio-inspired electronics, tissue engineering, drug delivery vehicles, and scaffolds for wound healing and so on.

4.1.1 Biocompatible matrices and nanosized reinforcements/fillers

Figure 4.1 shows that the bionanocomposite comprises highly biocompatible polymers and nanosized fillers or reinforcements. The biodegradable polymers serve as the host matrices for nanofillers/reinforcements. The biopolymers usually degrade and are then removed completely from the human body. Within our body, the different metabolic reactions such as chain scission or hydrolysis help us in the removal process [8, 9]. These biopolymers are eliminated in the human body with appropriate acidity, humidity, oxygenation, and essential minerals and metals [9, 10]. The biopolymers are extracted from a wide range of renewable resources in different animals and plants and their products. Biodegradable polymers are also prepared via bacteria with small-sized molecules, for example, butyric acid/valeric acid-producing polyhydroxybutyrate and polyhydroxyvalerate. Moreover, petroleum-derived biopolymers can be developed with sources including poly(-caprolactone), poly(butylene succinate) and poly[(butylene succinate)-co-adipate] etc [11].

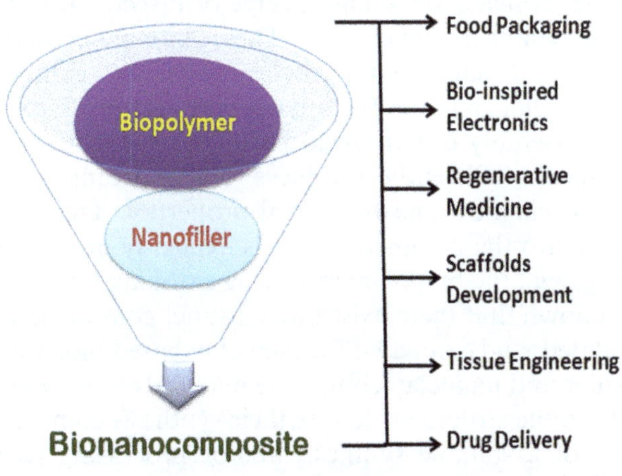

Figure 4.1. An illustration of key components used in synthesizing bionanocomposites offering interesting applications in different areas.

Aliphatic polyesters and aliphatic-aromatic copolyesters are the most utilized petroleum-based biopolymer products. Biopolymers that show complete degradation and are extracted from renewable sources are sought to develop multifunctional bionanocomposites with mass scaling in industries. In general, a variety of biopolymers like starch, chitin, chitosan, poly (lactic acid), cellulose, lignin, halloysite, protein, polysaccharides and so on are employed for synthesizing versatile bionanocomposites. The other key component of bionanocomposites is nanosized fillers or reinforcements with one or more dimensions below 100 nm. The incorporation of nanosized reinforcements into biopolymer matrices is capable of providing potential functionality to bionanocomposites. According to reported literature, multifunctional and advanced bionanocomposites extensively use nanofillers to achieve desired and suitable physical as well as chemical and mechanical properties. Previously, the nanofillers of inorganic and organic types with different structures, shapes, and sizes have been utilized with a biopolymer matrix. The organic type of nanofillers includes graphene, carbon nanotubes, nanorods, silica nanocrystals, cellulose-based nanocrystals and nanowhiskers, along with hydroxyapatite nanofillers etc. Cellulose-based nanofillers are called green fillers and are identified as one of the most prospective fillers or reinforcements in developing bionanocomposites [12, 13]. Inorganic nanofillers like nanostructures of metals, i.e., Ag, Cu, Zn, and Cd with their oxides, are also actively exploited to synthesize bionanocomposites in different applications.

4.2 Synthesis and processing techniques of bionanocomposites

Following the literature, there exist specific processing methods to prepare and develop efficient multifunctional bionanocomposite materials. The synthesis of bionanocomposites utilizes two major parts, i.e., nanosized particles and biocompatible polymer-based matrices. In general, nanosized particles are carefully incorporated within the used polymer, acting as a matrix to develop bionanocomposites. Nanoparticles which show a high degree of dispersion behavior are sought after for such nanocomposite materials. These bionanocomposites containing homogeneously dispersed nanosized particles essentially exhibit enhanced and distinct characteristics that only the biopolymers cannot produce. It is noteworthy that an appropriate assembly of nanosized particles interacting strongly with their host biopolymer matrix efficiently produces bionanocomposites with superior physical, chemical, mechanical and biological properties. The particular kind and size of nanoparticles into the polymer matrix is explicitly important to achieve the desired functionality, e.g., the biopolymers having exfoliated single platelets (~1 nm) of nanoclays. It is known that there exist three distinct composite structures such as intercalated, flocculated, and exfoliated for nanoclay based bionanocomposites. The exfoliated biopolymer and nanoclay composite materials are preferred among three thermodynamically stable structures despite their synthesis complexity [8]. For such reasons, the choice of a suitable synthesis and/or processing technique is highly dependent on the fact that the nanosized particles must be well dispersed within the biopolymer matrix resulting in bionanocomposites with required properties.

After ensuring the necessary dispersion of nanosized particles into the matrix, one should also examine that nanosized particles' initial structure is intact after the complete process. Under unusual processing conditions, the nanosized particles are very prone to losing their exact structural properties, which eventually leads to unexpected functionality of bionanocomposites. To achieve the most efficient bionanocomposites, the various parameters of processing technique can be optimized in such a way that the quality of the biopolymer matrix and nanosized particles remain the same or provide the least possible variations in different properties. Therefore, the selected processing technique's effectiveness relies on two vital parameters, i.e., competence with environment and ease of integration with present industrial platforms. Multifunctional bionanocomposites can be synthesized and processed through such techniques as *in situ* polymerizations, solution casting, and melt processing.

Apart from the above primary processing techniques, a few other novel synthesis methods have been reported, including electro-spinning and process methodology employing supercritical conditions such as carbon dioxide. These process techniques show remarkable potential and have emerged to produce bionanocomposites with multifold properties. The supercritical conditions pertaining to carbon dioxide are known as $T_c = 31.1$ °C and $P_c = 73.8$ bar. In practice, it is very much feasible to attain such supercritical values. The supercritical carbon dioxide may be utilized in two distinct ways where it plays a role as a foaming agent and/or a medium during the processing of bionanocomposites. For *in situ* polymerization and/or melt processing techniques, the supercritical carbon dioxide-based solvent is derived from greener source extracts, whereas other solvents use organic sources [14, 15]. This makes supercritical carbon dioxide a more viable option considering its environment-friendly nature in the long run. The potential of such a solvent is seen in biopolymer and nanoclay composite materials where supercritical carbon dioxide playing one of the two roles (i.e., foaming agent/medium) essentially increases the interlayer distance of the matrix. As a result, the nanosized particles are easily dispersed into the biopolymer matrix. Among the above-mentioned special processing techniques, melt processing is of great importance due to its incorporation into industries for mass scaling. It can be perceived that an individual biopolymer matrix involving, more importantly, a certain type of nanosized particles ultimately determines the appropriate process technique.

4.2.1 *In situ* polymerization

First, the nanosized particles are added to prepared monomer solvents followed by thorough mixing. Afterward, in order to start *in situ* polymerization, the mixed solution is treated at a definite temperature by exposing to heat/ radiation etc. *In situ* polymerization is known to be a facile and rapid processing technique to synthesize different bionanocomposites.

4.2.2 Solution casting method

In this processing technique, the required biopolymer is first made into a proper solvent medium. This is followed by mixing and dispersing the nanosized particles.

The incorporation of nanoparticles can be performed by adding them directly to the previous biopolymer-based solution. On the other hand, one might also prefer to prepare an individual solution of nanosized particles, which is then thoroughly mixed with the biopolymer solution to synthesize bionanocomposites. Ray *et al* extensively discuss the preparation of nanocomposites. It is shown that the clays are initially pre-swell using a suitable solvent under ambient conditions [16]. Owing to weak forces between the clays' stacks, it is relatively easy to disperse the clays into solvents. After swelling the clays in the solvent, it is added to the biopolymer solution and mixed carefully. Following this, intercalation of biopolymer chains occurs by dislocating the solvent inside the stack layers of clay, which is finally adsorbed on top of silicate layers' surface. The phenomenon of the biopolymer intercalation within the interlayers of clay under the presence of solution is primarily derived due to the excess of entropy from the desorption of solvent molecules. This arises in order to take care of the reduction in entropy related to the restrained intercalated biopolymer chains. At the final stage, the bionanocomposites with the integrated intercalated structure are developed after removing the solvents.

4.2.3 Melt processing

The popular melt processing method employs total mixing and dissolution of the biopolymer and nanosized particles. Both the biopolymer and nanosized particles are used in molten states. After preparing the mixture of biopolymer with the particles, it is heated at elevated temperatures usually higher than that of the biopolymer softening point, statically or less than shear value [17, 18]. For example, considering clay-based bionanocomposites, such a processing technique reveals significant benefits compared to the above discussed *in situ* intercalative polymerization or solution casting method. This melt processing method uses no organic solvents and hence endorses its environment-friendly nature. Moreover, this processing method is also greatly in compliance with ongoing bionanocomposite industrial level techniques, including well-established extrusion and injection molding processes. In contrast to the *in situ* polymerization method, the melt processing of bionanocomposite is very versatile and provides feasibility to achieve intercalation in most biopolymers. Various melt processing techniques remarkably affect the strength of intercalation of biopolymer with nanosized particles while synthesizing the bionanocomposites. Such a thermodynamic interaction in the case of clay/biopolymer nanocomposites can be either stronger or weaker according to the biopolymer chain movement, resulting in the formation of a quality interface between bulk melt and silicate interlayers [17, 19]. Also, the well-dispersed nanoparticles are achieved depending on the used biopolymer. A suitable biopolymer usually facilitates an apt dispersion of nanosized particles.

The selection of a processing technique among the above is mainly based on achieving a high level of nanoparticle dispersion within the biopolymer matrices. In general, while synthesizing polymer/clay bionanocomposites, the layered silicate platelets are converted into single platelet via the exfoliation route. This is necessary to ensure well-dispersed silicate platelets in the biopolymer matrix. The stacked silicate platelets can also break and possibly divide into small unstable intercalated and flocculated structures. For melt processing of bionanocomposites, enthalpy energy of the interaction among nanosized particles and individual platelet layers is considered one of the vital parameters that allow a high degree of nanoparticle dispersion inside the biopolymer matrix. In addition, other melt processing parameters such as temperature etc, also depict a significant impact on the level of dispersion of nanoparticles. With the required amount of enthalpy energy of polymer and nanoparticles, it is much easier to synthesize melt-processed bionanocomposites. However, improper enthalpy energy, whether in excess or deficiency, usually lead to poor dispersion of nanosized particles producing unwanted micro composite materials. Therefore, the high-quality bionanocomposites are prepared under optimum process parameter conditions and enthalpy energy of polymer–nanoparticles interactions through melt processing. In this regard, Hunter *et al* discuss the details of polymer and clay bionanocomposites [20]. It has been shown that the intercalation and/or exfoliation processes are likely to be related to shear phenomenon. During such processes, many tactoids containing particles with size ranging from 8–10 μm are located far from each other under the influence of both the mechanical and chemical forces. As an unusual behavior, this again converts those tactoids into relatively smaller ones. Following previous conventional literature, it is believed that there exists a steady movement of chains of a biopolymer essentially towards galleries of the clay [18, 19]. Such a movement of biopolymer chains evidently increases the distance between adjacent galleries known as *d*-spacing. The expansion of biopolymer chains is limited when it surpasses the van der Waals force, which causes the platelets to detach from each other completely. In contrast, Hunter *et al* describe the exfoliation process in a somewhat different manner [20]. According to the reports, the exfoliation process is carried out by taking off strip by strip from small-sized stacks and then converting them into separate silicate platelets. Since the melt processing technique employs the applications of inherent mechanical shearing force as well as temperature, the bionanocomposites can face minor deterioration after complete processing in some specific cases. For instance, the melt processing technique's undesired effect is seen for poly(lactic acid) or polylactide (PLA) based nanocomposite materials. PLA shows some degradation under unusual thermal, oxidation or hydrolytic conditions. This effect eventually reduces the molecular weight of the utilized biopolymer primarily because of redundant polymer chain openings. On the other hand, such unwanted biopolymer degradation becomes more pronounced in the case of organically modified clays based bionanocomposite materials. For clay/biopolymer nanocomposites, a sufficiently large shear force is applied for a longer time to take off a strip of layered silicate platelets. During melt processing technique, irrespective of the extruder or internal mixer, a large shear force for such a long span of time will cause excess biopolymer degradation resulting in the formation of unexpected bionanocomposites.

However, such a large shear force is very useful for some nanostructures like carbon nanotubes (CNTs) in terms of improved dispersion behavior. Due to the extended span of shear force, there is a high probability that the mixed nanostructures are likely to be physically deformed, losing their initial structural properties. Also, melt processing bionanocomposite performed at the elevated temperature noticeably diminishes the viscosity of biopolymer. Under optimum conditions of the enthalpy energy of interactions among particles and temperature, particularly in the case of clay/polymer composites, one can deliver a controlled flow of the biopolymer chains from the bulk melt phase into the galleries. Additionally, it reduces the shearing effect of the polymer on silicates at the same time. The production of good bionanocomposites needs optimized processing conditions, e.g. enthalpy, temperature and time etc, are required for most thermally sensitive biopolymers. Therefore, the melt processing technique is very helpful when employed with appropriate synthesis parameters to provide maximum separation of tactoids/agglomerations from the nanoscale's well-dispersed particles.

4.3 Various bionanocomposite based on the type of matrices and reinforcements

4.3.1 Starch derived bionanocomposites

As an alternative to fossil resources, starch-based resources are very useful in practical fields apart from food industries. Starch as an active source outperforms due to the low cost, ease of availability along with complete recycling with no hazardous extracts. Also, starch as other polymers is highly biocompatible but is confined and lacks poor processing, has weak mechanical properties, issues of prolonged stability, and reactivity with water. However, there are consistent efforts for development and fundamental understanding to overcome such critical issues. Native starch is usually found as granules in seeds, roots including tube-shaped maize, wheat, potato, and rice etc, with distinct genesis. These granules exhibit multi-level structures ranging from 1–100 μm. Such structures usually contain amorphous and semi-crystalline shells arranged alternately known as growth rings, crystalline and amorphous lamellae called periodicity, that possess macromolecular chains [21–24]. Starch has D-glucose units as in a polysaccharide, termed as homoglucan or glucopyranose. These consist of two important biomacromolecules known as amylose and amylopectin. Amylose is comprised of a relatively low number of carbohydrate branches based on α-bonds [1–4] and can have a molecular weight in the range 10^5–10^6 with a degree of polymerization (DP) up to 600 [21]. In the case of amylopectin, there is a very high content of multiple-branched polymers with a large molecular weight ~10^7–10^9. Apart from this, starch granules also contain minute traces of proteins, lipids and phosphorus according to the natural polymer resource [22, 23]. The concentration of amylose in a botanical source can help enhance the thermal, rheological, and other properties [25–29]. Further, during starch processing, it is usually transferred in the form of molten, termed as plasticized or thermoplastic starch. Such a conversion of native granular starch is called the gelatinisation/melting process.

In order to realize practical applications, different processing techniques, as discussed previously, are utilized for plasticized starch-based materials. Under optimized moisture content, melting temperature, starch is processed with plasticisers of non-volatile nature like polyols including glycerol, sorbitol, glycol, etc [30–36], nitrogen-based compounds such as urea, ammonium derived, amines, etc [37–43], or citric acid (CA) [44, 45]. One can further improve the quality of the final starch-based product in terms of mechanical or water resistance properties by modifying it chemically, i.e., post-treatments with hydroxylation [46, 47] and acetylation [48, 49]. Such chemical improvisations are depicted by replacing starch with ester or ether groups for the hydroxyls. From another point of view, one can also prepare starch-based composite systems via blending into other biopolymers, e.g., PLA, polycaprolactone (PCL), poly(butylene succinate adipate) (PBSA), and poly(vinyl alcohol) (PVA) etc [50–52]. Moreover, starch-based biocomposite materials are also developed after reinforcing biopolymers with different fibrous fillers, nanostructures and lignin fillers etc [53], which aid in producing nanocomposites with excellent physical, chemical and biological properties. In most cases, starch based bionanocomposite materials use phyllosilicates as reinforcement due to their facile availability, inexpensive processing, flexibility, and environment friendly with non-hazardous nature. Phyllosilicates are also peculiarly known as layered silicates with varying structure, texture, and/or morphology as well as sepiolite type fibrous structure, and halloysite with spheroidal forms [54, 55]. Since phyllosilicates contain vital clay minerals, micas, chlorite, serpentine, etc, they are sought after as fillers for multifunctional bionanocomposites. The reinforcement of phyllosilicates significantly enhances the tensile strength, Young's modulus, storage modulus, glass transition temperature (T_g), thermal stability, moisture resistance, oxygen barrier property and biodegradation rate etc [56, 57]. The observed modifications in physical and other properties are attributed to improved structural integrity due to homogeneously dispersed silicate layers within the host matrix, the strong coupling of nanofiller with starch matrix, and large surface-to-volume ratios nanostructured fillers [58–60].

Most of the other polymers, including the recently utilized starch matrix, are also commonly reinforced with carbonaceous nanofillers, including graphene, CNTs, graphite, and carbon black (CB) in different forms [61–63]. This is done to achieve novel functional properties such as electrical conductivity and electroactivity etc. Starch/CNT reinforced bionanocomposites are very promising for biological applications such as sensors, bone cell stimulators, etc, for various clinical trials [64, 65]. It is known that the biocompatibility of CNTs is debatable and still requires more critical study [61, 66]. CNTs are essentially found in one of two forms, i.e., single-wall carbon nanotubes (SWCNTs) and multi-wall carbon nanotubes (MWCNTs). MWCNTs are more preferred because of their low cost and natural abundance. In addition, they also offer a relatively high aspect ratio, good mechanical, thermal with remarkable electrical properties [67, 68]. The dispersion of CNTs and adhesion to the surface in the strach matrix is not that easy due to the starch's hydrophilic nature. Nevertheless, the addition of CNTs as nanofillers into a starch matrix can notably enhance the functional properties of bionanocomposite materials from nanofiller–matrix interactions [61–63, 69, 70], ensuring appropriate chemical modification of CNTs. Figure 4.2 demonstrates the synthesis of starch, chitosan and graphene bionanocomposites [71]. Starch matrix is also reinforced with metalloid

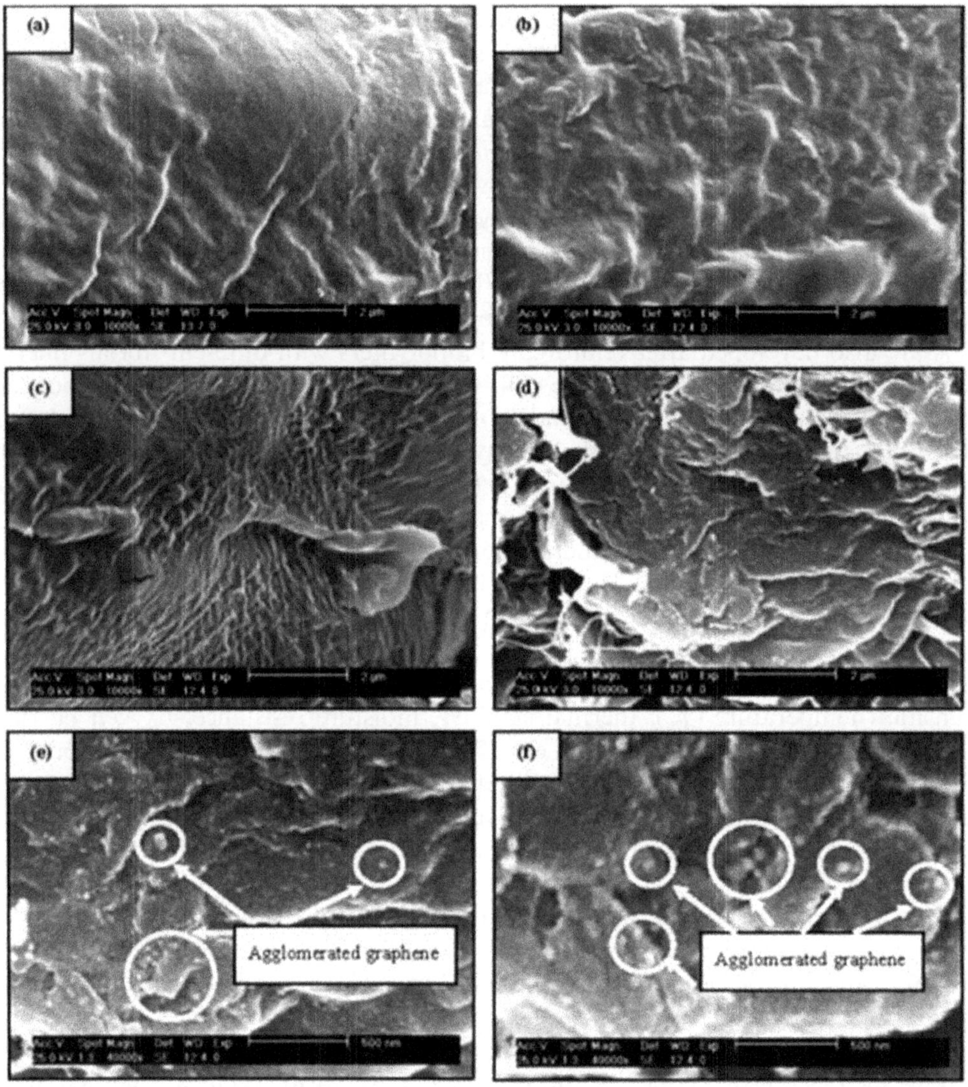

Figure 4.2. Scanning electron microscopy (SEM) images of (a) chitosan film, (b) starch film, (c) chitosan with 1.5 wt% graphenes, (d) starch with 1.5 wt% graphenes, (e) chitosan with 3 wt% graphenes, and (f) starch with 3 wt% graphenes. Reprinted with permission from [71], copyright (2014) John Wiley & Sons.

oxides, i.e., SiO_2 and Sb_2O_3, metal oxides such as ZnO, TiO_2, and $ZrO_2{\cdot}nH_2O$, and metal chalcogenides viz. CdS, CdSe. When these active nanofillers are incorporated into the starch matrix, excellent physical, chemical and biological properties can be perceived. The highly multifunctional bionanocomposites based on such nanofillers can lead to great implications in various fields. Depending on the type of nanofillers, such novel bionanocomposites are useful in photovoltaic solar cells, light-emitting diodes, photodiodes, and gas sensors etc [72]. It is important to mention that a proper amount of nanofiller should be added into the matrix to ensure good dispersion. An excess concentration of nanofillers usually leads to aggregations and/ or agglomeration of nanoparticles [73–75], highly undesired for the development of bionanocomposites. In addition, layered double hydroxides (LDHs) have reinforced starch nanocomposites with better mechanical properties along with good water resistance [76] but suffer from weak thermal stability. LDH structure primarily comprises brucite-like layers exhibiting edge-sharing $M(OH)_6$ octahedra [77, 78]. In order to obtain intercalation in a starch matrix with LDH, carboxymethyl cellulose sodium (CMC) as a stabilizer is used, offering desired dispersion [76].

4.3.2 Clay bionanocomposites

In clay based bionanocomposites, the clay is mainly constituted from inorganic silicate component. Clay bionanocomposites commonly use the natural as well as synthetic smectites containing the layered charged silicates. However, a few reports investigate clay systems with structure of non-lamellar nature, e.g. tubular halloysite, imogolite, and other repeatedly usable fibrous clays, including sepiolite and palygorskite. Multifunctional bionanocomposites employ such silicate clay structure usually as fillers of nanometer scale. In particular, owing to superior morphological features and surface textures of sepiolite and palygorskite structures, it is of fibrous nature and is well known to facilitate desired physical, chemical and biological properties. The fibrous nature of such silicate structures when reinforced into biopolymer matrices show formation of strong hydrogen bonds due to silanol group (Si–OH) located externally on the surface of clay systems. Sepiolite and palygorskite, which are fibrous clays, exhibit crystalline structure of type talc-like ribbons with axis parallel to that of the fiber axis. These are treated as basic structure blocks irregular with structural cavities usually called tunnels and are placed at the inner surface of silicate layer which extend further towards the direction of clay fiber growth, i.e. along the c-axis [79–81]. These tunnels looking like structures that alternatively move along the external surfaces of fibrous clays are referred to as the channels.

Sepiolite has the unit cell formula ($Si_{12}O_{30}Mg_8(OH)_4(H_2O)_4{\cdot}8H_2O$), which belongs to the hydrated magnesium silicate structure. This is comprised of the structural block made up of two tetrahedral silica sheets embedded into an innermost sheet of magnesium oxide-hydroxide. These tetrahedral silicon layers have periodic inversion inducing discontinuous silica sheets which endorse Si–OH bond existence onto the exterior plane of the fibrous silicate. Therefore, the presence of silanol groups in various organic species, e.g. coupling agents and polymers, aid in the development of organoinorganic materials having nanosized structures [82–84]. On the other hand, palygorskite or attapulgite and sepiolite are almost identical in nature because of similar morphologies. Both are essentially differing in terms of excess concentration of aluminum that substitutes magnesium within the octahedral layers. The sepiolite tunnels exhibit larger cross sectional area than that of palygorskite. Owing to smaller tunnel size of palygorskite structures, only molecules like water and methanol of small size can move along and through these tunnels [82]. With every synthesis of clay based bionanocomposite materials, they can have slightly modified morphology as well as composition. The length of sepiolite fibrous structure is normally in the range of ~1–2 μm and can be more in length for some other fibers of different origins [85]. Usually, the length of palygorskite fibers is relatively higher than that of sepiolite. It has been found to have lengths typically <5 μm and palygorskites fibre can have also average size more than 20 μm, especially for hydrothermal origin fiber [86]. In the case of clay systems, sepiolite and palygorskite silicates tunnels as well as channels posses two distinct kinds of water molecules. The first type of water molecules is of coordinated nature which is bonded to divalent Mg ion located at the octahedral corners of the sheet. The second one is referred as the water molecules of zeolitic type which primarily help in filling up the intracrystalline cavity areas. In clay systems, the coordinated water and the silicate layers are attached with each other larger bond strength. Due to their strong bonding nature, it is quite difficult to remove such water molecules from the host system and hence, higher temperature treatments (above 400 °C) are generally required for removal under dynamic vacuum conditions. On the contrary, zeolitic type water molecules can be eliminated by only simple vacuum treatments and/or process aided with temperature approximately 100 °C. During the coordinated water removal, the standard structure tunnels or channels tend to disintegrate and the process is called structural folding [87].

In addition, there also exists a layered clay system like the montmorillonite which is one of the most common forms of clay nanofillers utilized in synthesis and development of biopolymer/clay bionanocomposites. Such clay based nanocomposite materials employ exfoliated processed silicate layers. However, bionanocomposites developed with clay fibers cannot go through the exfoliation process. This implies that the bionanocomposites based on sepiolite and palygorskite do not exhibit any aggregation behavior and are well dispersed when mixed with the polymer matrix. In particular, the layered silicates, i.e. smectites and vermiculites, differ from the clay fibers in terms of the silanol groups. The fibrous clays contain relatively higher density of silanol groups, almost two Si–OH groups/nm^2. The presence of silanol group permits both the hydrogen bonding as well as van der Waals interactions at the exterior surface of polymer silicate. Hence, one can utilize even low-polar polymers with fibrous clays when surface treated with appropriate organic surfactants [88]. The organically modified fibrous clays are obtained using grafting method. Generally, with the help of silanes and other coupling agents, organic groups can be easily grafted over silicate surfaces via formation of covalent bonds [82, 89, 90]. This can in turn facilitate the production of bionanocomposites with superior adhesion and ability to cope with any other polymeric matrices with enhanced mechanical properties [91]. Figure 4.3 shows the developed montmorillonite clay and CNT hybrid materials acting as nanofillers [92]. The fibrous clay based bionanocomposites are processed primarily with adsorption, and covalent grafting of polymers onto the exterior surface of clay is employed infrequently [93–95]. Mostly, bionanocomposites utilizing clay fibers are synthesized in the forms of low density foams for purposes like insulation, cushioning, packaging, scaffolds etc, and as thin film prepared for uses in different fields, e.g. packaging, membranes, coatings and catalysis, electronic devices for medical applications etc [96–100].

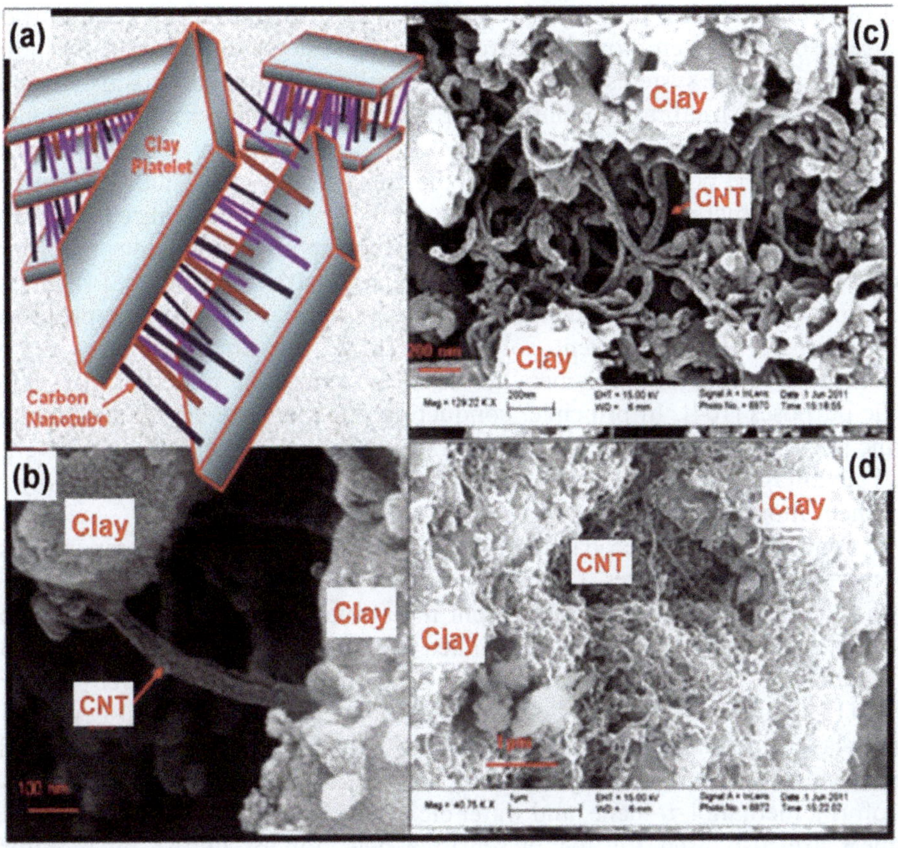

Figure 4.3. (a) Schematic diagrams of montmorillonite clay and CNT hybrid materials. (b)–(d) SEM images of clay–CNT hybrids were recorded at different magnification values. Reprinted with permission from [92], copyright (2012) American Chemical Society.

4.3.3 Conducting polymer based bionanocomposites

Bionanocomposites based on electrically conducting polymer find potential in next generation hybrid functional materials for a variety of industrial applications. Such bionanocomposites are promising because of synergistic size effects, biodegradable nature along with required plasticity [101, 102]. These bionanocomposites are mainly comprised of biopolymers and conducting polymers with embedded metallic nanosized particles [103]. Usually, conducting polymers are used to improve the electrical sensitivity, speed, and stability of bioelectronic devices. Conducting polymers can be of various types depending on the electric charge, e.g. delocalized π electrons, electrically conducting nanosized particles and cations/anions. In particular, there can be five kinds of conducting polymers based on π electrons, i.e. polyacetylene (PA), polythiophene (PT), polypyrrole (PPy), polyphenylene, and polyaniline (PANi). The natural occurring polymers like chitosan, collagen, fibroin, and gelatin can also be converted into conducting polymers [104]. In addition to novel use of conducting polymers in tissue engineering and regenerative purposes, they are also actively employed in cardiovascular systems and electrically induced targeted drug release systems [104, 105]. The conducting polymers are also sought in clinical fields for treating lagophthalmos affected patients where nerve conduits based on conducting polymers can be developed to stimulate nerve regeneration. The conjugated π polymers are one of the most and widely studied electrically conducting polymers having free electrons [106]. These delocalized π-electrons transport within the unsaturated backbone without any constraints in order to establish an electrical way for the moving charge carriers [107, 108]. For tissue engineering, the natural biopolymers like polyurethane (PU), poly(ε-caprolactone) (PCL), chitosan (CS), collagen, polylactide (PLA) etc are modified with these conjugated π conducting polymers to develop composite materials for various specific purposes [104]. In principle, conducting polymers are very much similar to organic polymers in terms of mechanical and processing capabilities. However, the added advantages of electrical as well as optical properties of conducting polymers make them more demanding as metal and semiconductor systems.

The conducting polymer based bionanocomposites have been prepared using carbon based nanostructures. Carbon is capable of providing unmatched physical and chemical properties since it is present in various forms ranging from graphite, carbon nanotube (single and multi-walled), diamond, and amorphous carbon. Multifunctional bionanocomposites are developed by mixing well dispersed MWCNTs solution with the host conducting polymer matrix such as PLA by spray layer-by-layer method. This can be used to fabricate electric components like transducers which can actively respond to different organic volatile vapors of chloroform, methanol, toluene, and water etc. These hybrid CNTs based conducting polymers are also used for highly sensitive detection of DNAs by monitoring electrical conductivity. Carbon in the form of fullerene is a nanosized spherical or elliptical ball-like structure in which the molecule contains only carbon atoms.

The fullerene carbon renders various applications such as in medicine, heat resistance, light sensitive materials as antimicrobial agents, proton conductors etc. The fullerenes are mostly available in powder form and when reinforced within the polymer matrices enhance different properties like proton conductivity, thermo-mechanical stability while suppressing thermo-oxidative degradation biopolymers. Graphene is another variety of carbon in its two-dimensional form, which has been extensively studied after reinforcing into polymers for synthesizing functional bionanocomposites. After appropriate modifications, reduced graphene oxide with large-scale preparation and graphene foams have been hybridized with biopolymers, and doped by nitrogen, metals etc, to obtain multipurpose composite materials. Figure 4.4 depicts the graphene and PANi bionanocomposites synthesized for supercapacitors application [109]. The conducting polymer based bionanocomposites also popularly use nanofillers of metal like Ag, Au, Cu and metal oxide such as SnO_2, ZnO, TiO_2, CuO etc. Depending on the individual properties of nanofillers, along with specific electrical conductivity, other active features such as catalytic properties can be perceived. Use of metal nanofillers within conducting polymers not only enhances the structural stability of synthesized bionanocomposites but also

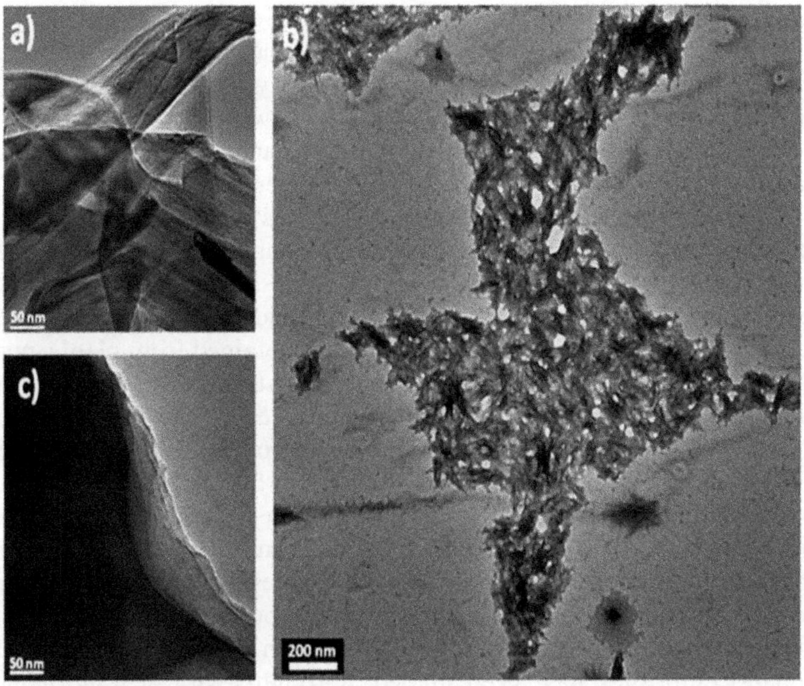

Figure 4.4. Transmission electron microscopy (TEM) images showing (a) structure of graphene platelets, (b) graphene and PANi bionanocomposites, and (c) graphene interconnection with PANi network ensuring complete embedment. Reprinted from [109], copyright (2011), with permission from Elsevier.

results in the excellent phenomenon of surface plasmon resonance [110]. Such an important phenomenon observed in conducting polymers and metal composite systems are essential for accessing body metabolites and also constituents of biological fluids.

4.3.4 Polysaccharides bionanocomposites

Polysaccharides are basically a group of large-sized molecules of carbohydrates usually found in many edible food items. This includes mainly polysaccharides in the form of chitin, cellulose, chitosan, starch, glycogen etc. Recent studies have revealed that the naturally occurring polysaccharides like cellulose contain amorphous and crystalline regions. Depending on requirement and field of applications, amorphous or crystalline polysaccharides are obtained after optimizing synthesis and treatment parameters. In this way, one can perceive nanocrystals of polysaccharides in various interesting structures such as rods, whiskers, platelets etc [111–115]. Polysaccharides nanocrystals have now become one of the most promising alternatives to conventional inorganic nanoparticles. These polysaccharides nanocrystals are completely organic in nature and hence offer great advantages in terms of enhanced biocompatibility and biodegradability, relatively facile processing, similar nanosized effects, higher mechanical properties and inexpensive nature. Also, their natural abundance is an extremely added benefit for mass scaling in different industries [115]. In contrast to other biopolymers such as protein and lipid, the polysaccharide is more stable. This is primarily due to their being irreversibly denatured through different heat treatments [116]. Although polysaccharides show potential for robust matrix material owing to their various structures and molecular weights, they suffer from brittle nature, weak thermal and water vapor barrier properties. In addition, the hydrophilic nature of polysaccharides usually hinders their successful implementation in industry platforms [117, 118]. Therefore, in order to improve the physical, mechanical and chemical properties of polysaccharides, the notion of adding fillers is utilized extensively. In practice, these fillers can be divided into two prime categories: organic and inorganic. Organic fillers include fibers obtained from plants, micro and nanocrystalline cellulose, other cellulose based nanostructures including nanocrystals, nanofibrils and whiskers. The polysaccharides based bionanocomposites utilizing such organic fillers are useful in biological applications, e.g. tissue engineering scaffolds, biofabrication, and wound healing etc. Secondly, there are inorganic fillers like montmorillonite, calcium carbonate, silver nanoparticles, and carbon based nanostructures, i.e. graphene oxides, carbon nanotubes, carbon nanorods etc.

The bionanocomposites based on polysaccharides containing such inorganic fillers are mainly deployed in pharmaceuticals, the food industry, textile field, and paper industry etc [119–123]. The most popular form of polysaccharides, chitosan based bionanocomposites, have been studied thoroughly with such inorganic nanoparticles. The silver nanoparticles (Ag NPs) have been exploited much as a promising nanofillers due to their antimicrobial properties and low toxicity [124]. Ag NPs based chitosan bionanocomposites are developed in the form of hydrogel beads with improved swelling ability over that of chitosan alone [125]. These Ag NPs containing hydrogels have exhibited excellent antimicrobial activity based on the results of gram-negative (*Escherichia coli*) and gram-positive (*Staphylococcus aureus*) as per agar diffusion investigations. Due to remarkable antibacterial properties, such hydrogels are useful in drug delivery with controlled release [125]. Another demanding form of polysaccharides, i.e. linear structured cellulose based bionanocomposites, find great attention due to their abundance of natural sources like cotton and wood pulp etc [126–128]. Cellulose can be obtained in many chemical derivations and is prepared via various solvents including N-methyl morpholine N-oxide, lithium chloride/1,3-dimethyl-2-imidazolidinone, lithium chloride/N,N-dimethylacetamide and phosphoric acid [129–133]. The cellulose in different forms of nanostructures has been developed into such forms as rod-like shapes, whiskers, nanocrystals. Using such cellulose nanostructures, different kefir an based bionanocomposites are synthesized for food packaging application with eco-friendly nature. The bionanocomposites prepared using carboxymethyl cellulose, starch and reinforced with cellulose nanocrystals have shown excellent mechanical, thermal, optical and barrier behavior in the field of food packaging [118, 134–139]. Such bionanocomposites possessing enhanced properties are perceived due to strong interfacial interactions among hydrogen bonds attached to functional moieties of cellulose nanocrystals fillers and matrix of starch-carboxymethyl cellulose [140]. It is known that although the bionanocomposites films of carboxymethyl cellulose offer good barrier properties for O_2, CO_2 and lipids, the water vapor barrier is very weak since they are chemically hydrophilic in nature containing OH and COOH groups [141, 142]. Various studies have been conducted after incorporation of hydrophobic nanostructures which significantly improve the water vapor barrier properties of these bionanocomposites films [143]. Further, graphene derived nanostructures such as nanoplatelets are also particularly utilized as nanofiller for realization of cellulose based bionanocomposites having better mechanical, thermal, electrical and gas barrier properties [144, 145]. Interestingly, polysaccharide bionanocomposites are also very useful in removing wastes of heavy metals coming from different industries. These heavy metals mainly include Cd(II), Ni(II), Cu(II), Zn(II), Pb(II), and Cr(II) ions which are very hazardous for our environment. The mechanism of heavy metal removal is called biosorption, i.e. the adsorption of metal ions with biocompatible materials such as polysaccharides. In order to remove such toxic heavy metal ions from wastewater, polysaccharide based homopolymers, composites, blends and copolymer etc, are usually synthesized. For example, a polysaccharide such as chitin with three-dimensional structure and sufficient porosity is capable of adsorbing ~288 mg g^{-1} uranium at *pH* 6 having uranium concentration of 76 mg l^{-1}. The chitin provides excellent adsorption capacity which is essentially associated with sponge type structure of chitin that offers enhanced network surface area resulting in improved metal–cation interactions. This nanofibrous chitin was nanofibrils synthesized via wet-grinding followed by compression of chitin microparticles suspension [146]. The chitin has rigid molecular structure as well as high sorption capacity, which gives easy access to the metal binding sites. The high adsorption capacity is obtained due to well dispersed chitin nanofibrils having better porosity and larger surface area. In addition, the chitin nanofibers functionalized with thiol through linking cysteine molecules is capable of producing sites for adsorption of As(III) ion. Such thiol functionalized nanofibers along with larger surface help to reach remarkable biosorption of such hazardous heavy metal ions. The analysis performed with sodium arsenite (Na_3AsO_3) in distilled water solution at *pH* 7 revealed maximum adsorption capacity as 138 mg g^{-1} compared to chitin nanofibers without thiol function groups [147]. Therefore, polysaccharide based bionanocomposites with proper modification have been proven to be an effective way for removal of many other toxic metal ions in wastewater.

4.3.5 Bionanocomposites from polypeptide

Polypeptide based biocompatible composite material is a relatively new and emerging class of hybrid nanocomposites which is growing promptly for a range of industrial applications. Polypeptides show fascinating conformational transitions under the influence of different process parameters such as temperature, solvent, *pH*, and highly dependent on the type of surfactant used. There exists good literature dealing with conformational transitions including poly(γ-benzyl-L-glutamate) (PBLG) helix–coil transition and also discussing the character of PBLG secondary transitions [148–150]. For example, polytyrosine is capable of demonstrating the helix–coil type transition in dimethylsulfoxide (DMSO) when added with di-chloroacetic acid [151]. On the other hand, poly(Nε-carbobenzyloxy-L-lysine) (PCBL) undergoes a distinct and opposite kind of transition than that of helix, i.e. coil type in m-cresol with change in temperature [152]. Polypeptide in the form of poly(β-benzyl-L-aspartate) exhibits a different type of conformational transition in m-cresol [153]. It has been shown that the change in pH value can induce such transitions in PBLG, PCBL, etc, because of deprotected side chains. [154]. For polypeptides, long chained homopolypeptides in particular, are synthesized usually through the polymerization process of α-amino acid N-carboxyanhydrides (NCAs) [155]. Such a process is known to be the most inexpensive method. In an aqueous solution, the phosgenation of α-amino acid is achieved after the closing of NCA ring employing phosgene [156]. Use of phosgene, which is highly toxic in nature, generally produces an undesirable by-product of HCl in significant amounts and thus requires its total elimination from NCA solution. This removal is performed by recrystallization of NCA under an inert environment with appropriate solvents of anhydrous nature. Following this, a few more modified and alternative synthesis methods for preparation of polypeptide have been proposed [157].

Previously, homopolypeptide composite materials with silica have been developed with enhanced properties for various applications [158–160]. Such biocompatible composite materials are chemically very versatile due to sharp conformational transitions of polypeptide shell and specific properties of silica as core material [161]. These bionanocomposites also depict strict changes in structure depending on external stimuli source. Due to very large molecular weights of polypeptide, their silica based composites are usually developed with grafting to and from method, layer-by-layer assembly etc [162–166]. The polypeptide shells containing core with different physical and chemical properties like magnetic are very useful in particular applications where they act as gold supports for catalysis processes and viable carriers in drug delivery [167]. In addition, the elastin-like polypeptide and collagen based biocomposites have been synthesized in the form of scaffolds for engineering of bone tissues, in dental treatments with optimum biocompatibility, mechanical, porosity, and hydrophobic properties. Owing to the stimuli responsive nature of polypeptide based biocomposites, they also find potential applications in therapeutic molecules, actuators, biosensors or diagnostics and regenerative medicine etc [168, 169]. Charati *et al* developed gold nanorods and polypeptide bionanocomposites for controlled drug release. A near infrared light exposure induced local heating phenomenon leading to reversible volume and/or phase transitions (solid/liquid) is utilized in step-wise and regulated release of macromolecules (figure 4.5) [170]. Polypeptide bionanocomposites hold promising applications in wider fields.

4.3.6 Chitin and Chitosan derived bionanocomposites

Chitin is very much identical to cellulose structure. It is a linear structured polysaccharide primarily made up of 2-acetamido-2-deoxy-b-D-glucopyranose units [171]. Chitin has demonstrated potential in various fields including as a chelating agent, for wastewater treatment, as a drug carrier, and for wound-healing scaffolds

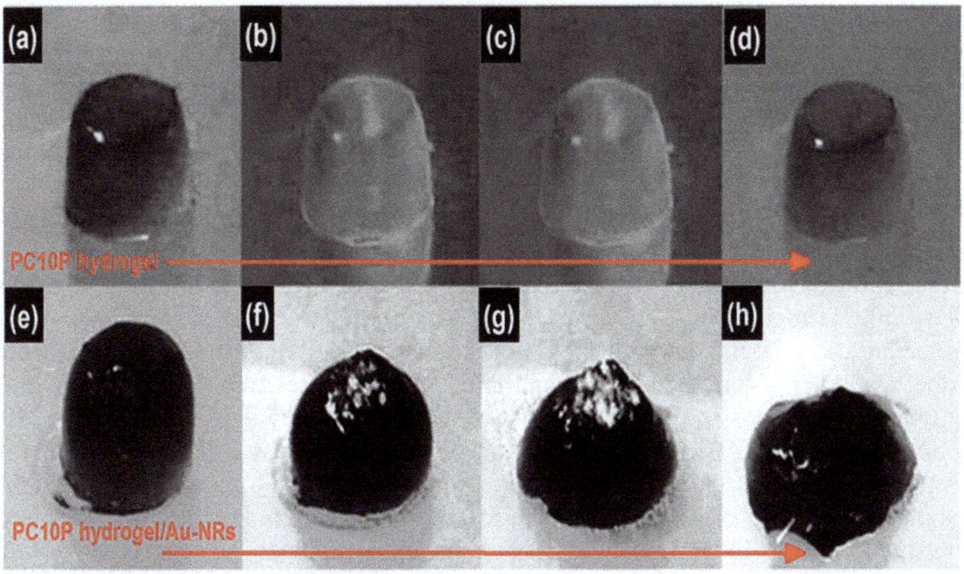

Figure 4.5. Optical images of triblock polypeptide PC10P hydrogels (a–d) without and (e–h) with Au nanorods indicating gel melting; (a), (e) under normal conditions, during exposure of NIR light (b), (c), (f), (g), and eventually (d), (h) depicts the hydrogel/Au nanorods melting by 10 min continuous NIR exposure. Reprinted with permission from [170], copyright (2010) John Wiley & Sons.

etc. In particular, chitin is weakly soluble in most of the organic solvents. It is due to the inherent hydrophobicity of chitin containing semicrystalline structures with extended hydrogen bonds. On the other hand, chitosan is usually derived via deacetylation and reverse polymerization of the host chitin [172]. Chitin in its physical appearance is very rigid and white in color comprised of primary constituents as large amounts of nitrogen based compounds. In practice, chitin is found in the exoskeleton and within the interior of invertebrate structures. Chitin functions in the same way as cellulose in plants cell walls and collagen in large-sized animals [173]. On the basis of distinct chain packing and polarity with an adjacent sheet, chitin shows polymorphism as α and β form of chitin. While α-chitin does not possess parallel arranged chains, β-chitin is known to be having molecular chains set parallel to each other. Recently, a few groups of researchers have claimed another new γ form of chitin [174].

Chitosan shows remarkable chemical properties such as rigid structure with high hydrophilicity, weak base in nature, high viscosity, salt formation after reacting with acids and ionic conductivity etc. There exist a few popular and demanding derivatives of chitosan. First, O- and N-carboxymethyl chitosan (CM-chitosan), the derivative of chitosan which easily dissolves in water. This finds excellent applications in *in vitro* diagnostics, theranostics, imaging of biological cells, biosensors, wound healing, and food packaging etc [175–180]. Such a derivative is amphoteric in nature reacting with both acid and base. O- and N-carboxymethyl form by reacting with sodium monochloracetate along with NaOH under optimized and controlled synthesis parameters [181, 182]. In the presence of a reducing agent, the reaction between chitosan and glyoxylic acid can also result in the formation of N-carboxymethyl chitosan [183]. There exist other chitosan derivatives and/or composite materials like trimethylchitosan ammonium, N-methylene phosphonic chitosans, chitosan 6-O-sulfate, lactic-glycolic acid-chitosan hydrogels, alkylated chitosans, carbohydrate-branched chitosans, cadmium sulfide (CdS) quantum dots chitosan etc. Such chitosan based bionanocomposites with multifunctional properties render different important applications. For instance, carboxymethyl chitosan offers remarkable antimicrobial activity and enhanced targeted delivery of drugs [184–186]. Trimethylchitosan ammonium, cationic derivative has shown great implementation in the paper production industry due to promising flocculating properties [187]. N-methylene phosphonic chitosans are anionic in nature and demonstrate superior solubility over wider *pH* values. They also form appropriate complex compounds with divalent metals such as Ca, Cu, Cd, Zn etc, useful for inhibiting unwanted corrosion [188, 189]. Luminsescent materials are very useful in imaging latent fingerprints for identification of an induvidual [190]. Chitosan based CdS quantum dots biocomposites showing strong luminescence property are found to be apt for detection of latent fingerprints in criminal investigations [191]. Such bionanocomposites are also very important and promising for fabrication of micro level electrochemical sensors in urea detection in human blood samples [192]. Chitosan based bionanocomposite films with enhaced antimicrobia properties are also developed for efficient food packaging and safety with increased storage life (figure 4.6) [193]. Therefore, depending on the type of chitosan derivative, these bionanocomposites are able to provide versatile practical applications in various fields of interest.

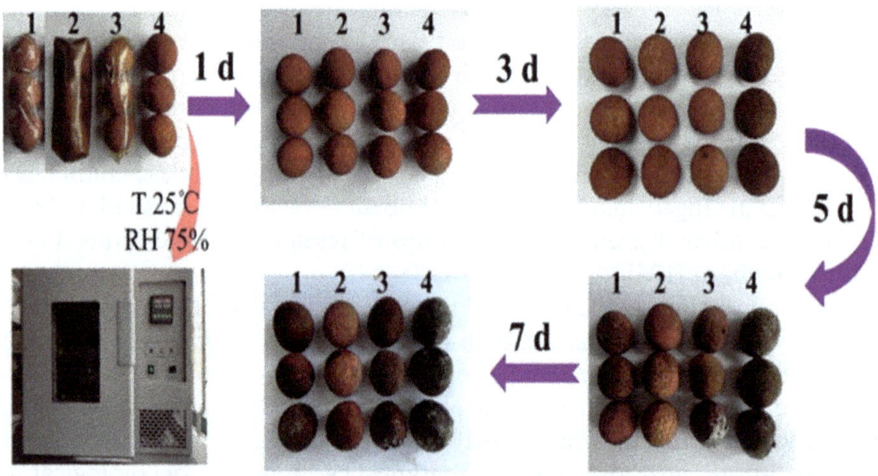

Figure 4.6. The storage results of litchis using CS-based films for food packaging. (Left to right) commercial PE clings wrap denoted as 1, CL2/LAP@AgNPs films as 2, pure CS films as 3 and control as 4. Results are obtained under similar environmental conditions with constant temperature and humidity chamber at 25 °C (75% RH). Reprinted from [193], copyright (2018), with permission from Elsevier.

4.3.7 lignocellulosic materials bionanocomposites

Lignocellulosic is one of the most abundant resources in nature. The primary constituents of lignocellulosic materials are natural occurring polymers which include cellulose, hemicelluloses, and lignin. It has been discussed in previous sections that the biopolymer cellulose occurs abundantly in Nature and is made up of polysaccharide structures with long chained molecules containing d-glucose building units [194]. The hydrogen bonds as well as van der Waals forces keep fibrous structures, i.e. microfibrils in contact with each other within the polymeric chains. Cellulose is naturally found in plants in different concentrations depending onto the type of species. Within the lignin matrix, it is usually packed with nano-sized fibrils. Such fibrils are highly crystalline in Nature and surrounded by amorphous domains [194–196]. Cellulose based systems show weak degradation *in vivo*, which is eliminated using enzymatic oxidation with peroxidase [197, 198]. On the other hand, hemicelluloses can be found within the walls of secondary cells walls. For inherent structures of plants, hemicellulose is an essential part similar to cellulose and lignin, providing excellent mechanical and transport behavior [199]. In general, hemicelluloses are the polysaccharides that are comprised of branched structures. These are identified by the presence of (1→4) linked repeated glucose building blocks, mannose or xylose unlike cellulose and pectin [200, 201]. However, both the hemicelluloses and cellulose exhibit free hydroxyl groups explicitly resulting in the intrinsic extreme hygroscopic properties of woods [196]. Owing to the remarkable reaction of water with hemicelluloses in wood, there has been developement of multifunctional hydrogels based on such materials offering a variety of potential industrial applications [199, 202]. Also, the biopolymer lignin naturally exists in plants with amorphous phases. Lignin predominatly acts as an important support for structure of plants. Lignin is comprised of phenolic-based structures which are of unsaturated nature but show aromatic behavior because of low hydrogen and high carbon content. It contains hydroxyl and methoxy groups as main constituents [203]. Lignin is a proven biomaterial with good antioxidant capability and exellent antiviral response against human immunodeficiency virus [204, 205]. Figure 4.7 depicts the similarities between the hierarchical lignocellulosic materials and bone structures. These hierarchical structures expand from nano to macro levels and contain minute pores which help in nutrient transportation [206]. Lignocellulose is also obtained from natural abundant bacterial cellulose. This type of cellulose is synthesis through the fermentation process with bacteria that produces acetic acid [207]. The bacterial cellulose is fibrous with hydrogen bonding, crystalline in nature, hydrophilic and has good mechanical properties [194, 208, 209].

Different types of reinforcement have been used to develop hydrogels, and bionanocomposites based on cellulose, hemicellulose and lignin as well as their modified derivatives are prepared for specific applications. The bionanocomposites have been prepared with pure as well as hydroxyapatite modified bacterial cellulose, microcrystalline cellulose and cellulose nanowhiskers reinforcements [210–213]. Bacterial cellulose has shown biological properties like osteoconduction which essentially render collagen-mimicking components for development of scaffolds [212, 214]. Lignocellulosic materials are prone to heat and can easily

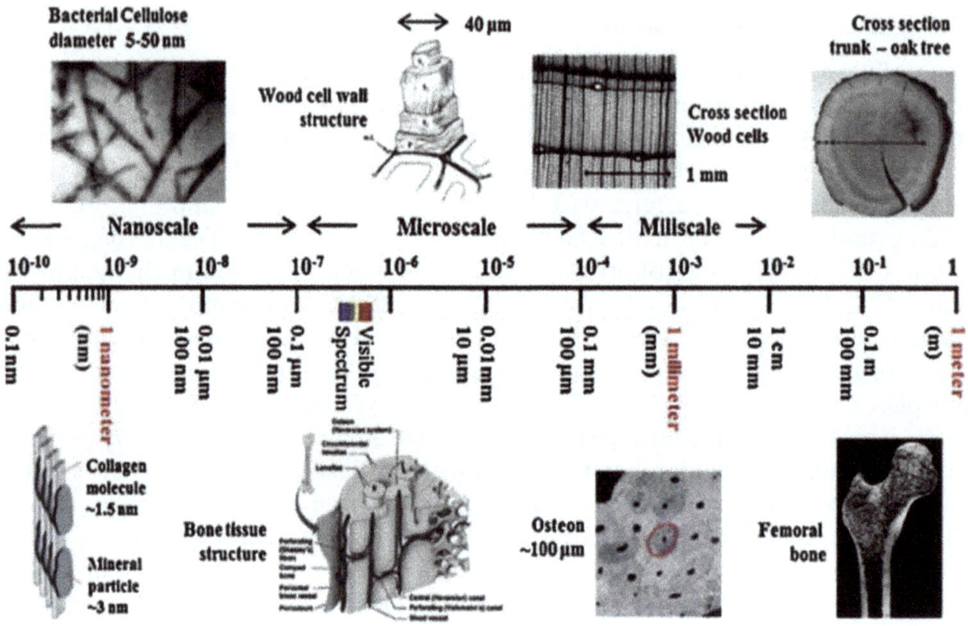

Figure 4.7. An illustration depicting the hierarchical structure of lignocellulosic, which resembles bone. Scale increasing from nano to macro level. Reproduced from [206], copyright (2013), with permission from Elsevier.

degrade at ~230 °C which limit them to a few kinds of matrices [215, 216]. Cellulose nanowhiskers have been combined with polylactic acid and polyethylene glycol to develop bionanocomposites exhibiting better tensile strength and modulus etc [217]. The cellulose and lignin are also modified through acetylation to prepare cellulose acetate. In particular, this can be used alone or by synthesizing blends and/or composites with biopolymers like starch to make scaffolds for tissue engineering, bone cements and vehicles for drug delivery [218–220]. Further, biocompatible hydrogels derived from cellulose are soluble in water and can be used as active components with distinct features such as swelling capacity and higher response ability towards stimuli sources [221]. The bacterial cellulose is also extensively utilized to synthesize hydrogels at nano levels. It exhibits surface area as high as 200 times compared to individual softwood cellulose. In contrast to plant based cellulose, such bacterial cellulose has greater water absorbing capability, better crystallinity and tensile strength etc [214, 222]. These celluloses from bacteria based hydrogels act like templates for developing biomimetic calcium deficient hydroxyapatite [223]. Therefore, lignocellulosic material bionanocomposites are now being extensively employed for various applications including wound dressing, tissue engineering and membranes for guided bone growth etc.

4.3.8 Bionanocomposites based on poly(lactic acid)

PLA biopolymers are prepared chemically using agriculture resources through the fermentation process [224, 225]. Compared to other discussed biopolymers, PLA is very much in demand in food packaging industries. This is due to the fact that such aliphatic polyester can be easily extracted from agro-resources resulting into the formation of monomers during fermentation of agricultural waste [226]. In order to avoid the conventional nonrenewable plastic from fossil resources, PLA is highly biocompatible and biodegradable, giving almost no harmful impact on our environment without any hazardous by-products [227]. PLA is primarily derived from naturally abundant starch. It is known that photosynthesis utilizes carbon dioxide for growth of starch sources in plants. The conversions of glucose into starch require carbon dioxide and eventually the production of PLA is carried out. Hence, in a way, the large manufacturing of PLA based industrial products can help reduce the amount of excess carbon dioxide in breathable air [228]. PLA contains lactic acid as a major constituent synthesized via the fermentation method from starch rich renewable agricultural resources [229]. Such a biopolymer offers excellent biocompatibility, inexpensive processing and hence PLA is easy to prepare through available industrial processing techniques [230, 231]. Owing to remarkable properties of PLA, it has emerged as a promising alternative for packaging purposes including fresh food, blister, dairy products and lamination filming etc [232]. A few large scale industries essentially produce poly (lactic acid) of high molecular weight through ring opening polymerization process with quick reaction time under moderate parameters of reaction [233].

Nowadays, there are many types of food borne diseases and infections caused by microorganism based contaminants present on the surface of uncooked food and other packaged edible products. This has evoked an awareness to find novel ways to eliminate the growth of micro level organisms over various surfaces including food packaging wraps. In practice, the consumption of infected food products can result in several stomach based diseases affecting viral human organs. In order to prevent such growth of microorganisms, food products are actively packaged containing different kinds of inhibitors such as antioxidants, oxygen scavengers, flavoring, moisture absorber, ultraviolet barrier and antimicrobials etc [234, 235]. Such active food packaging offering non-active biocide substances is very promising since it provides long food life by reducing the growth of micro level organisms. To prevent surface microorganisms, biocides with excellent antimicrobial activity are used in foods in direct ways and can also be employed as an outer space enclosing edible products. Food packages with antimicrobial properties help in increasing food life due to restrained growth of microorganisms [236]. The antimicrobial agents are of both inorganic and organic nature. Different organic acids, enzymes and polymers etc, form the organic class of antimicrobial materials, whereas biocompatible nanosized metals and their oxides lie within the inorganic antimicrobial category. Usually, inorganic antimicrobial materials are relatively more thermally stable than organic ones [237]. Most of the industries employ nanostructures of Cu, Au, Zn, Ag and Ti metals for food safety either by directly or by developing antimicrobial food packages. Among them, silver nanoparticles are of great interest owing to remarkable antimicrobial properties [237]. Silver based nanostructures have large surface area which provides efficient interaction amongst microbial cells and nanosized structures [238, 239]. In addition, PLA based bionanocomposites are also actively

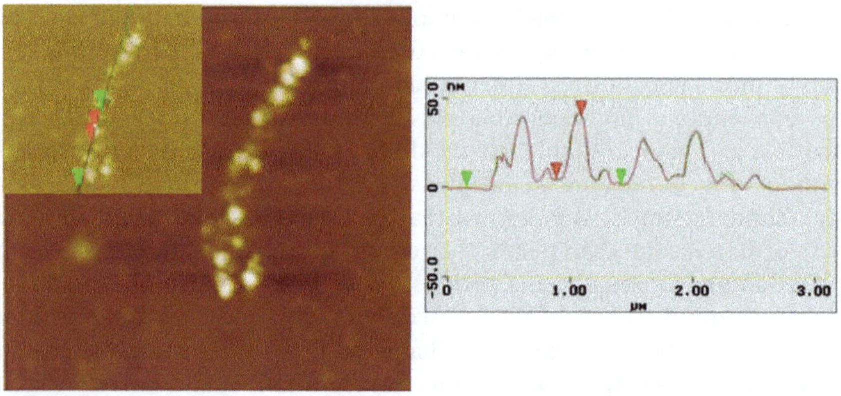

Figure 4.8. AFM images of bionanocomposites based on an anticancer drug, i.e. daunorubicin, combined with nano-TiO_2 and PLA for drug delivery (scan size: 3.7 µm × 3.7 µm). Reprinted with permission from [240].

used for novel drug release applications in clinical treatments. Figure 4.8 demonstrates the atomic force microscopy (AFM) images of developed bionanocomposites using PLA, nanosized TiO_2 and anticancer drug, daunorubicin, for efficient drug release [240].

4.4 Different properties of bionanocomposites

In general, the multifunctional properties of synthesized bionanocomposite materials decide their potential implementation in various applications. The physical properties of individual biopolymer matrices and nanofillers or reinforcements include size, shape, surface, compartmentalization, viscosity and so on. This also encompasses surface properties such as surface tension, surface characterization, charge–charge interaction, etc. The bionanocomposites usually have excellent mechanical properties such as good hardness, fatigue, fracture toughness and elastic modulus, etc. The reduced size of bionanocomposites enhances the chemical, biological and physical properties of materials significantly compared to their bulk counterparts. It is essentially due to the fact that nanosized components evoke interesting modifications, e.g. larger surface area, higher surface-to-volume ratio, quantum confinement effects, reduction of imperfections and remarkable phenomena including surface plasmon resonance (SPR) observed in metal nanostructures. We discuss different important properties of the bionanocomposite materials in the following sections (figure 4.9).

4.4.1 Biological properties

Bionanocomposite materials can degrade biologically when exposed to different environments. Biological damage occurs when a log, sawn product, or final product is not stored, handled, or designed properly. Growth of biological organisms such as bacteria, mold, stain, decay fungi, insects, and marine borers depends mainly on

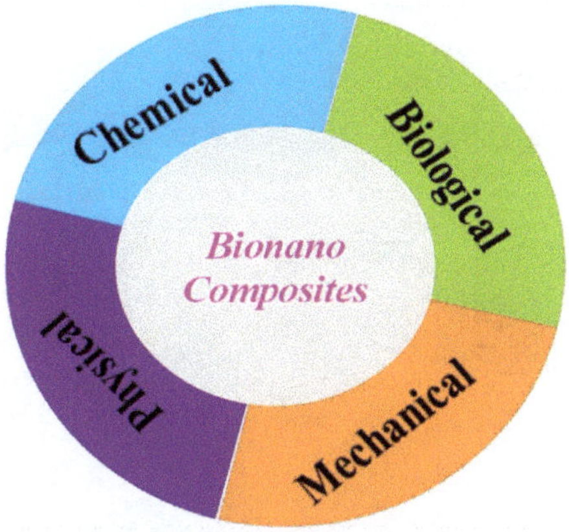

Figure 4.9. Various properties of multifunctional bionanocomposite materials.

temperature and moisture conditions of the environment around them. The continuous growth means a greater hazard when consumed by an individual. This section focuses on the biological organisms and their mechanism of degradation and necessary prevention measures to be taken. If degradation cannot be controlled by design or exposure conditions, then protection is obtained utilizing bionanocomposites with unique biological properties.

A living organism exhibits material structure to provide an environment for complicated chemistry for sustainment. Different chemical and physical reactions take place producing energy to maintain living functions and to renew those structural materials. These microbial organisms are infectious when they unknowingly enter the human body. The polymers obtained whether from synthesis or natural sources degrade during use with continuous loss of different properties such as mechanical strength, and overall integrity etc. The biodegradable polymeric materials are of utmost importance since they degrade within the body as a result of natural biological processes after intended functions, for example, elimination of a drug delivery system after accomplishment of active agent release. In the context of biodegradable polymers, it is essential to understand that the degradation is a chemical process triggered through stimuli sources such as light, heat, water, and ultrasound etc. The degradation of polymers and/or hydrogels occurs gradually with dissolution and diffusion processes. For example, biopolymers like polyanhydrides and polyorthoesters degrade only at the surface and are hence employed specifically in the drug delivery system. Most of the degradation processes observed in biopolymers are activated by the initial bond-breaking reactions. Such breakage of bonds into smaller molecular chains can finish the degree of deterioration. The degradation of biopolymers is usually induced due to different stimuli such as light, thermal sources, hydrolytic, oxidative, biodegradation, radiation, and also can be chemically triggered. The polymer degradation occurs by following one of the two possible mechanisms of erosion, i.e. surface or inhomogeneous erosion and bulk or homogeneous erosion (see figure 4.10) [241]. The erosion of outermost layers of polymer surface takes place relatively more

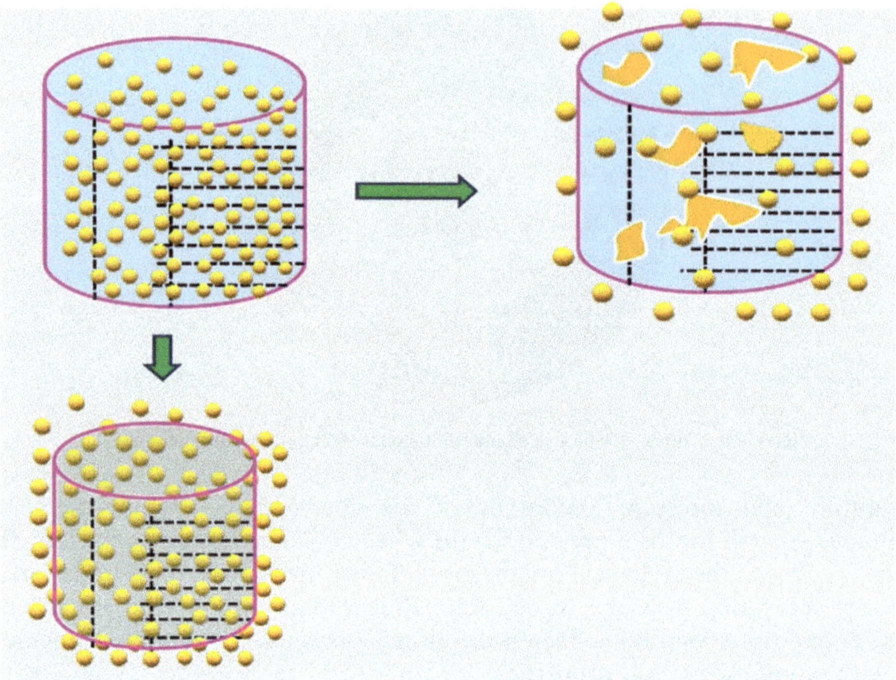

Figure 4.10. Drug deliveries from (a) bulk eroding and (b) surface eroding biodegradable systems. Reprinted with permission from [241].

rapidly than the bulk of polymer. This suggests the erosion effects on the polymer surface only, leaving the matrix interior unchanged. On the other hand, bulk eroding polymers degrade very gradually, whereas the system uptake of water is very quick compared to polymer degradation rate. Therefore, hydration occurs at a much faster rate within the entire system [242, 243].

4.4.2 Mechanical properties

The development of bionanocomposites with appropriate mechanical proprieties paves the way for its successful implementation in fabrication of biological components. The different mechanical parameters include Young's modulus, tensile strength, and toughness enhanced by tuning the fillers or reinforcements at the nanometer scale. For example, cellulose nanostructures such as nanocrystals and whiskers having large specific area demonstrate improved mechanical properties. The linear mechanical strength of synthesized bionanocomposites is usually evaluated using dynamical mechanical analysis (DMA) at various temperature or frequency ranges. However, nonlinear mechanical behavior is realized using classical tensile or compressive tests employed previously.

An appropriate mechanical strength of bionanocomposite materials is very important. For example, in drug delivery, the vehicle material should have good integrity during its whole lifetime or use. The synthesized bionanocomposite does not become very useful if it is not designed to protect a sensitive therapeutic agent such as protein with apt mechanical strength for protection until released out of the system. Further, in hydrogels, there have been several modifications in the degree of cross-linking in order to attain required mechanical properties. Optimal changes in the degree of cross-linking form a strong yet elastic hydrogel. It is noteworthy to mention that a higher degree of cross-linking of the system results in a hydrogel with weak structure. In addition, the copolymerization process is also being implemented to develop hydrogels possessing excellent mechanical properties. Moreover, one can also use co-monomers which essentially increase the amount of hydrogen bonding present in the hydrogel.

4.4.3 The physical properties

The physical properties, e.g., size, shape and texture greatly affect performance of the bionanocomposites developed for specific applications. For the desired biological functionality, control over physical properties of the system is necessary and emerges from its biological sources. This is understood by considering the fact that bacteria can exist with a variety of sizes and shapes such as rods, spirals and ellipsoids etc. Such an available diversity in shapes of bacteria indicates the relevance of physical properties deciding the function of synthesized bionanocomposites. It is also interesting that the cells of human body such as platelets and erythrocytes exhibit an exclusive type of shapes and mechanical properties, helping them to achieve definite functions in organs. For example, erythrocytes present in the human body act to evade filtration in the spleen due to their distinct discoidal shape with good mechanical flexibility. Also, platelets possess disc-like shape which helps them to provide good adhesion function and rolling on vascular endothelium. Figure 4.11 depicts different natural occurring biological objects possessing specific shape, size and appearance. It is well known that human body cells usually utilize compartmentalization in order to manage different biochemical reactions. Moreover, the surface texture of cells may also be important in cellular function. In particular, surface roughness of macrophages may be important in their ability to recognize the size of objects [244]. Therefore, bionanocomposites with optimized physical properties are capable of rendering remarkable performance for different fields of application.

4.5 Applications of bionanocomposites

Bionanocomposites are actively employed in the development of food packaging, scaffolds, bio-sensing, implants, cancer diagnostics, cosmetics, biomedical devices and drug delivery systems etc. Bionanocomposites containing nanosized fillers or reinfrocements enable them and ensure their versatile applications in different industries. The biocompatibility and biodegradable nature of both the polymer matrix and nanofiller is very important while considering any biomedical applications [245–249]. Figure 4.12 demonstrates various potential applications of multifunctional bionanocomposites.

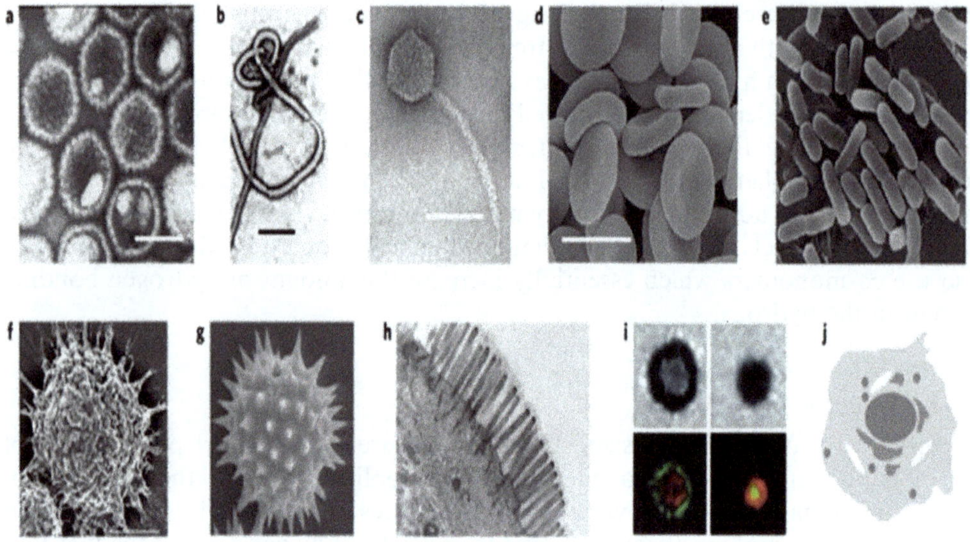

Figure 4.11. An illustration of biological objects in nature which show different physical properties (a), human herpesvirus 3; scale bar, 100 nm, (b), Ebola virus; scale bar, 500 nm (c), Enterobacteria phage λ; scale bar, 50 nm, (d), human erythrocytes; scale bar approximately 10 μm. (e), *Escherichia coli*; image size approximately 7 μm × 6 μm, (f), surface texture in alveolar macrophages73; scale bar, 5 μm, (g), pollen; image size approximately 50 μm × 45 μm, (h), intestinal villi; approximate magnification μ5,950, (i), the immunological synapse; T cell forming a synapse with a supported membrane containing GPI linked pMHC and ICAM, (j), a schematic of cellular compartmentalization showing several organelles surrounding the nucleus. The images clearly establish that nature uses physical parameters such as size, shape, texture and compartmentalization in designing life. Reprinted from [244], copyright (2009) with permission of Springer.

4.5.1 Cardiovascular stent

Bionanocomposites have been extensively implemented in cardiovascular stent synthesis and development. For such stents, scaffolds such as a small hollow mesh are placed in the artery to keep the lumen broad and unblocked. For now, the stent is carried out throughout sixty percent of the balloon angioplasty technique. These methods include stents mounted with balloons in the lumens placed at a particular position of interest, and volume is then increased significantly by inflating a balloon. Further, such an inflated stent is moved against the artery wall until the required level. After the complete procedure, the balloon is deflated and removed. The scaffold of hollow stents inserted into the body is of biocompatible materials such as 316 L stainless steel, or standard gold materials that give the required mechanical support to the arteries to keep the lumen in an open condition. However, there are other biodegradable stents made up of iron and magnesium-based alloys. These metals perform work properly and thereafter, degrade once new tissues are developed in that place [250, 251].

4.5.2 Ocular applications

Blindness, also termed vision impairment, is one of the major health related problems. Since it is an eye based issue, the capability of an individual to carry

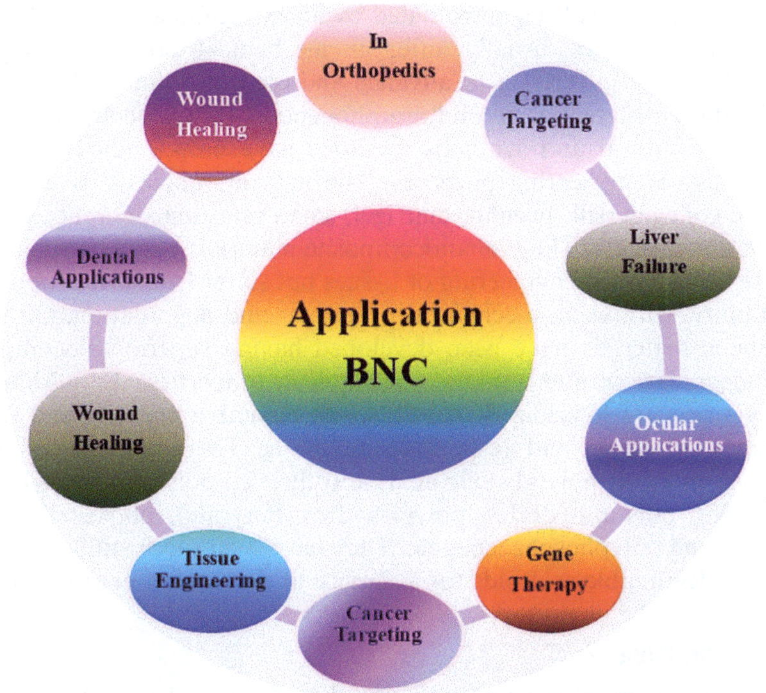

Figure 4.12. The potential applications of multifunctional bionanocomposites in a variety of industrial and research fields.

out everyday activities is highly affected. In this context, ocular drug delivery systems are popularly employed to clean the choroidal and conjunctival vessels. In the development of bionanocomposites, nanosized filler enhances the drug penetration, bioavailability and lowers the risks of toxicity in contrast to other commercially available conventional eye drops. Nevertheless, therapeutic based clinical approaches might be avoided since they can result in visual disorder of diabetic retinopathy, cataracts, glaucoma and retinal degeneration. For the clinical trials of glaucoma, a larger bioavailability of antiglaucoma drugs like timolol and brimonidine have been obtained after synthesizing hybrid polyamidoamine (PAMAM) dendrimer hydrogel/poly(lactic-co-glycolic acid) (PLGA) polymeric nanoparticles. Nanoparticles and drug-based formulations integrated into contact lenses for sustained release therapy have demonstrated enhanced corneal bioavailability as well as superior patient acquiescence [252–254].

4.5.3 Tissue engineering

Tissue engineering primarily utilizes a combination of cells that focus on the biochemical and physicochemical events which replace biological tissues. Tissue engineering employing three-dimensional scaffolds of biocompatible nature and biologically active appropriate bioreactor conditions are similar to functional structures. This term very much corresponds to the repair and/or replacement of an entire tissue which has been surrounded by an extracellular matrix (ECM). The ECM bionanocomposites usually offer a mechanical structured support to implanted cells and also interact to advance and control cellular adhesion, migration, proliferation, differentiation and morphogenesis. Bionanocomposite materials developed from natural and synthetic methods have been studied and tested as scaffolds for tissue engineering purposes. The natural sources derived polymeric materials are collagen, silk protein, matrigel, small intestinal submucosa, agarose, alginate and chitosan etc. The bionanocomposite materials based on such polymers demonstrate potential for engineering of tissues but suffer from critical problems of biocompatibility, with weak mechanical properties and degradation. On the other hand, synthetic materials have been developed having superior biocompatibility, controlled degradation and tunable mechanical properties. In addition, such polymeric systems are hybridized with different bioactive moieties and functional groups suggesting smart and responsive materials. There are various synthetic polymers such as PLA, poly(glycolic acid) and their co-polymers, poly(lactic acid-coglycolic acid), poly(anhydride), poly(4-hydroxybutyrate), poly(urethane), polyphosphoesters and polyphosphazenes etc. They have been successfully utilized in the fabrication of degradable scaffolds for a variety of tissues and organs [255–262].

4.5.4 Cancer targeting

Cancer drugs have emerged with promising benefits like drug solubilization and prolonged blood circulation. However, they are usually limited by efficacy, which is predominantly constrained by lack of ability to achieve high target absorption and control at sites having tumor cells. In the context of cancer treatment procedure, the therapeutic efficacy of antitumor drugs is very poor due to inadequate uptake by the cells. There is also severe drug accumulation within healthy tissues which results in adverse side effects preventing successful deployment in clinical trials. This demands the development of proficient delivery systems with high throughput. Such delivery systems for tumor drugs are capable of releasing the drug in a regulated manner. In practice, usually the notion of utilizing a specific ligand is regarded as a more appropriate strategy. Such specific ligands are able to identify the molecular signs of surface of cancer tumor cells. This, in turn, can provide better targeting of a tumor cell by conjugating antitumor drug carriers achieved through a particular ligand. In clinical trials, there is a variety of ligands for targeting tumor cells such as folic acid, peptides, transferrin, polysaccharides and monoclonal antibodies etc. They have been extensively studied by synthesizing hybrids with graphene and graphene oxide acting as the drug nanocarriers in treatment of cancer patients [185, 263–266].

4.5.5 Gene therapy

Human beings are regularly affected by diseases with genetic disorders. Such genetically induced diseases are treated with efficient gene therapies. Such treatments employ gene vectors which primarily preserve DNA from nuclease degradation. This helps significantly in cellular uptake of DNA with better transfection efficiency. Nevertheless, there are several critical issues inhibiting their successful execution such as improper, precarious and incompetent gene vectors. The development of appropriate vehicles for gene delivery is equally important. Previously, it has been demonstrated that single-stranded DNA (ssDNA) and RNA are effectively immobilized onto the surface of graphene and/or graphene oxide using non-covalent adsorption obtained via stacking and other interactions of electrostatic and molecular types. Such carbon based materials depict robustness in the development of active and efficient gene carriers. In this context, graphene essentially provides protection to oligonucleotides from enzymatic cleavage and delivers ssDNA into the cells. Graphene oxide has shown potential for gene delivery due to good cell internalization and excellent biomolecule properties. Bionanocomposites in the form of hydrogels have been developed using methacrylated gelatin after incorporating polyethylenimine (PEI) functionalized graphene oxide nanosheets. Following careful examination with 22-gauge needle, such hydrogels demonstrate improved injectable performances because of the high surface area of graphene oxide nanosheets.

Moreover, for unhealthy cardiac tissues, specific targeting at the delivery site can be efficiently achieved with the pro-angiogenic human vascular endothelial growth factor plasmid DNA (pDNAVEGF). It is known that nonviral nanoparticles show weak efficiency of transfection compared to viral systems. Graphene oxide nanosheets attached ionically to PEI are strongly combined with DNA. This primarily assists the nucleic acids to release easily once the cellular internalization is complete. For such purposes, graphene oxide nanosheets are one of the best choices for pDNAVEGF gene delivery in an improved way. These hydrogels reveal superior cellular proliferation in the case of HUVECs for proangiogenic activities. Also, it does not induce any major toxicity and/or inflammation while performing the *in vivo* investigations. In addition, the developed hydrogels loaded with graphene oxide and pDNAVEGF gene do help the locamyocardial neovascularization, decrease fibrosis and normalize cardiac function in the case of acute myocardial infarction. Such hydrogels promise more advances in the field of nonviral gene delivery. There are also other carbonous nanostructures such as nanoparticles and nanotubes which have been employed for synthesizing biomimetic nanocomposites. The synthetic native-like tissues can be developed with the help of improved interactions and regulations between nanostructure and polymer [267–269].

4.5.6 Drug delivery

In drug delivery, the release rate of different drugs out of their carriers is typically regulated through the diffusion process. This indicates the fact that after drug administration, it is not possible to control or change the quantity of drug to be released and the release behavior itself. In order to eradicate such drawbacks, the passive drug delivery technique seeks improved systems which should be capable of drug release with a certain amount at a desired point in time. In this regard, many efficient methods have been proposed for different drug carriers which are responsive to external or internal stimuli including body temperature, *pH*, a specific chemical reaction, ultrasound signals, magnetic and electric fields and light etc. There have been many studies discussing the use of carbon based nanostructures or inorganic like gold based drug delivery systems that actively respond to environmental stimulations.

For example, drugs attached to the drug carriers e.g. graphene oxide grouped with *pH* sensitive linkers show the controlled drug release under regulated *pH* value of environments. These alternative materials have emerged to be an effective way for drug release while eliminating excess release of drug in blood circulation. Liu *et al*, developed the phospholipid monolayer membrane functionalized graphene based biocompatible drug carriers which demonstrate regulated drug release depending on *pH* values along with a high drug loading capacity of 70%.[270] Also, Bai *et al*, [271] prepared the bionanocomposites using graphene oxide and poly(vinyl alcohol) as the hydrogel depicting gel–sol transition ascribed to their pH dependence. It assists in loading and selectively releasing drugs at particular physiological pH value [270, 272].

4.6 Conclusions

This chapter summarized bionanocomposites and their multidirectional applications in the field of science and technology that merge interdisciplinary material sciences, nanotechnology, and biology. Bionanocomposites are hybrid materials of biopolymers on the surface of inorganic and organic nanoparticles. Three synthetic techniques are used to make bionanocomposites: solution casting, *in situ* intercalative polymerization, and melt processing. These bionanocomposites are valuable, amazing, and important hybrid materials because they show interesting biological properties such as biocompatibility, biodegradability, low toxic effect on human health and the environment, excellent physical and chemical properties such as size, shape, morphology, surface properties, chemical functionality viscosity etc. Apart from this, bionanocomposites show tremendous mechanical properties such as good hardness, fatigue resistance, fracture toughness and elastic modulus, etc. These properties provide them with additional benefits in biomedical applications (tissue engineering, cancer-targeting, gene delivery, drug delivery systems etc). In recent decades, many biopolymer materials have been transformed into bionanocomposites, which play very important and critical roles in the biomedical field. Very recently, bionanocomposites based on natural biopolymers (including chitin, chitosan, cellulose, starch, and lactic acid) have been explored for different applications, and one such emerging area is drug and gene discoveries. However, the development of bionanocomposites for environmental applications still remains a challenge to researchers and scientists, but the importance will carry on increasing over the years due to the utilization and commercialization of goods based on various bionanocomposites. The main challenges are in their synthesis process so that we can scale up for large production of bionanomaterials, keeping in mind that low toxic chemicals should be used for their synthesis. However, the technological, industrial community still needs to make great efforts to achieve their biofunctioning and success in large-scale, economic balance, safety assessment, and life cycle analysis on incorporating bionanocomposites in clinical and biomedical applications, which are essential for providing insights and outlines for the future. Thus there is consensus for the employment of bionanocomposites in humans, and there is still a long-range of applications yet to be revealed which will provide a platform for the work of researchers and scientists with innovation and discoveries for the advantage of humans and the environment.

Acknowledgements

We thank Professor Rakesh Bhatnagar, Vice Chancellor, Banaras Hindu University, Varanasi for his interest in this work. Author JS acknowledge the Department of Science and Technology (DST), New Delhi and UGC New Delhi for financial support. Author JS also acknowledges BHU for providing a seed grant under BHU, IoE scheme.

References

[1] Ozin G A and Arsenault A 2015 *Nanochemistry: A Chemical Approach to Nanomaterials* (London: Royal Society of Chemistry)

[2] Dujardin E and Mann S 2002 Bio-inspired materials chemistry *Adv. Mater.* **14** 775–88

[3] Srivastava N, Singh J, Ramteke P W, Mishra P and Srivastava M 2015 Improved production of reducing sugars from rice straw using crude cellulase activated with Fe_3O_4/Alginate nanocomposite *Bioresour. Technol.* **183** 262–6

[4] Ruiz-Hitzky E, Aranda P, Darder M and Ogawa M 2011 Hybrid and biohybrid silicate based materials: molecular vs. block-assembling bottom–up processes *Chem. Soc. Rev.* **40** 801–28

[5] Ruiz-Hitzky E, Darder M and Aranda P 2005 Functional biopolymer nanocomposites based on layered solids *J. Mater. Chem.* **15** 3650–62

[6] Alexandre M and Dubois P 2000 Polymer-layered silicate nanocomposites: preparation, properties and uses of a new class of materials *Mater. Sci. Eng.: R: Rep.* **28** 1–63

[7] Bergaya F and Lagaly G 2013 *Handbook of Clay Science* (Amsterdam: Elsevier)

[8] Ray S S and Bousmina M 2005 Biodegradable polymers and their layered silicate nanocomposites: in greening the 21st century materials world *Prog. Mater. Sci.* **50** 962–1079

[9] Hule R A and Pochan D J 2007 polymer nanocomposites for biomedical applications *MRS Bull.* **32** 354–8

[10] Ahmed J and Varshney S K 2011 Polylactides—chemistry, properties and green packaging technology: a review *Int. J. Food Prop.* **14** 37–58

[11] Doi Y and Fukuda K 1994 *Biodegradable Plastics and Polymers* vol 12 (Amsterdam: Elsevier) 156

[12] Fortunati E, Armentano I, Zhou Q, Puglia D, Terenzi A and Berglund L A *et al* 2012 Microstructure and nonisothermal cold crystallization of PLA composites based on silver nanoparticles and nanocrystalline cellulose *Polym. Degrad. Stab.* **97** 2027–36

[13] Fortunati E, Armentano I, Zhou Q, Iannoni A, Saino E and Visai L *et al* 2012 Multifunctional bionanocomposite films of poly (lactic acid), cellulose nanocrystals and silver nanoparticles *Carbohydr. Polym.* **87** 1596–605

[14] Urbanczyk L, Ngoundjo F, Alexandre M, Jérôme C, Detrembleur C and Calberg C 2009 Synthesis of polylactide/clay nanocomposites by *in situ* intercalative polymerization in supercritical carbon dioxide *Eur. Polym. J.* **45** 643–8

[15] Jiang G, Huang H X and Chen Z K 2011 Microstructure and thermal behavior of polylactide/clay nanocomposites melt compounded under supercritical CO_2 *Adv. Polym. Tech.* **30** 174–82
[16] Ray S S and Okamoto M 2003 Polymer/layered silicate nanocomposites: a review from preparation to processing *Prog. Polym. Sci.* **28** 1539–641
[17] Vaia R A, Jandt K D, Kramer E J and Giannelis E P 1996 Microstructural evolution of melt intercalated polymer—organically modified layered silicates nanocomposites *Chem. Mater.* **8** 2628–35
[18] Vaia R A and Giannelis E P 1997 Lattice model of polymer melt intercalation in organically-modified layered silicates *Macromolecules* **30** 7990–9
[19] Vaia R A and Giannelis E P 1997 Polymer melt intercalation in organically-modified layered silicates: model predictions and experiment *Macromolecules* **30** 8000–9
[20] Hunter D L, Kamena K W and Paul D 2007 Processing and properties of polymers modified by clays *MRS Bull.* **32** 323–7
[21] Pérez S, Baldwin P M and Gallant D J 2009 Structural features of starch granules I *Starch* ed J BeMiller and R Whistler 3rd edn (San Diego, CA: Academic) pp 149–92
[22] Jane J-L 2009 Structural features of starch granules II *Starch* (Amsterdam: Elsevier) pp 193–236
[23] Pérez S and Bertoft E 2010 The molecular structures of starch components and their contribution to the architecture of starch granules: a comprehensive review *Starch-Stärke* **62** 389–420
[24] Buleon A, Colonna P, Planchot V and Ball S 1998 Starch granules: structure and biosynthesis *Int. J. Biol. Macromol.* **23** 85–112
[25] Liu H, Yu L, Xie F and Chen L 2006 Gelatinization of cornstarch with different amylose/amylopectin content *Carbohydr. Polym.* **65** 357–63
[26] Liu P, Xie F, Li M, Liu X, Yu L and Halley P J *et al* 2011 Phase transitions of maize starches with different amylose contents in glycerol–water systems *Carbohydr. Polym.* **85** 180–7
[27] Xie F, Yu L, Su B, Liu P, Wang J and Liu H *et al* 2009 Rheological properties of starches with different amylose/amylopectin ratios *J. Cereal Sci.* **49** 371–7
[28] Wang J, Yu L, Xie F, Chen L, Li X and Liu H 2010 Rheological properties and phase transition of cornstarches with different amylose/amylopectin ratios under shear stress *Starch-Stärke* **62** 667–75
[29] Li M, Liu P, Zou W, Yu L, Xie F and Pu H *et al* 2011 Extrusion processing and characterization of edible starch films with different amylose contents *J. Food Eng.* **106** 95–101
[30] Enrione J, Osorio F, Pedreschi F and Hill S 2010 Prediction of the glass transition temperature on extruded waxy maize and rice starches in presence of glycerol *Food Bioprocess Technol.* **3** 791–6
[31] Lourdin D, Coignard L, Bizot H and Colonna P 1997 Influence of equilibrium relative humidity and plasticizer concentration on the water content and glass transition of starch materials *Polymer* **38** 5401–6
[32] Forssell P M, Mikkilä J M, Moates G K and Parker R 1997 Phase and glass transition behaviour of concentrated barley starch-glycerol-water mixtures, a model for thermoplastic starch *Carbohydr. Polym.* **34** 275–82
[33] Da Róz A, Carvalho A, Gandini A and Curvelo A 2006 The effect of plasticizers on thermoplastic starch compositions obtained by melt processing *Carbohydr. Polym.* **63** 417–24

[34] Mathew A P and Dufresne A 2002 Plasticized waxy maize starch: effect of polyols and relative humidity on material properties *Biomacromolecules* **3** 1101–8
[35] Gaudin S, Lourdin D, Le Botlan D, Ilari J and Colonna P 1999 Plasticisation and mobility in starch-sorbitol films *J. Cereal Sci.* **29** 273–84
[36] Kirby A, Clark S, Parker R and Smith A 1993 The deformation and failure behaviour of wheat starch plasticized with water and polyols *J. Mater. Sci.* **28** 5937–42
[37] Ma X F, Yu J and Wan J 2006 Urea and ethanolamine as a mixed plasticizer for thermoplastic starch *Carbohydr. Polym.* **64** 267–73
[38] Ma X and Yu J 2004 The plastcizers containing amide groups for thermoplastic starch *Carbohydr. Polym.* **57** 197–203
[39] Ma X and Yu J 2004 The effects of plasticizers containing amide groups on the properties of thermoplastic starch *Starch-Stärke* **56** 545–51
[40] Ma X, Yu J and Ma Y 2005 Urea and formamide as a mixed plasticizer for thermoplastic wheat flour *Carbohydr. Polym.* **60** 111–6
[41] J-h Y, J-g Y and X-f M 2006 Study on the properties of ethylenebisformamide and sorbitol plasticized corn starch (ESPTPS) *Carbohydr. Polym.* **66** 110–6
[42] Jh Y, Jg Y and Xf M 2006 Preparation of a novel thermoplastic starch (TPS) material using ethylenebisformamide as the plasticizer *Starch-Stärke* **58** 330–7
[43] Yang J-H, Yu J-G and Ma X-F 2006 Preparation and properties of ethylenebisformamide plasticized potato starch (EPTPS) *Carbohydr. Polym.* **63** 218–23
[44] Shi R, Zhang Z, Liu Q, Han Y, Zhang L and Chen D *et al* 2007 Characterization of citric acid/glycerol co-plasticized thermoplastic starch prepared by melt blending *Carbohydr. Polym.* **69** 748–55
[45] Jiugao Y, Ning W and Xiaofei M 2005 The effects of citric acid on the properties of thermoplastic starch plasticized by glycerol *Starch-Stärke* **57** 494–504
[46] Chaudhary A, Miler M, Torley P, Sopade P and Halley P 2008 Amylose content and chemical modification effects on the extrusion of thermoplastic starch from maize *Carbohydr. Polym.* **74** 907–13
[47] Lafargue D, Pontoire B, Buléon A, Doublier J L and Lourdin D 2007 Structure and mechanical properties of hydroxypropylated starch films *Biomacromolecules.* **8** 3950–8
[48] Fringant C, Desbrieres J and Rinaudo M 1996 Physical properties of acetylated starch-based materials: relation with their molecular characteristics *Polymer* **37** 2663–73
[49] Jarowenko W 1986 Acetylated starch and miscellaneous organic esters *Modified Starches: Properties and Uses* ed Wurzburg O B (Boca Raton, FL: CRC Press) pp 55
[50] Averous L 2004 Biodegradable multiphase systems based on plasticized starch: a review *J. Macromol. Sci. Part C: Polym. Rev.* **44** 231–74
[51] Yu L, Dean K and Li L 2006 Polymer blends and composites from renewable resources *Prog. Polym. Sci.* **31** 576–602
[52] Wang X-L, Yang K-K and Wang Y-Z 2003 Properties of starch blends with biodegradable polymers *J. Macromol. Sci. Part C: Polym. Rev.* **43** 385–409
[53] Avérous L and Halley P J 2009 Biocomposites based on plasticized starch *Biofuels Bioprod. Biorefin.* **3** 329–43
[54] Bergaya F, Jaber M and Lambert J-F 2012 Clays and clay minerals as layered nanofillers for (bio) polymers *Environmental Silicate Nano-Biocomposites* (Berlin: Springer) 41–75
[55] Duquesne E, Moins S, Alexandre M and Dubois P 2007 How can nanohybrids enhance polyester/sepiolite nanocomposite properties? *Macromol. Chem. Phys.* **208** 2542–50

[56] Zeppa C, Gouanvé F and Espuche E 2009 Effect of a plasticizer on the structure of biodegradable starch/clay nanocomposites: thermal, water-sorption, and oxygen-barrier properties *J. Appl. Polym. Sci.* **112** 2044–56

[57] Magalhães N and Andrade C 2009 Thermoplastic corn starch/clay hybrids: effect of clay type and content on physical properties *Carbohydr. Polym.* **75** 712–8

[58] Huang M and Yu J 2006 Structure and properties of thermoplastic corn starch/montmorillonite biodegradable composites *J. Appl. Polym. Sci.* **99** 170–6

[59] Cyras V P, Manfredi L B, Ton-That M-T and Vázquez A 2008 Physical and mechanical properties of thermoplastic starch/montmorillonite nanocomposite films *Carbohydr. Polym.* **73** 55–63

[60] Ibrahim S M 2011 Characterization, mechanical, and thermal properties of gamma irradiated starch films reinforced with mineral clay *J. Appl. Polym. Sci.* **119** 685–92

[61] Famá L M, Pettarin V, Goyanes S N and Bernal C R 2011 Starch/multi-walled carbon nanotubes composites with improved mechanical properties *Carbohydr. Polym.* **83** 1226–31

[62] Cao X, Chen Y, Chang P R and Huneault M A 2007 Preparation and properties of plasticized starch/multiwalled carbon nanotubes composites *J. Appl. Polym. Sci.* **106** 1431–7

[63] Ma X, Yu J and Wang N 2008 Glycerol plasticized-starch/multiwall carbon nanotube composites for electroactive polymers *Compos. Sci. Technol.* **68** 268–73

[64] Harrison B S and Atala A 2007 Carbon nanotube applications for tissue engineering *Biomaterials* **28** 344–53

[65] Wang J 2005 Carbon-nanotube based electrochemical biosensors: a review *Electroanalysis* **17** 7–14

[66] Valdés M G, González A C V, Calzón J A G and Díaz-García M E 2009 Analytical nanotechnology for food analysis *Microchim. Acta* **166** 1–19

[67] Curran S A, Ajayan P M, Blau W J, Carroll D L, Coleman J N and Dalton A B *et al* 1998 A composite from poly (m-phenylenevinylene-co-2,5-dioctoxy-p-phenylenevinylene) and carbon nanotubes: a novel material for molecular optoelectronics *Adv. Mater.* **10** 1091–3

[68] Ajayan P M 1999 Nanotubes from carbon *Chem. Rev.* **99** 1787–800

[69] Liu Z, Zhao L, Chen M and Yu J 2011 Effect of carboxylate multi-walled carbon nanotubes on the performance of thermoplastic starch nanocomposites *Carbohydr. Polym.* **83** 447–51

[70] Famá L, Rojo P G, Bernal C and Goyanes S 2012 Biodegradable starch based nanocomposites with low water vapor permeability and high storage modulus *Carbohydr. Polym.* **87** 1989–93

[71] Ashori A 2014 Effects of graphene on the behavior of chitosan and starch nanocomposite films *Polym. Eng. Sci.* **54** 2258–63

[72] Godovsky D Y 2000 Device applications of polymer-nanocomposites. Biopolymers· PVA hydrogels *Anionic Polymerisation Nanocomposites* (Berlin: Springer) 163–205

[73] Yu J, Yang J, Liu B and Ma X 2009 Preparation and characterization of glycerol plasticized-pea starch/ZnO–carboxymethylcellulose sodium nanocomposites *Bioresour. Technol.* **100** 2832–41

[74] Ma X, Chang P R, Yang J and Yu J 2009 Preparation and properties of glycerol plasticized-pea starch/zinc oxide-starch bionanocomposites *Carbohydr. Polym.* **75** 472–8

[75] Liu D, Chang P R, Deng S, Wang C, Zhang B and Tian Y *et al* 2011 Fabrication and characterization of zirconium hydroxide-carboxymethyl cellulose sodium/plasticized Trichosanthes Kirilowii starch nanocomposites *Carbohydr. Polym.* **86** 1699–704

[76] Wu D, Chang P R and Ma X 2011 Preparation and properties of layered double hydroxide–carboxymethylcellulose sodium/glycerol plasticized starch nanocomposites *Carbohydr. Polym.* **86** 877–82
[77] Leroux F and Besse J-P 2001 Polymer interleaved layered double hydroxide: a new emerging class of nanocomposites *Chem. Mater.* **13** 3507–15
[78] Hofmeister W and Platen H V 1992 Crystal chemistry and atomic order in brucite-related double-layer structures *Crystallogr. Rev.* **3** 3–26
[79] Brauner K and Preisinger A 1956 Struktur und entstehung des sepioliths *Tscher. Miner. Petrogr.* **6** 120–40
[80] Santaren J, Sanz J and Ruiz-Hitzky E 1990 Structural fluorine in sepiolite *Clays Clay Miner.* **38** 63–8
[81] Bradley W 1940 The structural scheme of attapulgite *Am. Min.* **25** 405–10
[82] Ruiz-Hitzky E 2001 Molecular access to intracrystalline tunnels of sepiolite basis of a presentation given at Materials Discussion No. 3, 24–26 September 2000, University of Cambridge, UK *J. Mater. Chem.* **11** 86–91
[83] Ruiz-Hitzky E and Van Meerbeek A 1978 Mechanism of the grafting of organosilanes on mineral surfaces I. Nature and role of the hydrolysis products of the methylvinyldichlorosilane in the grafting of silicates in hydrochloric acid and isopropanol *Colloid. Polym. Sci.* **256** 135–9
[84] Ruiz-Hitzky E and Van Meerbeek A 2006 Clay mineral–and organoclay–polymer nanocomposite *Dev. Clay Sci.* **1** 583–621
[85] Kuang W, Facey G A, Detellier C, Casal B, Serratosa J M and Ruiz-Hitzky E 2003 Nanostructured hybrid materials formed by sequestration of pyridine molecules in the tunnels of sepiolite *Chem. Mater.* **15** 4956–67
[86] López-Galindo A, Viseras C, Aguzzi C and Cerezo P 2011 Pharmaceutical and cosmetic uses of fibrous clays *Developments in Clay Science* vol 3 (Amsterdam: Elsevier) 299–324
[87] Ahlrichs J, Serna C and Serratosa J 1975 Structural hydroxyls in sepiolites *Clays Clay Miner.* **23** 119–24
[88] Tartaglione G, Tabuani D, Camino G and Moisio M 2008 PP and PBT composites filled with sepiolite: morphology and thermal behaviour *Compos. Sci. Technol.* **68** 451–60
[89] Ruiz-Hitzky E, Aranda P and Serratosa J M 2004 *Clay-Organic Interactions: Organoclay Complexes and Polymer-Clay Nanocomposites* (New York: Marcel Dekker)
[90] Ruiz-Hitzky E 2004 Organic-inorganic materials: from intercalation chemistry to devices *ChemInform* **35** 15–49
[91] Ruiz-Hitzky E, Aranda P, Álvarez A, Santarén J and Esteban-Cubillo A 2011 Advanced materials and new applications of sepiolite and palygorskite *Developments in Clay Science* vol 3 (Amsterdam: Elsevier) pp 393–452
[92] Tang C, Hackenberg K, Fu Q, Ajayan P M and Ardebili H 2012 High ion conducting polymer nanocomposite electrolytes using hybrid nanofillers *Nano Lett.* **12** 1152–6
[93] Chivrac F, Pollet E, Schmutz M and Avérous L 2010 Starch nano-biocomposites based on needle-like sepiolite clays *Carbohydr. Polym.* **80** 145–53
[94] Darder M, Aranda P, Ferrer M L, Gutiérrez M C, del Monte F and Ruiz-Hitzky E 2011 Progress in bionanocomposite and bioinspired foams *Adv. Mater.* **23** 5262–7
[95] Darder M, López-Blanco M, Aranda P, Aznar A J, Bravo J and Ruiz-Hitzky E 2006 Microfibrous chitosan–sepiolite nanocomposites *Chem. Mater.* **18** 1602–10

[96] Sorrentino A, Gorrasi G and Vittoria V 2007 Potential perspectives of bio-nanocomposites for food packaging applications *Trends Food Sci. Technol.* **18** 84–95
[97] Ulbricht M 2006 Advanced functional polymer membranes *Polymer* **47** 2217–62
[98] Nussinovitch A 2009 Biopolymer films and composite coatings *Modern Biopolymer Science* (Amsterdam: Elsevier) pp 295–326
[99] Lee J K, Song I K and Lee W Y 1997 Design of novel catalyst imbedding heteropoly acids in polymer films: catalytic activity for ethanol conversion *J. Mol. Catal. A: Chem.* **120** 207–16
[100] Kim D-H, Viventi J, Amsden J J, Xiao J, Vigeland L and Kim Y-S *et al* 2010 Dissolvable films of silk fibroin for ultrathin conformal bio-integrated electronics *Nat. Mater.* **9** 511–7
[101] Mucha M, Wańkowicz K and Balcerzak J 2007 Analysis of water adsorption on chitosan and its blends with hydroxypropylcellulose *e-Polymers* **7** 16
[102] Aggas J R, Lutkenhaus J and Guiseppi-Elie A 2018 Chemiresistive and chemicapacitive devices formed via morphology control of electroconductive bio-nanocomposites *Adv. Electron. Mater.* **4** 1700495
[103] Tiwari A, Mishra A, Dhakate S R, Khan R and Shukla S 2007 Synthesis of electrically active biopolymer–SiO_2 nanocomposite aerogel *Mater. Lett.* **61** 4587–90
[104] Nezakati T, Seifalian A, Tan A and Seifalian A M 2018 Conductive polymers: opportunities and challenges in biomedical applications *Chem. Rev.* **118** 6766–843
[105] Jin G and Li K 2014 The electrically conductive scaffold as the skeleton of stem cell niche in regenerative medicine *Mater. Sci. Eng.* C **45** 671–81
[106] Gerard M, Chaubey A and Malhotra B 2002 Application of conducting polymers to biosensors *Biosens. Bioelectron.* **17** 345–59
[107] Park A R, Kim J S, Kim K S, Zhang K, Park J and Park J H *et al* 2014 Si–Mn/reduced graphene oxide nanocomposite anodes with enhanced capacity and stability for lithium-ion batteries *ACS Appl. Mater. Interfaces* **6** 1702–8
[108] Green R A, Baek S, Poole-Warren L A and Martens P J 2010 Conducting polymer-hydrogels for medical electrode applications *Sci. Technol. Adv. Mater* **11** 014107
[109] Gómez H, Ram M K, Alvi F, Villalba P, Stefanakos E L and Kumar A 2011 Graphene-conducting polymer nanocomposite as novel electrode for supercapacitors *J. Power Sources* **196** 4102–8
[110] Dubey N, Kushwaha C S and Shukla S 2020 A review on electrically conducting polymer bionanocomposites for biomedical and other applications *Int. J. Polym. Mater. Polym. Biomater.* **69** 709–27
[111] Filson P B, Dawson-Andoh B E and Schwegler-Berry D 2009 Enzymatic-mediated production of cellulose nanocrystals from recycled pulp *Green Chem.* **11** 1808–14
[112] Ahola S, Turon X, Osterberg M, Laine J and Rojas O 2008 Enzymatic hydrolysis of native cellulose nanofibrils and other cellulose model films: effect of surface structure *Langmuir* **24** 11592–9
[113] Kadokawa J-I, Takegawa A, Mine S and Prasad K 2011 Preparation of chitin nanowhiskers using an ionic liquid and their composite materials with poly (vinyl alcohol) *Carbohydr. Polym.* **84** 1408–12
[114] LeCorre D, Bras J and Dufresne A 2011 Ceramic membrane filtration for isolating starch nanocrystals *Carbohydr. Polym.* **86** 1565–72
[115] Lin N, Huang J and Dufresne A 2012 Preparation, properties and applications of polysaccharide nanocrystals in advanced functional nanomaterials: a review *Nanoscale* **4** 3274–94

[116] Avella M, De Vlieger J J, Errico M E, Fischer S, Vacca P and Volpe M G 2005 Biodegradable starch/clay nanocomposite films for food packaging applications *Food Chem.* **93** 467–74

[117] Othman S H 2014 Bio-nanocomposite materials for food packaging applications: types of biopolymer and nano-sized filler *Agric. Agric. Sci. Proc.* **2** 296–303

[118] Rhim J-W, Park H-M and Ha C-S 2013 Bio-nanocomposites for food packaging applications *Prog. Polym. Sci.* **38** 1629–52

[119] Xu Q, Chen C, Rosswurm K, Yao T and Janaswamy S 2016 A facile route to prepare cellulose-based films *Carbohydr. Polym.* **149** 274–81

[120] Mbey J-A, Hoppe S and Thomas F 2012 Cassava starch–kaolinite composite film. Effect of clay content and clay modification on film properties *Carbohydr. Polymers* **88** 213–22

[121] Sun Q, Xi T, Li Y and Xiong L 2014 Characterization of corn starch films reinforced with $CaCO_3$ nanoparticles *PLoS One* **9** e106727

[122] Alves V D, Costa N and Coelhoso I M 2010 Barrier properties of biodegradable composite films based on kappa-carrageenan/pectin blends and mica flakes *Carbohydr. Polym.* **79** 269–76

[123] Shankar S, Wang L-F and Rhim J-W 2016 Preparations and characterization of alginate/silver composite films: effect of types of silver particles *Carbohydr. Polym.* **146** 208–16

[124] Rai M, Yadav A and Gade A 2009 Silver nanoparticles as a new generation of antimicrobials *Biotechnol. Adv.* **27** 76–83

[125] Yadollahi M, Farhoudian S and Namazi H 2015 One-pot synthesis of antibacterial chitosan/silver bio-nanocomposite hydrogel beads as drug delivery systems *Int. J. Biol. Macromol.* **79** 37–43

[126] Ma H, Zhou B, Li H-S, Li Y-Q and Ou S-Y 2011 Green composite films composed of nanocrystalline cellulose and a cellulose matrix regenerated from functionalized ionic liquid solution *Carbohydr. Polym.* **84** 383–9

[127] Soheilmoghaddam M, Wahit M U and Akos N I 2013 Regenerated cellulose/epoxidized natural rubber blend film *Mater. Lett.* **111** 221–4

[128] Soheilmoghaddam M, Wahit M U, Mahmoudian S and Hanid N A 2013 Regenerated cellulose/halloysite nanotube nanocomposite films prepared with an ionic liquid *Mater. Chem. Phys.* **141** 936–43

[129] Heinze T and Liebert T 2001 Unconventional methods in cellulose functionalization *Prog. Polym. Sci.* **26** 1689–762

[130] Fink H P, Weigel P, Purz H J and Ganster J 2001 Structure formation of regenerated cellulose materials from NMMO-solutions *Prog. Polym. Sci.* **26** 1473–524

[131] Takaragi A, Minoda M, Miyamoto T, Liu H Q and Zhang L N 1999 Reaction characteristics of cellulose in the LiCl/1,3-dimethyl-2-imidazolidinone solvent system *Cellulose* **6** 93–102

[132] McCormick C L and Callais P A 1987 Derivatization of cellulose in lithium chloride and NN-dimethylacetamide solutions *Polymer* **28** 2317–23

[133] Northolt M, Boerstoel H, Maatman H, Huisman R, Veurink J and Elzerman H 2001 The structure and properties of cellulose fibres spun from an anisotropic phosphoric acid solution *Polymer* **42** 8249–64

[134] El Miri N, Abdelouahdi K, Barakat A, Zahouily M, Fihri A and Solhy A *et al* 2015 Bio-nanocomposite films reinforced with cellulose nanocrystals: rheology of film-forming solutions, transparency, water vapor barrier and tensile properties of films *Carbohydr. Polym.* **129** 156–67

[135] Ghanbarzadeh B, Almasi H and Entezami A A 2010 Physical properties of edible modified starch/carboxymethyl cellulose films *Innovat. Food Sci. Emerg. Technol.* **11** 697–702

[136] Chen Y, Liu C, Chang P R, Cao X and Anderson D P 2009 Bionanocomposites based on pea starch and cellulose nanowhiskers hydrolyzed from pea hull fibre: effect of hydrolysis time *Carbohydr. Polym.* **76** 607–15

[137] Oun A A and Rhim J-W 2015 Preparation and characterization of sodium carboxymethyl cellulose/cotton linter cellulose nanofibril composite films *Carbohydr. Polym.* **127** 101–9

[138] Alves J, Dos Reis K, Menezes E, Pereira F and Pereira J 2015 Effect of cellulose nanocrystals and gelatin in corn starch plasticized films *Carbohydr. Polym.* **115** 215–22

[139] Kamal M R and Khoshkava V 2015 Effect of cellulose nanocrystals (CNC) on rheological and mechanical properties and crystallization behavior of PLA/CNC nanocomposites *Carbohydr. Polym.* **123** 105–14

[140] El Miri N, Abdelouahdi K, Zahouily M, Fihri A, Barakat A and Solhy A *et al* 2015 Bio-nanocomposite films based on cellulose nanocrystals filled polyvinyl alcohol/chitosan polymer blend *J. Appl. Polym. Sci.* **132** 42004

[141] Donhowe I G and Fennema O 1993 The effects of solution composition and drying temperature on crystallinity, permeability and mechanical properties of methylcellulose films *J. Food Process. Preserv.* **17** 231–46

[142] Donhowe I G and Fennema O 1993 The effects of plasticizers on crystallinity, permeability, and mechanical properties of methylcellulose films *J. Food Process. Preserv.* **17** 247–57

[143] Li Y, Shoemaker C F, Ma J, Shen X and Zhong F 2008 Paste viscosity of rice starches of different amylose content and carboxymethylcellulose formed by dry heating and the physical properties of their films *Food Chem.* **109** 616–23

[144] Sheshmani S, Ashori A and Arab Fashapoyeh M 2013 Wood plastic composite using graphene nanoplatelets *Int. J. Biol. Macromol.* **58** 1–6

[145] Ebrahimzadeh S, Ghanbarzadeh B and Hamishehkar H 2016 Physical properties of carboxymethyl cellulose based nano-biocomposites with graphene nano-platelets *Int. J. Biol. Macromol.* **84** 16–23

[146] Liu D, Zhu Y, Li Z, Tian D, Chen L and Chen P 2013 Chitin nanofibrils for rapid and efficient removal of metal ions from water system *Carbohydr. Polym.* **98** 483–9

[147] Yang R, Su Y, Aubrecht K B, Wang X, Ma H and Grubbs R B *et al* 2015 Thiol-functionalized chitin nanofibers for As (III) adsorption *Polymer* **60** 9–17

[148] Karasz F E, O'Reilly J M and Bair H E 1964 Thermal helix-coil transition in poly-γ-benzyl-L-glutamate *Nature* **202** 693–4

[149] Watanabe H, Yoshioka K and Wada A 1964 Electrooptical and dielectric investigations on the conformation and the electrical properties of poly-γ-benzyl-L-glutamate in mixed solvents *Biopolymers* **2** 91–101

[150] Ackermann T and Neumann E 1967 Experimental thermodynamics of the helix–random coil transition. I. Influence of polymer concentration and solvent composition in the PBG–DCA–EDC system *Biopolymers* **5** 649–62

[151] Wen K J and Woody R W 1975 Conformational studies of poly (L-tyrosine). A helix–coil transition in dimethyl sulfoxide–dichloroacetic acid mixtures *Biopolymers* **14** 1827–40

[152] Omura I, Teramoto A and Fujita H 1975 Dielectric dispersion of polypeptide solutions. II. Helix-coil transition of poly (iε-carbobenzoxy-L-lysine) in m-Cresol *Macromolecules* **8** 284–90

[153] Wada A 1971 Dielectric evidence of chemical relaxation in the helix-coil transition of polypeptides *Chem. Phys. Lett.* **8** 211–3

[154] Huang J and Heise A 2013 Stimuli responsive synthetic polypeptides derived from N-carboxyanhydride (NCA) polymerisation *Chem. Soc. Rev.* **42** 7373–90

[155] Kricheldorf H and Penczek S 1990 *Models of Biopolymers by Ring-Opening Polymerization* (Boca Raton, FL: CRC Press) 46–62

[156] Fuchs F 1922 On N-carbonic acid-anhydride *Ber. Dtsch. Chem. Ges.* **55** 2943

[157] Rosu C, Selcuk S, Soto-Cantu E and Russo P S 2014 Progress in silica polypeptide composite colloidal hybrids: from silica cores to fuzzy shells *Colloid. Polym. Sci.* **292** 1009–40

[158] Dietz E, Fery N and Hamann K 1974 Polyreactions on pigmented surfaces. 4. Polymerization of n-carboxy-alpha-amino-acid anhydrides on surface of silicon dioxide *Angew. Makromol. Chem.* **35** 115–29

[159] Heise A, Menzel H, Yim H, Foster M D, Wieringa R H and Schouten A J *et al* 1997 Grafting of polypeptides on solid substrates by initiation of N-carboxyanhydride polymerization by amino-terminated self-assembled monolayers *Langmuir* **13** 723–8

[160] Fong B and Russo P S 1999 Organophilic colloidal particles with a synthetic polypeptide coating *Langmuir* **15** 4421–6

[161] Wang Y and Chang Y C 2003 Synthesis and conformational transition of surface-tethered polypeptide: poly (L-lysine) *Macromolecules* **36** 6511–8

[162] Kolb H C, Finn M and Sharpless K B 2001 Click chemistry: diverse chemical function from a few good reactions *Angew. Chem. Int. Ed.* **40** 2004–21

[163] Golas P L and Matyjaszewski K 2007 Click chemistry and ATRP: a beneficial union for the preparation of functional materials *QSAR Comb. Sci.* **26** 1116–34

[164] Wieringa R, Siesling E, Geurts P, Werkman P, Vorenkamp E and Erb V *et al* 2001 Surface grafting of poly (L-glutamates). 1. Synthesis and characterization *Langmuir* **17** 6477–84

[165] Wieringa R H and Schouten A J 1996 Oriented thin film formation by surface graft polymerization of γ-methyl L-glutamate N-carboxyanhydride in the melt *Macromolecules* **29** 3032–4

[166] Johnston A P, Cortez C, Angelatos A S and Caruso F 2006 Layer-by-layer engineered capsules and their applications *Curr. Opin. Colloid Interface Sci.* **11** 203–9

[167] Marcelo G, Muñoz-Bonilla A and Fernández-García M 2012 Magnetite–polypeptide hybrid materials decorated with gold nanoparticles: study of their catalytic activity in 4-nitrophenol reduction *J. Phys. Chem.* C **116** 24717–25

[168] Mano J F 2008 Stimuli-responsive polymeric systems for biomedical applications *Adv. Eng. Mater.* **10** 515–27

[169] Ahn S-K, Kasi R M, Kim S-C, Sharma N and Zhou Y 2008 Stimuli-responsive polymer gels *Soft Matter* **4** 1151–7

[170] Charati M B, Lee I, Hribar K C and Burdick J A 2010 Light-sensitive polypeptide hydrogel and nanorod composites *Small.* **6** 1608–11

[171] Hu X, Du Y, Tang Y, Wang Q, Feng T and Yang J *et al* 2007 Solubility and property of chitin in NaOH/urea aqueous solution *Carbohydr. Polym.* **70** 451–8

[172] Hudson S and Smith C 1998 Polysaccharides: chitin and chitosan: chemistry and technology of their use as structural materials *Biopolymers from Renewable Resources* (Berlin: Springer) pp 96–118

[173] Muzzarelli R A, Jeuniaux C and Gooday G W 1986 *Chitin in Nature and Technology* (Berlin: Springer)

[174] Atkins E 1985 Conformations in polysaccharides and complex *Carbohydr. J. Biosci.* **8** 375–87

[175] Hawary D, Motaleb M, Farag H, Guirguis O and Elsabee M 2011 Water-soluble derivatives of chitosan as a target delivery system of 99mTc to some organs *in vivo* for nuclear imaging and biodistribution *J. Radioanal. Nucl. Chem.* **290** 557–67

[176] Bava A, Cappellini F, Pedretti E, Rossi F, Caruso E and Vismara E *et al* 2013 Heparin and carboxymethylchitosan metal nanoparticles: an evaluation of their cytotoxicity *BioMed Res. Int.* **2013** 314091

[177] Xie M, Liu H-H, Chen P, Zhang Z-L, Wang X-H and Xie Z-X *et al* 2005 CdSe/ZnS-labeled carboxymethyl chitosan as a bioprobe for live cell imaging *Chem. Commun.* **44** 5518–20

[178] Adányi N, Levkovets I, Rodriguez-Gil S, Ronald A, Váradi M and Szendrő I 2007 Development of immunosensor based on OWLS technique for determining Aflatoxin B1 and Ochratoxin A *Biosens. Bioelectron.* **22** 797–802

[179] Wang G, Lu G, Ao Q, Gong Y and Zhang X 2010 Preparation of cross-linked carboxymethyl chitosan for repairing sciatic nerve injury in rats *Biotechnol. Lett.* **32** 59

[180] Luo Y, Teng Z, Wang X and Wang Q 2013 Development of carboxymethyl chitosan hydrogel beads in alcohol-aqueous binary solvent for nutrient delivery applications *Food Hydrocoll.* **31** 332–9

[181] Rinaudo M, Le Dung P, Gey C and Milas M 1992 Substituent distribution on O,N-carboxymethylchitosans by ^{1}H and ^{13}C NMR *Int. J. Biol. Macromol.* **14** 122–8

[182] Sandford P A, Zikakis J P and Brine C J 1992 *Advances in Chitin and Chitosan* (Amsterdam: Elsevier Applied Science)

[183] Le Dung P, Milas M, Rinaudo M and Desbrières J 1994 Water soluble derivatives obtained by controlled chemical modifications of chitosan *Carbohydr. Polym.* **24** 209–14

[184] Sun L, Du Y, Fan L, Chen X and Yang J 2006 Preparation, characterization and antimicrobial activity of quaternized carboxymethyl chitosan and application as pulp-cap *Polymer* **47** 1796–804

[185] Upadhyaya L, Singh J, Agarwal V and Tewari R P 2014 The implications of recent advances in carboxymethyl chitosan based targeted drug delivery and tissue engineering applications *J. Control. Release* **186** 54–87

[186] Upadhyaya L, Singh J, Agarwal V, Pandey A, Verma S P and Das P *et al* 2015 Efficient water soluble nanostructured ZnO grafted O-carboxymethyl chitosan/curcumin-nanocomposite for cancer therapy *Process Biochem.* **50** 678–88

[187] Domard A, Rinaudo M and Terrassin C 1989 Adsorption of chitosan and a quaternized derivative on kaolin *J. Appl. Polym. Sci.* **38** 1799–806

[188] Heras A, Rodriguez N, Ramos V and Agullo E 2001 N-methylene phosphonic chitosan: a novel soluble derivative *Carbohydr. Polym.* **44** 1–8

[189] Ramos V, Rodrıguez N, Dıaz M, Rodrıguez M, Heras A and Agullo E 2003 N-methylene phosphonic chitosan. Effect of preparation methods on its properties *Carbohydr. Polym.* **52** 39–46

[190] Kumar S, Rai S B and Rath C 2019 Latent fingerprint imaging using Dy and Sm codoped HfO_2 nanophosphors: structure and luminescence properties *Part. Part. Syst. Charact.* **36** 1900048

[191] Dilag J, Kobus H and Ellis A V 2009 Cadmium sulfide quantum dot/chitosan nanocomposites for latent fingermark detection *Forensic Sci. Int.* **187** 97–102

[192] Lian H-T, Liu B, Chen Y-P and Sun X-Y 2012 A urea electrochemical sensor based on molecularly imprinted chitosan film doping with CdS quantum dots *Anal. Biochem.* **426** 40–6

[193] Wu Z, Huang X, Li Y-C, Xiao H and Wang X 2018 Novel chitosan films with laponite immobilized Ag nanoparticles for active food packaging *Carbohydr. Polym.* **199** 210–8

[194] Klemm D, Schumann D, Kramer F, Heßler N, Koth D and Sultanova B (ed) 2009 Nanocellulose materials—different cellulose, different functionality *Macromolecular Symposia* (New York: Wiley Online Library)

[195] Chen W, Yu H and Liu Y 2011 Preparation of millimeter-long cellulose I nanofibers with diameters of 30–80 nm from bamboo fibers *Carbohydr. Polym.* **86** 453–61

[196] Stokke D D and Gardner D J 2003 Fundamental aspects of wood as a component of thermoplastic composites *J. Vinyl Add. Tech.* **9** 96–104

[197] Entcheva E, Bien H, Yin L, Chung C-Y, Farrell M and Kostov Y 2004 Functional cardiac cell constructs on cellulose-based scaffolding *Biomaterials* **25** 5753–62

[198] Vroman I and Tighzert L 2009 Biodegradable polymers *Materials.* **2** 307–44

[199] Gabrielii I, Gatenholm P, Glasser W, Jain R and Kenne L 2000 Separation, characterization and hydrogel-formation of hemicellulose from aspen wood *Carbohydr. Polym.* **43** 367–74

[200] Scheller H V and Ulvskov P 2010 Hemicelluloses *Annu. Rev. Plant Biol.* **61** 263–89

[201] Li X and Pan X 2010 Hydrogels based on hemicellulose and lignin from lignocellulose biorefinery: a mini-review *J. Biobased Mater. Bioenergy* **4** 289–97

[202] Karaaslan M A, Tshabalala M A, Yelle D J and Buschle-Diller G 2011 Nanoreinforced biocompatible hydrogels from wood hemicelluloses and cellulose whiskers *Carbohydr. Polym.* **86** 192–201

[203] Adler E 1977 Lignin chemistry—past, present and future *Wood Sci. Technol.* **11** 169–218

[204] Cazacu G, Pascu M C, Profire L, Kowarski A, Mihaes M and Vasile C 2004 Lignin role in a complex polyolefin blend *Ind. Crops Prod.* **20** 261–73

[205] Raschip I E, Hitruc E G and Vasile C 2011 Semi-interpenetrating polymer networks containing polysaccharides. II. Xanthan/lignin networks: a spectral and thermal characterization *High Perform. Polym.* **23** 219–29

[206] Fernandes E M, Pires R A, Mano J F and Reis R L 2013 Bionanocomposites from lignocellulosic resources: properties, applications and future trends for their use in the biomedical field *Prog. Polym. Sci.* **38** 1415–41

[207] Klemm D, Schumann D, Kramer F, Heßler N, Hornung M and Schmauder H-P *et al* 2006 Nanocelluloses as innovative polymers in research and application *Polysaccharides II* (Berlin: Springer) 49–96

[208] Millon L and Wan W 2006 The polyvinyl alcohol–bacterial cellulose system as a new nanocomposite for biomedical applications *J. Biomed. Mater. Res. Part* B **79** 245–53

[209] Miyamoto T, Takahashi S, Ito H, Inagaki H and Noishiki Y 1989 Tissue biocompatibility of cellulose and its derivatives *J. Biomed. Mater. Res.* **23** 125–33

[210] Svensson A, Nicklasson E, Harrah T, Panilaitis B, Kaplan D and Brittberg M *et al* 2005 Bacterial cellulose as a potential scaffold for tissue engineering of cartilage *Biomaterials* **26** 419–31

[211] Oksman K, Mathew A P, Bondeson D and Kvien I 2006 Manufacturing process of cellulose whiskers/polylactic acid nanocomposites *Compos. Sci. Technol.* **66** 2776–84

[212] Wan Y, Huang Y, Yuan C, Raman S, Zhu Y and Jiang H *et al* 2007 Biomimetic synthesis of hydroxyapatite/bacterial cellulose nanocomposites for biomedical applications *Mater. Sci. Eng.* C **27** 855–64

[213] Saska S, Barud H, Gaspar A, Marchetto R, Ribeiro S J L and Messaddeq Y 2011 Bacterial cellulose-hydroxyapatite nanocomposites for bone regeneration *Int. J. Biomater.* **2011** 175362

[214] Wan Y, Hong L, Jia S, Huang Y, Zhu Y and Wang Y *et al* 2006 Synthesis and characterization of hydroxyapatite–bacterial cellulose nanocomposites *Compos. Sci. Technol.* **66** 1825–32

[215] Paul M-A, Alexandre M, Degée P, Henrist C, Rulmont A and Dubois P 2003 New nanocomposite materials based on plasticized poly (L-lactide) and organo-modified montmorillonites: thermal and morphological study *Polymer* **44** 443–50

[216] Azizi Samir M A S, Alloin F and Dufresne A 2005 Review of recent research into cellulosic whiskers, their properties and their application in nanocomposite field *Biomacromolecules.* **6** 612–26

[217] Bondeson D and Oksman K 2007 Polylactic acid/cellulose whisker nanocomposites modified by polyvinyl alcohol *Compos. Part A: Appl. Sci. Manuf.* **38** 2486–92

[218] Alves N, Saiz-Arroyo C, Rodriguez-Perez M, Reis R and Mano J 2007 Microhardness of starch based biomaterials in simulated physiological conditions *Acta Biomater.* **3** 69–76

[219] Boesel L F, Mano J F and Reis R L 2004 Optimization of the formulation and mechanical properties of starch based partially degradable bone cements *J. Mater. Sci., Mater. Med.* **15** 73–83

[220] Jeon J and Puleo D 2008 Formulations for intermittent release of parathyroid hormone (1–34) and local enhancement of osteoblast activities *Pharm. Dev. Technol.* **13** 505–12

[221] Sannino A, Demitri C and Madaghiele M 2009 Biodegradable cellulose-based hydrogels: design and applications *Materials* **2** 353–73

[222] Krieger J 1990 New coating increases efficiency of lamps *Chem. Eng. News* **68** 35

[223] Hutchens S A, Benson R S, Evans B R, O'Neill H M and Rawn C J 2006 Biomimetic synthesis of calcium-deficient hydroxyapatite in a natural hydrogel *Biomaterials* **27** 4661–70

[224] Elsawy M A, Kim K-H, Park J-W and Deep A 2017 Hydrolytic degradation of polylactic acid (PLA) and its composites *Renew. Sustain. Energy Rev.* **79** 1346–52

[225] Souza V G L and Fernando A L 2016 Nanoparticles in food packaging: biodegradability and potential migration to food—a review *Food Packag. Shelf Life* **8** 63–70

[226] Tiimob B J, Rangari V K, Mwinyelle G, Abdela W, Evans P G and Abbott N *et al* 2018 Tough aliphatic-aromatic copolyester and chicken egg white flexible biopolymer blend with bacteriostatic effects *Food Packag. Shelf Life* **15** 9–16

[227] Lizundia E, Fortunati E, Dominici F, Vilas J L, León L M and Armentano I *et al* 2016 PLLA-grafted cellulose nanocrystals: role of the CNC content and grafting on the PLA bionanocomposite film properties *Carbohydr. Polym.* **142** 105–13

[228] Vink E T, Glassner D A, Kolstad J J, Wooley R J and O'Connor R P 2007 The eco-profiles for current and near-future NatureWorks® polylactide (PLA) production *Ind. Biotechnol.* **3** 58–81

[229] Abdulkhani A, Hosseinzadeh J, Ashori A, Dadashi S and Takzare Z 2014 Preparation and characterization of modified cellulose nanofibers reinforced polylactic acid nanocomposite *Polym. Test.* **35** 73–9

[230] Rasal R M, Janorkar A V and Hirt D E 2010 Poly(lactic acid) modifications *Prog. Polym. Sci.* **35** 338–56

[231] Rhim J W, Mohanty A K, Singh S P and Ng P K 2006 Effect of the processing methods on the performance of polylactide films: thermocompression versus solvent casting *J. Appl. Polym. Sci.* **101** 3736–42

[232] Ingrao C, Gigli M and Siracusa V 2017 An attributional Life Cycle Assessment application experience to highlight environmental hotspots in the production of foamy polylactic acid trays for fresh-food packaging usage *J. Clean. Prod.* **150** 93–103

[233] Hamdan A M and Sonomoto K 2011 Production of optically pure lactic acid for bioplastics *Lactic Acid Bacteria and Bifidobacteria* (Portland, OR: Academic Press)

[234] Otoni C G, Espitia P J P, Avena-Bustillos R J and McHugh T H 2016 Trends in antimicrobial food packaging systems: emitting sachets and absorbent pads *Food Res. Int.* **83** 60–73

[235] Sung S-Y, Sin L T, Tee T-T, Bee S-T, Rahmat A R and Rahman W A W A *et al* 2013 Antimicrobial agents for food packaging applications *Trends Food Sci. Technol.* **33** 110–23

[236] Ribeiro-Santos R, Andrade M and Sanches-Silva A 2017 Application of encapsulated essential oils as antimicrobial agents in food packaging *Curr. Opin. Food Sci.* **14** 78–84

[237] Carbone M, Donia D T, Sabbatella G and Antiochia R 2016 Silver nanoparticles in polymeric matrices for fresh food packaging *J. King Saud Univ.—Sci.* **28** 273–9

[238] de Azeredo H M C 2013 Antimicrobial nanostructures in food packaging *Trends Food Sci. Technol.* **30** 56–69

[239] Guo L, Yuan W, Lu Z and Li C M 2013 Polymer/nanosilver composite coatings for antibacterial applications *Colloids Surf.* A **439** 69–83

[240] Chen C, Lv G, Pan C, Song M, Wu C and Guo D *et al* 2007 Poly (lactic acid)(PLA) based nanocomposites—a novel way of drug-releasing *Biomed. Mater.* **2** L1

[241] Saini R K, Bajpai A K and Jain E 2018 Fundamentals of bionanocomposites *Biodegradable and Biocompatible Polymer Composites* (Cambridge: Woodhead Publishing) pp 351–77

[242] Alexis F 2005 Factors affecting the degradation and drug-release mechanism of poly(lactic acid) and poly[(lactic acid)-co-(glycolic acid)] *Polym. Int.* **54** 36–46 2005

[243] Grassie N 1985 *GS. Polymer Degradation and Stabilization* (Cambridge: Cambridge University Press) 1445

[244] Mitragotri S and Lahann J 2009 Physical approaches to biomaterial design *Nat. Mater.* **8** 15–23

[245] Rizvi S A and Saleh A M 2018 Applications of nanoparticle systems in drug delivery technology *Saudi Pharm. J.* **26** 64–70

[246] Sharma S, Narang J K, Ali J and Baboota S 2016 Synergistic antioxidant action of vitamin E and rutin SNEDDS in ameliorating oxidative stress in a Parkinson's disease model *Nanotechnology* **27** 375101

[247] Liang H, Zhang X-B, Lv Y, Gong L, Wang R and Zhu X *et al* 2014 Functional DNA-containing nanomaterials: cellular applications in biosensing, imaging, and targeted therapy *Acc. Chem. Res.* **47** 1891–901

[248] Fan Z, Fu P P, Yu H and Ray P C 2014 Theranostic nanomedicine for cancer detection and treatment *J. Food Drug Anal.* **22** 3–17

[249] Henriksen-Lacey M, Carregal-Romero S and Liz-Marzán L M 2017 Current challenges toward *in vitro* cellular validation of inorganic nanoparticles *Bioconjugate Chem.* **28** 212–21

[250] Cherian B M, Leão A L, de Souza S F, Costa L M M, de Olyveira G M and Kottaisamy M *et al* 2011 Cellulose nanocomposites with nanofibres isolated from pineapple leaf fibers for medical applications *Carbohydr. Polym.* **86** 1790–8

[251] Hermawan H, Dubé D and Mantovani D 2010 Developments in metallic biodegradable stents *Acta Biomater.* **6** 1693–7

[252] Duncan R and Gaspar R 2011 Nanomedicine(s) under the microscope *Mol. Pharm.* **8** 2101–41

[253] Li R, Jiang S, Liu D, Bi X, Wang F and Zhang Q *et al* 2011 A potential new therapeutic system for glaucoma: solid lipid nanoparticles containing methazolamide *J. Microencapsul.* **28** 134–41

[254] Vega E, Egea M A, Calpena A C, Espina M and García M L 2012 Role of hydroxypropyl-β-cyclodextrin on freeze-dried and gamma-irradiated PLGA and PLGA–PEG diblock copolymer nanospheres for ophthalmic flurbiprofen delivery *Int. J. Nanomed.* **7** 1357

[255] Khademhosseini A, Vacanti J P and Langer R 2009 Progress in tissue engineering *Sci. Am.* **300** 64–71

[256] Goldberg M, Langer R and Jia X 2007 Nanostructured materials for applications in drug delivery and tissue engineering *J. Biomater. Sci. Polym. Ed.* **18** 241–68

[257] Wang Y, Kim U-J, Blasioli D J, Kim H-J and Kaplan D L 2005 *In vitro* cartilage tissue engineering with 3D porous aqueous-derived silk scaffolds and mesenchymal stem cells *Biomaterials* **26** 7082–94

[258] Badylak S F, Record R, Lindberg K, Hodde J and Park K 1998 Small intestinal submucosa: a substrate for *in vitro* cell growth *J. Biomater. Sci. Polym. Ed.* **9** 863–78

[259] Marijnissen W J, van Osch G J, Aigner J, van der Veen S W, Hollander A P and Verwoerd-Verhoef H L *et al* 2002 Alginate as a chondrocyte-delivery substance in combination with a non-woven scaffold for cartilage tissue engineering *Biomaterials* **23** 1511–7

[260] Wang Y, Ameer G A, Sheppard B J and Langer R 2002 A tough biodegradable elastomer *Nat. Biotechnol.* **20** 602–6

[261] Barrera D A, Zylstra E, Lansbury P T Jr and Langer R 1993 Synthesis and RGD peptide modification of a new biodegradable copolymer: poly (lactic acid-co-lysine) *JACS* **115** 11010–1

[262] Ma P X 2004 Scaffolds for tissue fabrication *Mater. Today* **7** 30–40

[263] Nasongkla N, Shuai X, Ai H, Weinberg B D, Pink J and Boothman D A *et al* 2004 cRGD-functionalized polymer micelles for targeted doxorubicin delivery *Angew. Chem.* **116** 6483–7

[264] Daniels T R, Delgado T, Helguera G and Penichet M L 2006 The transferrin receptor part II: targeted delivery of therapeutic agents into cancer cells *Clin. Immunol.* **121** 159–76

[265] Dinauer N, Balthasar S, Weber C, Kreuter J, Langer K and von Briesen H 2005 Selective targeting of antibody-conjugated nanoparticles to leukemic cells and primary T-lymphocytes *Biomaterials* **26** 5898–906

[266] Augustine S, Singh J, Srivastava M, Sharma M, Das A and Malhotra B D 2017 Recent advances in carbon based nanosystems for cancer theranostics *Biomater. Sci.* **5** 901–52

[267] Lu C H, Yang H H, Zhu C L, Chen X and Chen G N 2009 A graphene platform for sensing biomolecules *Angew. Chem.* **121** 4879–81

[268] Liu J, Tao L, Yang W, Li D, Boyer C and Wuhrer R *et al* 2010 Synthesis, characterization, and multilayer assembly of pH sensitive graphene–polymer nanocomposites *Langmuir* **26** 10068–75

[269] Liu J, Yang W, Tao L, Li D, Boyer C and Davis T P 2010 Thermosensitive graphene nanocomposites formed using pyrene-terminal polymers made by RAFT polymerization *J. Polym. Sci., Part A: Polym. Chem.* **48** 425–33

[270] Liu J, Guo S, Han L, Wang T, Hong W and Liu Y *et al* 2012 Synthesis of phospholipid monolayer membrane functionalized graphene for drug delivery *J. Mater. Chem.* **22** 20634–40

[271] Bai H, Li C, Wang X and Shi G 2010 A pH-sensitive graphene oxide composite hydrogel *Chem. Commun.* **46** 2376–8

[272] Kim H, Namgung R, Singha K, Oh I-K and Kim W J 2011 Graphene oxide–polyethylenimine nanoconstruct as a gene delivery vector and bioimaging tool *Bioconjugate Chem.* **22** 2558–67

Chapter 5

Bionanomaterials for biosensor technology

Kingsley Eghonghon Ukhurebor, Charles Oluwaseun Adetunji, Ayodotun Oluwafemi Bobadoye, Uyiosa Osagie Aigbe, Robert Birundu Onyancha, Israel Uzuazor Siloko, Joseph Onyeka Emegha, Godstime Obiajulu Okocha and Isaac Chukwutem Abiodun

The application of bionanomaterials for biosensor machinery in the biomedical fields, as well as other domains, has become tremendously significant. Consequently, contemporary advancements in biological compositions and procedures have given rise to several discoveries of influential and wide-ranging investigative devices using biological sensing. Furthermore, several recorded advancements in bionanomaterials machinery have been of boundless assistance in developing biosensor machinery and have contributed meaningfully to advanced technology that has aided considerably in their improvement. Hence, this chapter provides a comprehensive overview of some inventions of bionanomaterials for biosensor machinery, specifically the nanostructured conducting polymeric bionanomaterials biosensor mechanisms vis-à-vis their biomedical applications.

5.1 Introduction

In the last few years, outstanding developments have been documented in the domain of nanoscience (NSc)/nanotechnology (NTech). Presently, the developments in NSc vis-à-vis nanomaterials (NMs) have been of tremendous support in the development of inventive machinery, which has significantly led to vast enhancement, measures, and products as well as the generation of critical inventive functionalities [1–4]. Accordingly, NSc has evolved biosensor technologies and biosensing-based systems in addition to their wide-ranging applications.

NSc holds numerous promising enhancements and developments, potentially acting as massive support for keeping and sustaining research in the biomedical, agricultural, and environmental fields. At the moment, there are numerous categories of biosensors that are employed for both the biomedical, agricultural, and environmental fields. Biosensors are essential monitoring and management

doi:10.1088/978-0-7503-3767-0ch5

mechanisms in intelligent systems. They are leading and ground-breaking diagnostic devices comprising biological sensing components with numerous applications and are currently gaining more usefulness in the biomedical, agricultural, and environmental fields and other aspects of human endeavours [1–4].

Consequently, even with these enormous benefits of biosensor mechanisms, there are still some issues, especially in inventing integrated biosensor mechanisms that could easily investigate various groups of biomedical, agricultural, and/or environmental issues. The stable built biosensor mechanisms that have been designed for considering the functional vis-à-vis the physical, chemical, biochemical, biological, and structural influence of biosensor mechanisms in the agricultural, biomedical and environmental domains still require some level of improvements. Hence, an adequate understanding of these biosensors' influence will play a crucial part in the agricultural, biomedical, and environmental domains. This will positively be of support in the extenuation of the continuous variation in the ecosystem, especially as it relates to climate change; which is considerably contributing to ecological hazards and other critical functionalities in the atmosphere/ecosystem [5–9], for example, the uneven radio waves proliferation in the atmosphere [10–13].

The current progressions in biosensors machinery and their momentous applications from nano-structured ingredients (NMs to be specific) are becoming of enormous significance to several researchers [14–16], especially those involved in the NSc domains. Reportedly, there are numerous bionanomaterials (BNMs) applications for biosensor machinery basically intended for biomedical purposes, and the advancement in this aspect has become tremendously significant [14]. Accordingly, this has assisted in the intensification of numerous discoveries of influential and wide-ranging investigative devices employing biological sensing components as biosensor mechanisms [2].

Topical progressions in biological compositions (in the form of BNMs) and measures have improved biosensor mechanisms, making most biosensors such as NMs and microbe built-biosensors have inclusive potential applications [14, 15]. Supposedly, these biosensor applications rely on sensing principles or transducers [2]. Therefore, it is imperative to integrate multi-crossed procedures in evolving biosensors that could be employed for further diverse benefits [2]. There is no doubt that BNMs machinery's progression has been of inestimable assistance in the revolution and renovation of biosensor machinery and contributes meaningfully to progressive technologies that are considerably enhancing their development.

Hence, this chapter presents an overview of some diverse BNMs for biosensor technology and their biomedical applications. In the other remaining sections of this chapter, the following are momentarily discussed: section 5.2 provides the historical developments and advances of biosensor machinery, BNMs for biosensor machinery and their biomedical applications are presented in section 5.3, prospects of BNMs for biosensor machinery are presented in section 5.4, while section 5.5 provides the conclusion and suggestions for future developments in the application of BNMs for biosensor machinery.

5.2 Historical developments and advances in biosensor machinery

5.2.1 Historical developments of biosensor machinery

From the time of the first established biosensor known as the glucose ($C_6H_{12}O_6$)/ chemical biosensor in 1956, by Clark and Lyons and others [17, 18], there are now numerous biosensors which are established for several purposes, commercially and otherwise. Fascinatingly, the biosensor came into the public domain with the first commercialized biosensor known as 'Yellow Spring Instruments (YSI)' in 1975 [16]. Presently, most of the contemporary biosensors have a broader range of applications that offer further sensitivities, swiftness, specifications, perceptibility, and developmental results as against the earlier conventional ones such as Clark's $C_6H_{12}O_6$ biosensors (also known as the Clark electrode) [1, 19], which was primarily designed to competently sense or detect the quantity of oxygen context circulation in the blood [17–19].

Ever since the discovery of Clark's $C_6H_{12}O_6$ biosensor (the Clark electrode), which was just an oxygen detector, numerous biosensors have been invented, with the first being the upgrading of the oxygen detector by covering or coating the $C_6H_{12}O_6$-sensitive enzyme film with a prevailing electrode. This additionally improved the functionality of Clark's $C_6H_{12}O_6$ biosensor to performing as a blood sugar biosensor, which was employed for sensing, detecting or discovering and measuring the quantity of blood $C_6H_{12}O_6$. In continuance to this advancement was the application of a layer of urease enzyme for detecting urine, urea in blood, etc [2, 16–19]. Subsequently, there are several historical events of biosensors to date, and there are numerous database reports on topics in biosensor mechanisms to date.

Generally, biosensor mechanisms are grouped into two broad categories, which are based on biological detecting (sensing) constituents and transduction means (transducers) [2, 16, 19]. The detecting constituent encompasses immunosensors or antibodies, enzymes, microbes, organic organelles, and tissues, whereas the transduction means is centred on the physiochemical distinction ensuing from the sensing constituents. According to Reyes De Corcuera and Cavalieri [20], the various known transducers in biosensor mechanism are the optical (such as 'absorbance, chemiluminense, and fluorescence'), electrochemical (such as 'conductometric, amperometric and potentiometric'), piezoelectric (such as 'ultrasonic and acoustic'), and calorimetric biosensors.

Also, biosensors can be grouped based on the order, date, or period of production; 'the first-generation biosensors (FGBs), the second-generation biosensors (SGBs) and the third-generation biosensors (TGBs)' [2, 17, 18]. A brief historical hierarchy of the development of biosensor mechanisms is illustrated in figure 5.1.

FGBs: They are the diffident means, encompassing the unwavering detection of either the increase of an enzymatically formed product or weakening of a substrate of oxidation-reduction enzymes employing an ordinary intermediary for the transmission of electrons. Examples of the FGBs are the $C_6H_{12}O_6$ biosensors [17, 18].

SGBs: They use non-natural oxidation-reduction intermediaries such as quinones, potassium ferricyanide ($C_6N_6FeK_3$), and ferrocene ($C_{10}H_{10}Fe$) for the transmission of electrons, which increase the biosensor sensitivity and duplicability. Examples of the SGBs are the self-monitoring amperometric $C_6H_{12}O_6$ biosensors [17, 18].

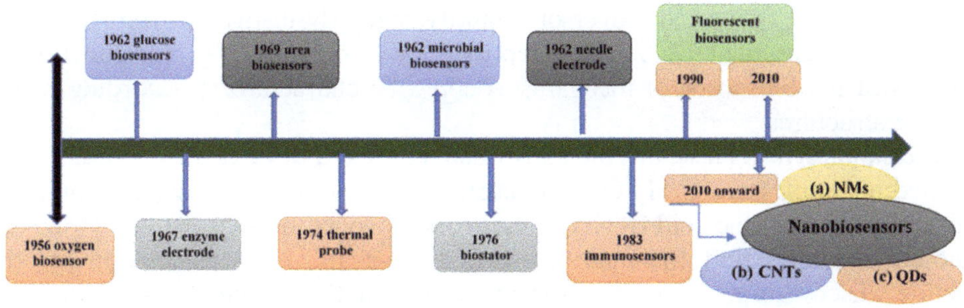

Figure 5.1. A brief hierarchy of the development of biosensor mechanisms (a) NMs: nanomaterials, (b) CNTs: carbon nanotubes, (c) QDs: quantum dots.

TGBs: These are supposedly the latest group in which the oxidation-reduction enzymes are restrained (immobilized) on the surface of the electrode (conductor) in such a way that direct transmission of electrons is allowed amongst the enzyme and transducer [17, 18], they employ biological or organic conducting substances such as '*tetrathiafulvalnetetracynoquinodi methane (TTF-TCQN)*' [21].

Topical progressions in integrated electronics (IEs) have been of assistance in the moderation of intricate electronic systems into nano sizes (mm^2 sizes). This prospect transpires in the execution of intricate and sophisticated instrumentation in affordable and transferrable devices for swift detection of damaging and noxious agents [3, 4]. Hence, NSc is becoming meaningfully advantageous in the creation of biosensors. The advancement of the most NMs for biosensor machinery vis-à-vis the applications of NSc has contributed meaningfully to the enhancement of agriculture, environmental management, and biomedical applications [1–4, 22]. Presently, the growth in the field of NSc has led to the disposition of NMs for the development of several affordable and portable biosensors that are unwaveringly assisting in evolving the agricultural, environmental, and biomedical fields as well as in the integration of these biosensor mechanisms into arrangements and devices for several commercial and other applications [2–4, 22].

Reportedly, NMs are advantageous in the invention of biosensor mechanisms [16]. The progressions in the field of NSc have led to enhanced performances of biosensor mechanisms, especially sensitivities, swiftness, specifications, and perceptibility, as well as in the production of reduced detection ranges of investigation [1–4, 23, 24]. NMs are advantageous in enhancing the biosensor's definite surface; this aids the control (immobilization) of enhanced quantities of bioreceptor mechanisms. Ordinarily, NMs are equipped with suitable roles, employing direct functionalization or covering (coating) with competent polymers, deprived of disturbance from their particular structures. Nevertheless, according to some studies, this feature is subject to their chemical formation and configuration [1–4].

5.2.2 Functioning principles of biosensor mechanisms

Ordinarily, biosensors could function internally or externally in living organisms; wherein, the target is the characteristic variable(s) to which the mechanism is employed to sense, detect, discover or quantify regularly instigated from the living organism's environment [2, 25]. As reported by Ukhurebor [2], the functioning principles of the biosensor of mechanisms could be characterized according to the following structures:

Targeted analytes: These are the constituents targeted to be detected, discovered, or sensed; examples are $C_6H_{12}O_6$ biosensors, oxygen biosensors, deoxyribonucleic acid (DNA)/ribonucleic acid (RNA) biosensors, nitrogen biosensors, etc. However, it should be noted that the analytes should have affinity or attraction for the detecting, discovering, or sensing surface to which they could respond or react electrochemically, chemically, and otherwise [2, 25].

Bioreceptors: These are the deactivated or neutralized medium (an immobilized/restrained soft or hard biocomponent) specific regular selectivity, which is to be exposed to the targeted constituent, habitually interfaced to the transducer [2, 25]. The recognized bioreceptors groups are; enzymes (such as peroxidases, oxidoreductases, polyphenol oxidases, aminooxidases, etc) [25], tissues, microbes, DNA, antibody, biomimetics, [1, 3, 27], NMs [14–16].

Sensing, detecting, or discovering (transduction) procedures: These replicate the type of sensing, discovering, or detection biosensors accomplish; this entails the physical, chemical, structural, biological, or biochemical adaptation principles [11, 12, 16–18]. Typically, the procedures are based on the behavioural attributes of the transducers. Contemporary procedures include: electrical, electrochemical, NMs, optical, piezoelectric, photoelectric, photoelectrochemical, and thermometric sensing, detecting or discovering procedures.

Nature of the organic or biological components employed: The nature of the organic or biological components layered over the transducer, which is habitually in neutralized or deactivated states, is also essential in biosensor mechanisms' structures.

Generation: The order, period, or date when the biosensor was established and brought to the public domain is also an imperative structure of biosensor mechanisms [2, 19]. This implies that biosensors produced, developed, and released into the public domain over a given duration with similar features belong to the same or a particular generation. Correspondingly, like other devices such as electronic machinery, the modern ones are often more sophisticated than the past ones; the superiority could be defined explicitly in terms of precision, energy consumption capacity, refinement of the integration scale, multifunctionality, dimensions, etc.

In all these structures mentioned above, it should be noted that biosensors are not just sensing or detecting devices (sensors/detectors), but they also perform some critical and analytical functions which are based on their application domains. For instance, as analytical devices, biosensors could be employed in detecting the exact existence of specific bioparticles, microbes, biological structures, or any other biological analytes. As stated previously, biosensor mechanisms function on the principle of signal transduction or cell signalling, in a procedure comprising the transmission of the physical, chemical, structural, biochemical, or biological signals that replicate molecular measures from a cell or constituent in such a means that is quantifiable [2, 18, 19, 26, 27].

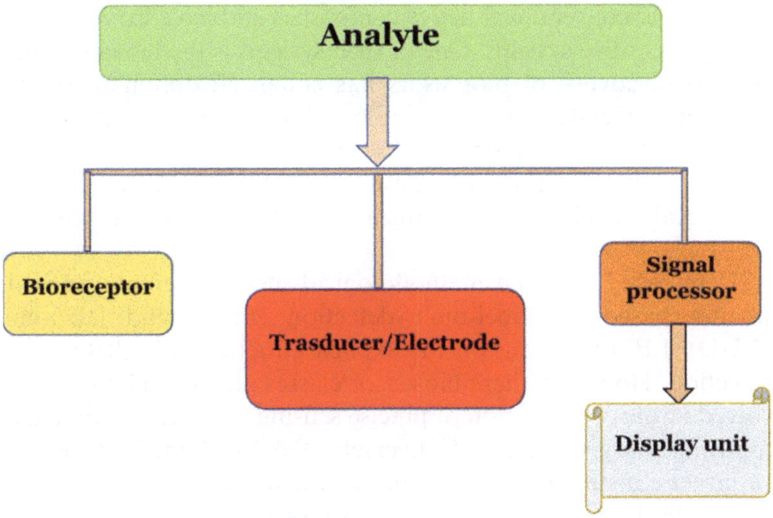

Figure 5.2. A prototypical biosensor mechanism, showing the primary components in biosensor mechanisms.

Figure 5.2 shows the foremost known components in biosensor mechanisms. The figure depicts a prototypical biosensor block diagram with the following components [2, 26]:

- The analyte; which is the constituent that is targeted to be detected, discovered, or sensed;
- The bioreceptor; which is the biorecognition constituent;
- The transducer; which is the physical, chemical, structural, biological or biochemical mechanism that translates or decodes distinctions in the target biophysical parameters such as $C_6H_{12}O_6$ or oxygen to a physically quantifiable output signal and/or the other way around;
- The signal processor; this is the electronic device that process and amplifies the signals;
- The output unit; which is also known as the display unit, where the final output is presented.

Biosensor mechanisms are further advanced and enhanced in their sensitivity and selectivity when likened to other usual categories of analytical technologies. Some of the momentous benefits and advantages of biosensors are fast and continuous measurement, condensed application of reagents, eradication of calibration and re-calibration, reasonable accuracy, rapid response duration, capability for measuring non-polar particles that other conventional machinery could barely evaluate [2, 26].

5.2.3 Advances in biosensor machinery

According to Kabra *et al* [28], the reduction in dimensions of constituent part particles to smaller units often referred to as nanometric scale, and its supplementary integration for the preparation of other useful composites such as BNMs, nano-energetic, etc have raised the potential of conventional active composites and have led to the growth and advancement of innovative systems. One of such systems is the biosensor mechanisms.

Generally, the discovery of biosensors has enhanced dominant significance in several aspects of our endeavours. Its exploitation has accomplished momentous application in the agricultural, biomedical sciences, as well as environmental science domains [2]. Undoubtedly, this has assisted in the advancement of precise and dominant analytical machinery in the utilization of biological detecting constituents [1–3, 29–31].

Turner [32] reported that the methodological methods employed in biosensor mechanisms are based on label-built detection (LBD) and label-unrestricted detection (LUD). LBD is reliant on the explicit structures of label parameters for targeting detection. However, these biosensor classes are dependable, since they are usually involved in the combination of precise sensing constituents that are invented with the controlled target protein. Conversely, the LUD method permits for the detection of target constituents that are not characterised or hard to label [33, 34]. Contemporary interdisciplinary procedures in biotechnology as well as electronics technology, especially IEs have paved the way for developing LUD biosensor mechanisms for the detection of several methods with various applications in the agricultural, biomedical, and environmental sciences domains [1–4].

Developments in electrochemical biosensors with reasonable quantity approaches focussed on the extent of detection, the investigation's duration, and the entailed compactness apply to user markets for affordable biosensors intended for $C_6H_{12}O_6$ and pregnancy appraisals through anti-human chorionic gonadotrophic hormone control (immobilization) strip with the lateral-flow procedure [32].

As reported by Vigneshvar *et al* [30], the management of analytes employing NMs and polymers is dynamic for the enhancement of the extent of detection and sensitivity of biosensors. Consequently, the lateral-flow procedure allows the direct transmission of samples to a predicted spot to generate accurate connections as an alternative to haphazard connections. Similarly, it has assisted in bio-fabrication enhancement employing either non-contact assembled, or contact assembled modelling. The application of NMs such as silver (Ag), gold (Au), and silicon (Si) assembled bio-fabrication has assisted in the production of inventive procedures. Similarly, covering of the polymers with NMs has brought enormous improvements in contact assembled electrochemical sensing [1, 3, 34]. One of the leading advantages of these classes of electrochemical sensors is their specificity and sensitivity along with real-time inquiry. However, some restrictions, such as the recuperating ability or long-term process of polymers and/or other ingredients, could cause a reduction in the cost and make such biosensors far beyond one's reach.

At the moment, there are numerous NMs such as Au, Ag, Si, copper (Cu), etc, as well as carbon NMs like graphite, graphene, and CNTs, which have been used for developing biosensors mechanisms [23, 30, 34–41]. Carbon NMs-based ingredients give vast specificity and sensitivity for developing electrochemical and other classes of biosensor mechanisms, while Au NMs possess more possibilities compared to other metallic and metallic-oxide NMs use in biosensor mechanisms such as Ag. Also, owing to their permanence against corrosion, they are not harmful when used for biomedical purposes. Essentially, procedures of BNMs for biosensor mechanisms are not without some limitations and challenges, which need to be effectively addressed when being employed for biomedical purposes [42].

Also, as reported by Ding *et al* [43], BNMs-based signal magnification methods have several possible benefits as well as some limitations and challenges. Nevertheless, BNMs are considered as dynamic ingredients in bio-diagnostic devices, fundamentally evolving the sensitivity and extent of detection for the discovery of sole/single element/particle [1, 3, 30, 32].

Therefore, it is remarkable to say that the evolution of platinum-based NMs for electrochemical magnification with sole/single label response for detecting the condensed concentration of DNA [30, 44]. Similarly, Niu *et al* [45] in their study stated that semiconductor QDs and iron oxide nanocrystals which have some magnetic and optical physiognomies that could be competently linked with cancer or tumour targeting ligands, such as peptides, monoclonal antibodies or trivial particles or elements that are aimed for cancer or tumour antigens with reasonable specificity and affinity [30].

Consequently, QDs machinery is beneficial for understanding cancer or tumour micro-environment for their treatment as well as for the transference of nano-biomedical purposes [23]. Also, the use of cantilever dimensions biosensor mechanisms such as 'milli-cantilever, micro-cantilever, and nano-cantilevers biosensors' are homogeneously analysed critically as a result of their vast benefits and applications [30].

The contemporary, fast and exciting evolution in CNTs has tremendously influenced the biomedical fields owing to the fact that CNTs are very sensitive to exposure to bioparticles as sensing parameters for biosensor mechanisms [16]. Subsequently, some researchers have employed much effort in the last few years globally to develop innovative biosensor mechanisms with reasonable sensitivity for the swift detection or sensing of targeted substrates. However, this chapter will concentrate fundamentally and briefly on some BNMs for biosensor mechanisms as well as some of their biomedical applications.

5.3 Bionanomaterials for biosensor machinery and their biomedical applications

Nanoparticles (NPs), which possess exceptional properties that make them advantageous in biological applications such as drug delivery, regenerative medicine, etc, are known as BNMs [1, 16, 24, 30]. These NMs are explored for several biomedical benefits, such as biosensors and tissue engineering [30]. BNMs have been evolving for various applications such as biosensing, drug delivery, and biotechnology/bioengineering.

The necessity of dimensions and biocompatibility made scientists explore more about BNMs to develop more exceptional functional possessions to apply them in biomedical applications. Presently, there are diverse categories of BNMs such as polymeric BNMs, metal/metal-oxide-based BNMs, protein-based BNMs, DNA/RNA-based BNMs, liposomal-based BNMs, dendrimer-based BNMs, semiconductor-based BNMs, etc [1, 16, 24, 30].

It has been reported that most of the present-day biological NMs (BNMs) for biosensor machinery development are primarily from biological compositions and procedures, which has given rise to several discoveries of robust and extensive investigative devices using biological sensing constituents [16].

Some of the biomedical applications of some developed BNMs biosensors as summarized from previous studies are:

- For investigating the quantity of $C_6H_{12}O_6$ in the biological sample and for diagnosing diabetes [1, 3].
- The dynamic investigative procedure for measuring glycated haemoglobin and diagnosing diabetes [1, 3, 31].
- For cardiovascular and investigating wide-ranging diseases [1, 3, 45, 46].
- For developing drugs and for visual/optical treatments [3, 45].
- For the control of biomolecular and reformatory treatments [1, 47].
- For evolving tumour/cancer biomarker, biosensing, bioimaging, and cancer/tumour therapy [37, 48, 49].
- For remedial therapeutic applications intended for disease/infection treatments and used for multi-layered aims such as biomedical mechanisms as well as analytical devices [1, 3, 4, 35, 36, 40–42, 44, 46, 50].
- For biological process consideration in addition to numerous molecular arrangements within cells [51–53].

Nevertheless, due to the broad nature of the BNMs for biosensor machinery, this chapter will concentrate briefly on discussing some of the nanostructured conducting polymeric (NSCP) BNMs biosensor mechanisms vis-à-vis their biomedical applications.

5.3.1 NSCP bionanomaterials biosensor mechanisms and their biomedical applications

As a result of the enormous applications of NSCP NMs in diverse domains, they have been given appropriate attention in recent times [1]. Consequently, NSCP has risen as one of the utmost auspicious constituents in several biomedical benefits, such as biosensing, tissue engineering applications, microelectronics, conversion of energy, actuators, polymeric cells, and several other biological applications due to their extraordinary stability, excellent conductivity, exceptional biocompatibility as well as their simple preparation techniques and excellent electrical features that could interpret biochemical statistics into electrical signals [1, 24, 54–57]. As reported by Soylemez *et al* [58], NSCP also has some functional groups (FGs) that offer extreme enzyme loading using the interface amongst the enzyme constituents and the polymers' FGs. Hence, restricted outline biosensors can be realized.

NSCP NMs have enormous application in the bioengineering domains due to their intense matrixes for the efficiency of numerous BNMs; they assist in improving the proficiencies as biosensors [1]. Moreover, some recent reports suggest that the combinations of metal/metal-oxide-based BNMs with NSCP assist in enhancing their sensitivity, compatibility, and stability as biosensors [24]. Accordingly, some procedures have been designated for evolving homogeneous nanostructures (NSs) thin layer metal/metal-oxide-based BNMs on the NSCP surfaces [1].

Presently, NSCP NMs serve as an exceptional building block for evolving vastly sensitive biosensors due to their exceptional properties that integrate with some other NMs resulting in the considerable surface area, flexible immobilization of biological particles quantum effect [59]. Some artificial procedures were designated for the synthesis of NSCP NMs, together with template-based procedures, template-unrestricted synthesis, and physical procedures such as electrospinning [60–64].

Fundamentally, polyaniline nanostructures (PNSs), which possess innovative sensitivity and tremendous response duration due to the progressive, dynamic surface area and the condensed depth of the penetration target of the particles, when compared to conventional ones, are one of the exceptional NSCP applications that have been established with the support of prototype-based polymerization within the domain of micro-permeable zeolites, permeable membranes, and chemical path composed with self-organized supra-molecules (stabilizers) [65–67]. Hence, there is an enormous diffusion of particles into the framework, making them relevant as biosensors.

The combination of metal/metal-oxide and coupled polymers to produce BNMs is projected to strengthen the electrical conductivity [68, 69]. One of the foremost topical critical deliberations has shown that Au and Ag NMs can be implanted into a polymeric film, which essentially improved the surface area to adjust the various biological particles. Lately, there has been extensive consideration in the classification of electrode modification applying to NMs as well as NSCP [1, 69–75].

5.3.1.1 NSCP-integrated electrochemical biosensor mechanisms

Some of the utmost topical established NSCP-integrated electrochemical biosensors and their biomedical applications as summarized and revised from previous studies are briefly discussed in the following.

5.3.1.1.1 NSCP NM for electrochemical detection of glucose and hydrogen peroxide

Due to the wide-ranging present-day nature of diabetes mellitus and the severe health complications universally, the problems arising from diabetes mellitus have been medically described to be more detrimental than diabetes itself [1, 76]. Hence, evolving specific and fast measures for its timely diagnosis is an imperative issue that should be given optimal consideration.

Diagnostic evaluations that have been described for the treatment of diabetes are typically based on the extent of $C_6H_{12}O_6$ present in the blood [77–79]. Supposedly, $C_6H_{12}O_6$ biosensors could be categorized as enzymatic and enzyme-unrestricted biosensors [77–80]. The emphasis here will briefly be on the applications of NSCP NMs for developing extremely delicate $C_6H_{12}O_6$ biosensors.

Saini *et al* [67], in their study, prepared PNSs applying sodium dodecyl sulphate ($NaC_{12}H_{25}SO_4$) as $C_6H_{12}O_6$ and hydrogen peroxide (H_2O_2) biosensor. The $NaC_{12}H_{25}SO_4$ serves as a suitable structure-guiding agent for synthesising the regimented NSCP composed of context protonated amine-like PNSs. Employing these NSCP NMs having enormous exact surface extent could increase the conductivity of PNSs and assist in controlling the high filling of horseradish peroxidase and $C_6H_{12}O_6$ oxidase to avoid many complications. Also, these NSCP NMs increase the quantity of conveyed electrons and the conversant reaction. These enhanced PNSs act as electrical and visual/optical biosensors with great potential for fast reaction duration, wide-ranging linear extent as well as decent selectivity, firmness, and duplicability [1].

In the same way, Yang *et al* [76] reported the fabrication and application of poly (3,4-ethylenedioxythiophene; which is the organosulphur composite with a chemical formula of $C_2H_4O_2C_4H_2S$) nanofibers (NFs) for electrochemical discovery of $C_6H_{12}O_6$ based on the captivation of the $C_6H_{12}O_6$ oxidase enzyme into the poly EDOT NFs via the 'galvanostatic polymerization technique' at platinum (Pt) electrode. This biosensor has been described to have enormous sensitivity and electrochemical stability, as well as the reduced extent of detection when compared to the g $C_6H_{12}O_6$ oxidase enzyme-integrated poly EDOT film biosensors' in relationship to their vast surface area.

Soganci *et al* [81] attempt to alter the 'graphite rod electrode' with a super-NSCP NM that consists of an 'amine substituted thienyl-pyrrole derivative' that is based on the electrochemical polymerization (ECP) technique. According to El-Said *et al* [1], this super-NSCP NM is categorized by the existence of free 'amine groups' that permits the covalent bonding of the electrode and the biorecognition particles (such as $C_6H_{12}O_6$ oxidase). This biosensor has demonstrated efficiency in the detection of $C_6H_{12}O_6$ in beverages. Also, Munteanu *et al* [82] demonstrated that a dual-electrochemical biosensor combined with 'optical-microscopy' as an opto-electrochemical biosensor could be useful for the detection of $C_6H_{12}O_6$ and H_2O_2. Supposedly, this biosensor's operational principle is based on osmium (Os, Ir) complex-based redox polymer applications. Thus, its oxidation state can be transformed when the $C_6H_{12}O_6$ and H_2O_2 are networking with the enzyme, and such networking depends primarily on time [1].

5.3.1.1.2 NSCP NM for cell-based chip

Customarily, owing to the fact that cells are considerably more intricate than the entirety of their machinery, it is stimulating to comprehend cell actions based solely on the amount of the nucleic acid or presence of protein levels [83]. Presently, there are reports about some electrically conductive outlines employed for producing cell-based chips to improve the bond, propagation, and separation of some categories of cells such as neurons [83–88]. Notwithstanding, the emphasis here will momentarily focus on NSCP-enhanced electrodes' applications in evolving cell-based chips vis-à-vis their biomedical applications.

Lee *et al* [85] produced an electrochemical conducting framework that consists of 'pyrrole N-hydroxyl succinimidyl ester and pyrrole copolymer', where they improved the 'copolymer' with a 'nerve growth factor (NGF)' which was helpful for the immobilizations of 'pheochromocytoma cells (PC12 cells)'. Allegedly, the cells have prolonged neurites consistently to that for cells that are cultured utilizing NGF.

El-Said *et al* [84] applied a 'thin layer of polyaniline emeraldine base' shielded 'indium–tin oxide/In_2O_5Sn (ITO) electrode as a cell-based chip. Correspondingly, the metal/metal oxide electrodes (PNSs emeraldine base/ITO electrode) displayed excellent electrochemical activity at a neutral (unbiased) pH level in the absence of co-depositing acidic counterion. Also, the established electrode was employed as a cell-based chip for a hasty and easy procedure for determining the cell electrochemical features, cell ability, cell bond, cell growth, as well as for monitoring of the implications of several anticancer treatments on the cell ability. In furtherance, they also used an *in situ* electrochemical combination of polypyrrole nanowires (NWs) and nano-porous alumina samples (NPAS), which also displayed the formation of remarkably well-organized porous alumina substrate (PAS) and the growth of the ester and pyrrole (PPy) NWs inside the NPAS via direct electrochemical oxidation of the PPy monomer [89]. The activities, morphology, bonding, and the cell's growth and the biocompatibility of PPy NWs/NPAS in the direction of both the study of cancerous complications were improved compared to other substrates. Supposedly, this is because PPy NWs/NPAS exhibit an enhanced cell bonding and growth, which has further proved the ability of PPy NWs/NPAS as a biocompatibility electroactive polymer substrate that can be useful for both dynamic and cancer cell cultures.

Strover *et al* [90] conducted another beneficial study where they combined 'pyrrole' and 'thiophene moieties' in their monomer for the production of polyPyThon-based molecular brushes. A film from this NSCP NM was placed on an Au substrate and employed as the support for the 'electrical stimuli-responsive surfaces of human fibroblasts cells.'

Hence, the cell-based chips' applications are an auspicious substitute for the use of animals due to the apparent deficiencies in animal models' applications, since they are heretical to animals' rights, complicated, expensive, as well as having reduced consequences for human environmental and biological science. Also, the applications of cell-based chips as biosensors for the management of the effects of anticancer medications or the management of the modification of the nervous cells revealed some advantages such as:

- Increasingly extra sophisticated illustration of circulation, absorption, excretion, metabolism, and harmfulness techniques.
- Exhibition of great possibilities in improving the prediction of medication proficiency and safety.
- Enhanced consideration of the medication interface machinery in humans.

5.3.1.1.3 Molecularly imprinted NSCP-based biosensor mechanisms

Molecularly imprinted (MI) NSCP NM is one of the utmost sensitivities and selective ingredients employed for the development of modern-day biosensors [91]. The fabrication technique of the MI-NSCP NM entails the application of some foremost mechanism such as; 'the embossed particles, functional monomers (FMNs) and cross-connector particles.' In the fabrication process of the MI-NSCP NM and its applications wherein the imprinted particles are combined with the FMNs to generate some reaction positions. The polymerization processes are somehow carried out with a cross-connector. The prototype particles are separated from the resulting polymers to generate imprinted cavities, possibly rebinding the prototype particles throughout the recognition progression. The selection mechanisms of the MI-NSCP NM to particles are connected to their equivalent chemical groups and the connections amongst the prototype particles and imprinted groups that are being exposed on the form as well as the stiffness of the prototype particles. Thus, these cavities could be used for enantiomeric purposes. MI-NSCP NM has been employed for electrochemical recognition of various targets [92–95].

The reduction of 'cyanocobalamin (which is among the octonary B-complex vitamins that could have effect on the mechanisms of the brain and the complete nervous system)' levels duplicates some health challenges like 'haematological and neurological syndromes' [1, 96, 97].

In the study conducted by Singh *et al* [98], they described the fabrication of biomimetic imprinted NSCP NM that comprises a sheet of condensed graphene oxide decked via multi-coated CNTs and methyl blue constituents and functionalized with poly acryloylurea. The established biosensor was employed for extreme trace detection of cyanocobalamin based on differential-pulse voltammetry (DPV) procedure, which showed a proportionality with the concentration limit ranging from 0.021 to 1.44 ng ml^{-1} with a limit of detection (LOD) of about 0.0056 ng ml^{-1} and basically without any interference in the authentic samples. Consequently, the amplified electrochemical conductivity of the biosensor was due to some interactions.

The fabrication of an IM NSCP-enhanced slick carbon electrode as electrochemical nonylphenol ($C_{15}H_{24}O$) biosensor was carried out by Liu *et al* [93]. The IM NSCP electrode consists of the surface of acrylamide-functionalized multi-walled CNTs as a transference surface, $C_{15}H_{24}O$ as a prototype constituent, methacrylic acid ($C_4H_6O_2$) as FMNs as well as ethylene glycol dimethacrylate ($C_{10}H_{14}O_4$) as a cross relating mediator, and the polymerization was supported based on the thermal polymerization technique. The established biosensor displayed a linear limit of concentration ranging from 0.1 to 30 μM with an LOD of about 0.02 μM.

5.3.1.1.4 NSCP NM for some other modern biosensor mechanisms

Presently, there is much conducted and ongoing research about the wide-ranging use of NSCP NMs for the production and development of biosensor mechanisms that have numerous advantageous influences due to the combination of their FGs during their production and development [1]. The applications of NSCP together with their compounds and their biosensor benefits to the diverse biological targets like nucleic acids (DNA/RNA), neurotransmitter, adenosine triphosphate (ATP), etc, cannot be overemphasized.

El-Said *et al* [99] developed poly[4-aminothiophenol] (PATP) NSs layered with Au nanodots (Au-NDs) patterned In_2O_5Sn (ITO) electrode, applying a simple procedure. The improved Au-NDs patterned In_2O_5Sn (ITO) electrode were established via an evaporated heat of pure Au metal on top of an In_2O_5Sn (ITO) surface employing a polystyrene monolayer. Subsequently, they used these Au-NDs as a model for self–assembly immobilization of ATP constituents trailed applying the ECP of ATP in generating the PATP. This enhanced electrode was employed for checking and managing the concentration of the combination of adenine ($C_5H_5N_5$) and guanine ($C_5H_5N_5O$) using LOD of 500 nM and 250 nM congruently. Similarly, the enhanced electrode was demonstratively employed for sensing $C_5H_5N_5$ and $C_5H_5N_5O$ in humans.

A selective electrochemical dopamine biosensor using polyimide (PI) and polyimide-boron nitride (PI-BN) compounds as a perceptive membrane for discovering dopamine was designed by Aksoy *et al* [100]. The application of BN constituents into the PI matrix led to the advancement of the sensitivity and selectivity and the rapid transmission of the electron (reversibility), with LOD of about 4×10^{-8} m.

Some pathogenic gram-adverse microbes could cause corneal ulcers and inability to see within two days; one of such pathogenic gram-adverse microbes is the '*Pseudomonas aeruginosa.*' Reportedly, pyocyanin (PYO) is the biomarker that has demonstrated enormous capability for their discovery and management [1].

Polyaniline/Au NSs (Au-NSs)/In_2O_5Sn (ITO) electrode as PYO biosensor in a culture of PNSs was prepared by Elkhawaga *et al* [78]. It was revealed that polyaniline/Au-NSs/In_2O_5Sn (ITO) electrode sensitivity nature toward PYO biomarker is greater than that of either bare In_2O_5Sn (ITO) electrode or Au-NSs/ In_2O_5Sn (ITO) electrode with LOD of about 500 nm. The improvement of the activity of electrochemical of polyaniline/Au-NSs/In_2O_5Sn (ITO) enhanced the electrode in the direction of the PYO linked to the existence of positive charges on its surface, which amplified the rate of transmission of the negative charged PYO based on the electrostatic force of attractive tremendously.

Also, Khalifa *et al* [101] applied polyaniline/Au-NSs/In_2O_5Sn (ITO) electrode for the diagnosis of '*Pseudomonas aeruginosa*' from fifty samples recovered from persons identified with corneal ulcers employing the 'square wave voltammetry (SWV)' method. Hence, their electrode was believed to be one of the fastest, economical, exact, and most selective PYO biomarker sensors in '*Pseudomonas aeruginosa*' for the corneal ulcer problems as a result of the SWV method, when compared to other conventional procedures such as the screen-printed electrode, automatic identification procedure, etc for the characteristic evaluation and identification of *Pseudomonas aeruginosa.*

Recently, the use of a zika virus (flavivirus) biosensor has been given appropriate recognition for development due to the virus-related infection in children (infants). Consequently, Tancharoen *et al* [102] developed a novel category of zika virus electrochemical biosensors, encompassing surface imprinted polymers/graphene oxide composites. The LOD of the biosensor conforms with that of the 'reverse transcription-polymerase chain reaction (RT-PCR) procedure'. Moreover, they can detect the zika virus in the presence of the dengue virus and serum samples.

Allegedly, another cellular metabolite with the potential to cause some severe health maintenance situations is lactate ($C_3H_6O_3^-$) [103]. Consequently, Pappa *et al* [103] designed a micrometer-scale polymer-based transistor model biosensor (MSPTB), which can be employed for the detection of $C_3H_6O_3$. The electron-transmission (n-type) biological polymer's application assimilated hydrophilic lateral chains, which boosted the ion injection, helped the enzyme unification and acted as a sequence redox centre. This established MSPTB showed rapid, sensitive, and selective metabolite possibilities.

5.4 Prospects of bionanomaterials for biosensor machinery

The pursuit and necessity for employing BNMs for biosensor machinery designed for instantaneous investigation with cost-effectiveness involve bio-fabrication, which has now paved the way for identifying the cells for effecting animal activities with the detection extent of realistic accuracy for a single constituent part.

The progression in biosensor mechanisms for the detection of biological warfare agents such as bacteria, virus, and pollutants are now occasionally employed for some techniques which today have enormous benefits in military operations [55].

Presently, integrating biological mechanisms in diagnostic devices, in the biomedical field, has become a requirement for the initial diagnosis of several diseases. The material physiognomies such as electrical, physical, chemical, structural, biological, or biochemical of BNMs are so sensitive to exposure to bioparticles, which has led to several research investigations. Although BNMs for biosensor machinery have been broadly used due to their enhanced performance, there are still some hands-on apprehensions, especially their applications. Hence, to effectively commercialize BNMs for biosensor machinery, several hurdles still need to be overcome; such requirements are the modifications of BNMs for biosensor machinery qualified with dramatic transformation as well as outstanding advancements and developments.

Supposedly, biosensors should be designed to work under multiplex and complex conditions [104]. However, some accomplishment has been demonstrated in this regard with some level for the potential for advancing their biomedical benefits.

The combination of BNMs and NSCP with different biosensor mechanisms has helped develop hybrid devices that have now enhanced their capabilities. Additionally, technological progression has been of tremendous assistance in biosensors using BNMs approaches that contribute to the biomedical, agricultural, and environmental science domains. Correspondingly, the hybridization of PNSs and BNMs offers excellent potential in the study of biosensors as a result of the enhancement of its electron conductivity and its ability to serve as a platform for the immobilization of the biological parameters. Hence, critical accelerated efforts and technological aspects on the development of various BNMs for utilization in biosensor mechanisms for various applications should be prospectively explored [105–111].

5.5 Conclusion

Owing to the present capacious research that covers NSc, BNMs for biosensor machinery as well as their biomedical applications have received significant consideration. Consequently, the exceptionality of BNMs is supreme when compared to any conservative material. Nevertheless, there are some limitations and challenges; for instance, there is a deficiency of macroscopic measures of manufactured BNMs that hardly suit the measure required for biomedical and industrial applications.

Hence, this chapter has provided a comprehensive overview of the topical developments and advancements in BNMs for biosensor machinery, specifically the NSCP BMNs biosensor mechanisms vis-à-vis their biomedical applications. Also, the prospects of BNMs for biosensor machinery are briefly discussed.

From evidence drawn from the reviews carried out in this chapter, it is evident that momentous research studies are still desirable to widen the scope of BNMs for biosensor machinery for diverse impending applications. Suggestively, since structural inconsistency and inaccurate fabrication have stalled dynamic and consistent application of BNMs for biosensor machinery in wide-ranging technology, the complete potential and the critical role of these BNMs for biosensor machinery could be accomplished when the limitations and challenges they encounter are thoroughly addressed in impending researches. Subsequently, imminent research perception should be anchored on enhancing and improving existing invention approaches on innovative ones. Accordingly, this would guarantee full exploitation and comprehension of the potential possessed by these BNMs for biosensor machinery.

Acknowledgments

The authors express their sincere gratitude to their respective affiliated institutions, the editors, anonymous reviewers, IOP Publishing team, and authors whose research materials and publications were used as support in the course of writing this chapter.

References

[1] El-Said W A, Abdelshakour M, Choi J H and Choi J W 2020 Application of conducting polymer nanostructures to electrochemical biosensors *Molecules* **25** 1–11

[2] Ukhurebor K E 2020 The role of biosensor in climate smart organic agriculture towards agricultural and environmental sustainability ed R S Meena *Agrometeorology* (London: IntechOpen) (doi: 10.5772/intechopen.93150)

[3] Stine K J 2019 Biosensor applications of electrodeposited nanostructures *Appl. Sci.* **9** 1–40

[4] Shao Y, Wang J, Wu H, Liu J, Aksay I A and Lin Y 2010 Graphene based electrochemical sensors and biosensors: a review *Electroanalysis* **22** 1027–36

[5] Nwankwo W and Ukhurebor K E 2019 An x-ray of connectivity between climate change and particulate pollutions *J. Adv. Res. Dynam. Control Syst.* **11** 3002–11

[6] Ukhurebor K E, Aigbe U O, Olayinka A S, Nwankwo W and Emegha J O 2020 Climatic change and pesticides usage: a brief review of their implicative relationship *AU-EJIR.* **5** 44–9

[7] Nwankwo W, Olayinka S A and Ukhurebor K E 2020 Green computing policies and regulations: a necessity? *Int. J. Sci. Technol. Res.* **9** 4378–83

[8] Ukhurebor K E, Azi S O, Aigbe U O, Onyancha R B and Emegha J O 2020 Analysing the uncertainties between reanalysis meteorological data and ground measured meteorological data *Measurement* **165** 108110

[9] Ukhurebor K E, Mishra P, Mishra R R and Adetunji C O 2020 Nexus between climate change and food innovation technology: recent advances ed P Mishra, R R Mishra and C O Adetunji *Innovations in Food Technology* (Singapore: Springer Nature) pp 289–99 (https://doi.org/10.1007/978-981-15-6121-4_20)

[10] Ukhurebor K E and Umukoro O J 2018 Influence of meteorological variables on uhf radio signal: recent findings for EBS, Benin City, South-South, Nigeria *IOP Conf. Ser.: Earth Environ. Sci.* **173** 012017

[11] Ukhurebor K E, Olayinka S A, Nwankwo W and Alhasan C 2019 Evaluation of the effects of some weather variables on UHF and VHF receivers within Benin City, South-South region of Nigeria *J. Phys.: IOP Conf. Ser.* **1299** 012052

[12] Ukhurebor K E and Azi S O 2019 Review of methodology to obtain parameters for radio wave propagation at low altitudes from meteorological data: new results for Auchi area in Edo State, Nigeria *J. King Saud Univ.—Sci.* **31** 1445–51

[13] Ukhurebor K E and Nwankwo W 2020 Estimation of the refractivity gradient from measured essential climate variables in Iyamho-Auchi, Edo State, South-South region of Nigeria *Indones. J. Electr. Eng. Comput. Sci.* **19** 276–84

[14] Anzar N, Hasan R, Tyagi M, Yadav N and Narang J 2020 Carbon nanotube—a review on synthesis, properties and plethora of applications in the field of biomedical science *Sensors Int.* **1** 100003

[15] Power A C, Gorey B, Chandra S and Chapman J 2019 Carbon nanomaterials and their application to electrochemical sensors: a review *Nanotechnol. Rev.* 19–41

[16] Sireesha M, Babu V J, Kiran A S K and Ramakrishna S 2018 A review on carbon nanotubes in biosensor devices and their applications in medicine *Nanocomposites* **4** 36–57

[17] Clark L Jr and Lyons C 1962 Electrode systems for continuous monitoring in cardiovascular surgery *Ann. N. Y. Acad. Sci.* **102** 29–45

[18] Turner A P F, Karubeand I and Wilson G S 1987 *Biosensors Fundamentals and Applications* (Oxford: Oxford University Press)

[19] Arora N 2013 Recent advances in biosensors technology: a review *Octa J. Biosci.* **1** 147–50

[20] Reyes De Corcuera J I and Cavalieri J 2003 Prototype instruments for laboratory and on-line measurement of lipoxygenase activity *Food Sci. Technol. Int.* **9** 5–9

[21] Borgmann S, Schulte A, Neugebauer S and Schuhmann W 2011 Amperometric biosensors *Advances in Electrochemical Science and Engineering: Bioelectrochemistry* vol 13 (New York: Wiley)

[22] Nwankwo W, Olayinka A S and Ukhurebor K E 2020 Nanoinformatics: why design of projects on nanomedicine development and clinical applications may fail? *Proc. of the 2020 Int. Conf. in Mathematics, Computer Engineering and Computer Science (ICMCECS)* (Lagos: IEEE Xplore) pp 1–7

[23] Long R, Guo Y, Xie L, Shi S, Xu J and Tong C *et al* 2020 White pepper-derived ratiometric carbon dots for highly selective detection and imaging of coenzyme A *Food Chem.* **315** 126171

[24] Zhou Q and Tang D 2020 Recent advances in photoelectrochemical biosensors for analysis of mycotoxins in food *TrAC—Trends Anal. Chem.* **124** 115814

[25] Kahn K and Plaxco K W 2010 Principles of biomolecular recognition *Recognition Receptors in Biosensors* ed M Zourob (New York: Springer) pp 3–46

[26] Mehrotra P 2016 Biosensors and their applications—a review *J. Oral Biol. Craniofacial Res.* **6** 153–9

[27] Bharat B 2009 Biomimetics: lessons from nature–an overview *Phil. Trans. R. Soc.* A **367** 1445–86

[28] Kabra S, Gharde S, Gore P M, Jain S, Khire V H and Kandasubramanian B 2020 Recent trends in nanothermites: fabrication, characteristics and applications *Nano Express* **1** 032001

[29] Rodriguez-Mozaz S, Alda M J and Marco M P 2005 Biosensors for environmental monitoring: a global perspective *Talanta* **65** 291–7

[30] Vigneshvar S, Sudhakumari C C, Senthilkumaran B and Prakash H 2016 Recent advances in biosensor technology for potential applications—an overview *Front. Bioeng. Biotechnol.* **4** 1–9

[31] Salek-Maghsoud A, Vakhshiteh F, Torabia R, Hassani S, Ganjali M R, Norouzi P, Hosseini M and Abdollahi M 2018 Recent advances in biosensor technology in assessment of early diabetes biomarkers *Biosens. Bioelectron.* **99** 122–35

[32] Turner A P 2013 Biosensors: sense and sensibility *Chem. Soc. Rev.* **42** 3184–96

[33] Citartan M, Gopinath S C, Tominaga J and Tang T H 2013 Label-free methods of reporting biomolecular interactions by optical biosensors *Analyst* **138** 3576–92

[34] Sang S, Wang Y, Feng Q, Wei Y, Ji J and Zhang W 2015 Progress of new label-free techniques for biosensors: a review *Crit. Rev. Biotechnol.* **15** 1–17

[35] Senveli S U and Tigli O 2013 Biosensors in the small scale: methods and technology trends *IET Nanobiotechnol.* **7** 7–21

[36] Guo X 2013 Single-molecule electrical biosensors based on single-walled carbon nanotubes *Adv. Mater.* **25** 3397–408

[37] Shen M Y, Li B R and Li Y K 2014 Silicon nanowire field-effect-transistor based biosensors: from sensitive to ultra-sensitive *Biosens. Bioelectron.* **60** 101–11

[38] Li M, Li R, Li C M and Wu N 2011 Electrochemical and optical biosensors based on nanomaterials and nanostructures: a review *Front. Biosci.* **3** 1308–31

[39] Zhou Y, Chiu C W and Liang H 2012 Interfacial structures and properties of organic materials for biosensors: an overview *Sensors* **12** 15036–62

[40] Ko P J, Ishikawa R, Sohn H and Sandhu A 2013 Porous silicon platform for optical detection of functionalized magnetic particles biosensing *J. Nanosci. Nanotechnol.* **13** 2451–60

[41] Lamprecht C, Hinterdorfer P and Ebner A 2014 Applications of biosensing atomic force microscopy in monitoring drug and nanoparticle delivery *Expert. Opin. Drug Deliv.* **11** 1237–53

[42] Hutter E and Maysinger D 2013 Gold-nanoparticle-based biosensors for detection of enzyme activity *Trends Pharmacol. Sci.* **34** 497–507

[43] Ding L, Bond A M, Zhai J and Zhang J 2013 Utilization of nanoparticle labels for signal amplification in ultrasensitive electrochemical affinity biosensors: a review *Anal. Chim. Acta* **797** 1–12

[44] Kwon S J and Bard A J 2012 DNA analysis by application of Pt nanoparticle electrochemical amplification with single label response *J. Am. Chem. Soc.* **134** 10777–9

[45] Niu X, Zhong Y, Chen R, Wang F, Liu Y and Luo D A 2018 'Turn-on' fluorescence sensor for Pb^{2+} detection based on graphene quantum dots and gold nanoparticles *Sens. Actuators* **B 255** 1577–81

[46] Farzin L, Shamsipur M, Samandari L, Sadjadi S and Sheibani S 2020 Biosensing strategies based on organic-scaffolded metal nanoclusters for ultrasensitive detection of tumor markers *Talanta* 214

[47] IKhimji I, Kelly E Y, Helwa Y, Hoang M and Liu J 2013 Visual optical biosensors based on DNA-functionalized polyacrylamide hydrogels *Methods* **64** 292–8

[48] Sode K, Yamazaki T, Lee I, Hanashi T and Tsugawa W 2016 Biocapacitor: a novel principle for biosensors *Biosens. Bioelectron.* **76** 20–8

[49] Peng F, Su Y, Zhong Y, Fan C, Lee S T and He Y 2014 Silicon nanomaterials platform for bioimaging, biosensing, and cancer therapy *Acc. Chem. Res.* **47** 612–23

[50] Valentini F, Galache F L, Tamburri E and Palleschi G 2013 Single walled carbon nanotubes/polypyrrole-GOx composite films to modify gold micro-electrodes for glucose biosensors: study of the extended linearity *Biosens. Bioelectron.* **43** 75–8

[51] Kunzelmann S, Solscheid C and Webb M 2014 Fluorescent bio-sensors: design and application to motor proteins *EXS.* **105** 25–47

[52] Oldach L and Zhang J 2014 Genetically encoded fluorescent biosensors for live-cell visualization of protein phosphorylation *Chem. Biol* **21** 186–97

[53] Randriamampita C and Lellouch A C 2014 Imaging early signalling events in T lymphocytes with fluorescent biosensors *Biotechnol. J.* **9** 203–12

[54] Kumar H and Rani R 2013 Development of biosensors for the detection of biological warfare agents: its issues and challenges *Sci. Prog.* **96** 294–308

[55] Arlett J L, Myers E B and Roukes M L 2011 Comparative advantages of mechanical biosensors *Nat. Nanotechnol.* **6** 203–15

[56] Navya P N, Kaphle A, Srinivas S P, Bhargava S K, Rotello V M and Daima H K 2019 Current trends and challenges in cancer management and therapy using designer nanomaterials *Nano Converg* **6** 23

[57] Kim J Y and O'Hare D 2018 Monolithic nano-porous polymer in microfluidic channels for lab-chip liquid chromatography *Nano Converg.* **5** 19

[58] Soylemez S, Kanik F E, Uzun S D, Hacioglu S O and Toppare L 2014 Development of an efficient immobilization matrix based on a conducting polymer and functionalized multiwall carbon nanotubes: synthesis and its application to ethanol biosensors *J. Mater. Chem.* B **2** 511–21

[59] Dhand C, Singh S P, Arya S K, Datta M and Malhotra B D 2007 Cholesterol biosensor based on electrophoretically deposited conducting polymer film derived from nanostructured polyaniline colloidal suspension *Anal. Chim. Acta* **602** 244–51

[60] Nandi M A, Gangopadhyay R B and Bhaumik A 2007 Mesoporous polyaniline having high conductivity at room temperature *Microporous Mesoporous Mater.* **109** 239

[61] Moulton S E, Innis P C, Kane-Maguire L A P, Ngamna O and Wallace G G 2004 Polymerisation and characterisation of conducting polyaniline nanoparticle dispersions *Curr. Appl Phys.* **2004** 402–6

[62] Mazur M, Tagowska M, Pałys B and Jackowska K 2003 Template synthesis of polyaniline and poly (2-methoxyaniline) nanotubes: comparison of the formation mechanisms *Electrochem. Commun.* **5** 403

[63] Lee K P, Gopalan A, Komathi S and Raghupathy D 2010 Polyaniline-based nanocomposites: preparation, properties and applications ed S C Tjong and Y W Mai *Physical Properties and Applications of Polymer Nanocomposites* 1st edn (Cambridge: Woodhead Publishing)

[64] Huang J and Kaner R B 2004 A general chemical route to polyaniline nanofibers *J. Am. Chem. Soc.* **126** 851–5

[65] Che S, Bennett A E G, Yokoi T, Sakamoto K, Kunieda H, Terasaki O and Tatsumi T 2003 A novel anionic surfactant templating route for synthesizing mesoporous silica with unique structure *Nat. Mater.* **2** 801–5

[66] Sawall D D, Villahermosa R M, Lipeles R A and Hopkins A R 2004 Interfacial polymerization of polyaniline nanofibers grafted to Au surfaces *Chem. Mater.* **16** 1606
[67] Saini D, Chauhan R and Basu T 2011 Fabrication of biosensors based on nanostructured conducting polymer (NSCP) *Int. Res. J. Biotechnol* **2** 145–56
[68] Moreno K J, Moggio I, Arias E, Llarena I, Moya S E, Ziolo R F and Barrientos H 2009 Silver nanoparticles functionalized *in situ* with the conjugated polymer (PEDOT:PSS) *J. Nanosci. Nanotechnol.* **9** 3987–92
[69] Melendez R G, Moreno K J, Moggio I, Arias E, Ponce A, Llanera I and Moya S E 2010 On the influence of silver nanoparticles size in the electrical conductivity of PEDOT:PSS *Mater. Sci. Forum* **644** 85–90
[70] Hussain I, Brust M, Papworth A J and Cooper A I 2003 Preparation of acrylate-stabilized gold and silver hydrosols and gold-polmer composite films *Langmuir* **19** 4831–5
[71] Cong H, Radosz M, Towler B F and Shen Y 2017 Polymer-inorganic nanocomposite membranes for gas separation *Sep. Purif. Technol.* **55** 281–91
[72] Feng Y, Yang T, Zhang W, Jiang C and Jiao K 2008 Enhanced sensitivity for deoxyribonucleic acid electrochemical impedance sensor: gold nanoparticle/polyaniline nanotube membranes *Anal. Chim. Acta* **616** 144–51
[73] Balamurugan A and Chen S M 2009 Silver nanograins incorporated PEDOT modified electrode for electrocatalytic sensing of hydrogen peroxide *Electroanalysis.* **21** 1419–23
[74] Dutse S W, Yusof N A, Ahmad H, Hussein M Z and Zainal Z 2012 An electrochemical DNA biosensor for Ganodermaboninense pathogen of oil palm utilizing a new ruthenium complex, [Ru(dppz)2(qtpy)] *Int. J. Electrochem. Sci.* **7** 8105–15
[75] Paulraj P, Janaki N, Sandhya S and Pandian K 2011 Single pot synthesis of polyaniline protected silver nanoparticles by interfacial polymerization and study its application on electrochemical oxidation of hydrazine *Colloids Surf.* A **377** 28–34
[76] Yang G, Kampstra K L and Abidian M 2014 High performance conducting polymer nanofiber biosensors for detection of biomolecules *Adv. Mater.* **26** 4954–60
[77] Zhu H, Li L, Zhou W, Shao Z and Chen X 2016 Advances in non-enzymatic glucose sensors based on metal oxides *J. Mater. Chem.* B **4** 7333–49
[78] Elkhawaga A A, Khalifa M M, El-badawy O, Hassan M A and El-Said W A 2019 Rapid and highly sensitive detection of pyocyanin biomarker in different *Pseudomonas aeruginosa* infections using gold nanoparticles modified sensor *PLoS One* **14** e0216438
[79] Lee J H, El-Said W A, Oh B K and Choi J W 2014 Enzyme-free glucose sensor based on Au nanobouquet fabricated indium tin oxide electrode *J. Nanosci. Nanotechnol.* **14** 8432–8
[80] Salazar P, Rico V and González-Elipe A R 2016 Nickel-copper bilayer nanoporous electrode prepared by physical vapor deposition at oblique angles for the non-enzymatic determination of glucose *Sens. Actuators B.* **226** 436–43
[81] Soganci T, Soyleyici H C, Demirko D O, Ak M and Timur S 2018 Use of super-structural conducting polymer as functional immobilization matrix in biosensor design *J. Electrochem. Soc.* **165** 22–6
[82] Munteanu R E, Ye R, Polonschii C, Ru A, Gheorghiu M, Gheorghiu E, Boukherroub R, Schuhmann W, Melinte S and Gáspár S 2019 High spatial resolution electrochemical biosensing using reflected light microscopy *Sci. Rep.* **9** 15196
[83] Yea C H, Lee B, Kim H H, Kim S U, El-Said W A, Minc J H, Oh B K and Choi J W 2008 The immobilization of animal cells using the cysteine-modified RGD oligopeptide *Ultramicroscopy* **2008** 1144–7

[84] El-Said W A, Yea C H, Choi J W and Kwon I l-K 2009 Ultrathin polyaniline film coated on an indium–tin oxide cell-based chip for study of anticancer effect *Thin Solid Film* **518** 661–7

[85] Lee J Y, Lee J W and Schmidt C E 2009 Neuroactive conducting scaffolds: nerve growth factor conjugation on active ester-functionalized polypyrrole *J. R. Soc. Interface* **6** 801–10

[86] Elkholy A E, Heakal F E T and El-Said W A 2019 Improving the electrocatalytic performance of Pd nanoparticles supported on indium/tin oxide substrates towards glucose oxidation *Appl. Catal. A: Gen.* **580** 28–33

[87] El-Said W A, Yea C H, Kwon I-K and Choi J W 2009 Fabrication of electrical cell chip for the detection of anticancer drugs and environmental toxicants effect *Biochip. J.* **3** 105–12

[88] El-Said W A, Yea C H, Kim H and Choi J W 2009 Fabrication of self-assembled RGD layer for cell chip to detect anticancer drug effect on HepG2 cells *Curr. Appl. Phys.* **9** 76–80

[89] El-Said W A, Yea C H, Jung M, Kim H C and Choi J W 2010 Analysis of effect of nanoporous alumina substrate coated with polypyrrole nanowire on cell morphology based on AFM topography *Ultramicroscopy* **2010** 676–81

[90] Strover L T, Malmström J, Laita O, Reynisson J, Aydemir N, Nieuwoudt M K, Williams D E, Dunbar P R, Brimble M A and Travas-Sejdic J 2013 A new precursor for conducting polymer-based brush interfaces with electroactivity in aqueous solution *Polymer* **54** 1305–17

[91] Rico-Yuste A and Carrasco S 2019 Molecularly imprinted polymer-based hybrid materials for the development of optical sensors *Polymers* **11** 1173

[92] Liu L, Zhu X, Zeng Y, Wang H, Lu Y, Zhang J, Yin Z, Chen Z, Yang Y and Li L 2018 An electrochemical sensor for diphenylamine detection based on reduced graphene oxide/ Fe_3O_4-molecularly imprinted polymer with 1,4-Butanediyl-3,30-bis-l vinylimidazolium dihexafluorophosphate Ionic liquid as cross-linker *Polymers* **10** 1329

[93] Liu B, Yan J, Wang M and Wu X 2018 Electrochemical sensor based on molecularly imprinted polymer for determination of nonylphenol *Int. J. Electrochem. Sci.* **13** 11953–60

[94] Essousi H, Barhoumi H, Bibani M, Ktari N, Wendler F, Al-Hamry A and Kanoun O 2019 Ion-imprinted electrochemical sensor based on copper nanoparticles-polyaniline matrix for nitrate detection *J. Sens.* **2019** 4257125

[95] Öndes B and Soysal M 2019 Determination of diuron by using electrochemical sensor based on molecularly imprinted polymer film *J. Electrochem. Soc.* **166** 395–401

[96] Samari F, Hemmateenejad B, Rezaei Z and Shamsipur M 2012 A novel approach for rapid determination of vitamin B12 in pharmaceutical preparations using BSA-modified gold *Anal. Methods* **4** 4155–60

[97] Nakos M, Pepelanova I, Beutel S, Krings U, Berger R G and Scheper T 2017 Isolation and analysis of vitamin B12 from plant samples *Food Chem.* **216** 301–8

[98] Singh R, Jaiswal S, Singh K, Fatma S and Prasad B B 2018 Biomimetic polymer-based electrochemical sensor using methyl blue adsorbed reduced graphene oxide and functionalized multiwalled carbon nanotubes for trace sensing of cyanocobalamin *ACS Appl. Nano Mater.* **1** 4652–60

[99] El-Said W A and Choi J W 2014 Electrochemical biosensor consisted of conducting polymer layer on gold nanodots patterned indium tin oxide electrode for rapid and simultaneous determination of purine bases *Electrochim. Acta* **123** 51–7

[100] Aksoy B, Pafsahan A, Güngör Ö, Köytepe S and Seçkin T 2017 A novel electrochemical biosensor based on polyimide-boron nitride composite membranes *Int. J. Polym. Mater. Polym. Biomater.* **66** 203–12

[101] Khalifa M M, Elkhawaga A A, Hassan M A, Zahran A M, Fathalla A M, El-Said W A and El-Badawy O 2019 Highly specific electrochemical sensing of *Pseudomonas aeruginosa* in patients suffering from corneal ulcers: a comparative study *Sci. Rep.* **9** 18320

[102] Tancharoen C, Sukjee W, Thepparit C, Jaimipuk T, Auewarakul P, Thitithanyanont A and Sangma C 2019 Electrochemical biosensor based on surface imprinting for zika virus detection in serum *ACS Sens.* **4** 69–75

[103] Pappa A M, Ohayon D, Giovannitti A, Maria I P, Savva A, Uguz I, Rivnay J, McCulloch I, Owens R M and Inal S 2018 Direct metabolite detection with an n-type accumulation mode organic electrochemical transistor *Sci. Adv.* **4** eaat0911

[104] Dias A D, Kingsley D M and Corr D T 2014 Recent advances in bioprinting and applications for biosensing *Biosensors* **4** 111–36

[105] Ukhurebor K E, Aigbe U O, Onyancha R B, Nwankwo W, Osibote O A, Paumo H K, Ama O M, Adetunji C O and Siloko I U 2021 Effect of hexavalent chromium on the environment and removal techniques: a review *J. Environ. Manage.* **280** 111809

[106] Adetunji C O and Ukhurebor K E 2021 Recent trends in utilization of biotechnological tools for environmental sustainability ed C O Adetunji, D G Panpatte and Y K Jhala *Microbial Rejuvenation of Polluted Environment Microorganisms for Sustainability* vol 27 (Singapore: Springer Nature) pp 239–63 (https://doi.org/10.1007/978-981-15-7459-7_11)

[107] Solanki S, Pandey C M, Gupta R K and Malhotra B D 2020 Emerging trends in microfluidics based devices *Biotechnol. J.* **15** 1900279

[108] Augustine S, Singh J, Srivastava M, Sharma M, Dasa A, Bansi D and Malhotra B D 2017 Recent advances in carbon based nanosystems for cancer theranostics *Biomater. Sci.* **5** 901–52

[109] Chauhan R, Singh J, Sachdev T, Basu T and Malhotra B D 2016 Recent advances in mycotoxins detection *Biosens. Bioelectron.* **81** 532–45

[110] Luong I-D, Roy I, Malhotra B D and Luong J H T 2021 Analytical and biosensing platforms for insulin: a review *Sens. Actuators Rep.* **3** 100028

[111] Ukhurebor K E, Nwankwo W, Adetunji C O and Makinde A S 2021 Artificial intelligence and internet of things in instrumentation and control in waste biodegradation plants: recent developments *Microbial Rejuvenation of Polluted Environment. Microorganisms for Sustainability* vol 27 ed C O Adetunji, D G Panpatte and Y K Jhala (Singapore: Springer Nature) pp 265–79

Chapter 6

Bionanomaterials: concept of nanomedicine

Kalpana Madgula and Venkata Sreenivas Puli

A rapidly changing global scenario demands diagnostics and therapeutics to be readily accessible and translated to clinical settings. Next generation nanotechnology is dedicated towards producing advanced nanomaterials relevant to diverse medical fields comprising bioimaging, therapeutics, targeted drug delivery and wound healing. Bionanomaterials are biocompatible materials in nanoscale dimensions, such as nanoparticles (NPs) of silver and gold, quantum dots, liposomes and so on. They can also be functionalized to make them biodegradable, stimuli-responsive or on-demand target delivery entities to harness their efficiency towards targeted applications. This book chapter mainly focusses on design strategies, current challenges and future directions for bionanomaterials in nanomedicine.

6.1 Introduction

Bionanomaterials have been considered to be materials at molecular level wholly or partially combined with materials of biological (e.g. antibodies, proteins/enzymes, DNA (deoxyribonucleic acid), RNA (ribonucleic acid), lipids, oligosaccharides, viruses, and cells) nature and in the nanoscale dimensions for biological function. In addition to this, nanomaterials in various forms are also engineered to deliver bioactive substances to the cells and continuously improved medical applications either in the form of devices or nanomedicine as in drug delivery, tissue engineering, disease diagnosis, treatment and monitoring. Further vectors or nanocarriers, i.e., in genetic modification, plasmid DNA or viral DNA and RNA serve as carriers to deliver genes that were cloned into the marked cells and similar to molecules or devices intended for drug delivery in pharmacology. The nanocarriers serve the purpose [1] of delivering active compounds, for example genes, proteins, medications or contaminants to the targeted areas of cells or to the other components such as organelles, cytoplasm or nucleus that are functioning within the cell or to the disease sites in the tissues while avoiding the loss of their activity and retaining the biological activity of these constituents before their accumulation in the targeted

doi:10.1088/978-0-7503-3767-0ch6

areas or cells. Sometimes, the nanovectors associated or loaded with therapeutic substances (or outer) surface are functionalized for a desired function, and to accomplish this they can also exist in various forms based on structure, composition or function, i.e., nanoconjugates, Janus particles, nanosomes, nanoscale mono/ multilayer liposomes or multifunctional NPs with dynamic nanoplatforms for molecular engineered biopharmaceuticals (as in figure 6.1(a)) [2]. The broad classification also includes NPs from biocompatible polymers, linear and branched (e.g. polyethylene glycol (PEG), polylactic acid (PLA), and dendrimers), lipid base carriers such as liposomes and micelles, and replication defective viral particles (RDVPs) as well. An RDVP is characterized by the presence of functioning defects in the viral genome, which is essential for viral particle replication or synthesis and assembly. Thus, RDVP viruses are expressed with missing gene product while proliferating in the accompanying cell lines; whereas in typical normal cells do not replicate into progeny virions, while expressing viral gene products sometimes serving as important probes to check host immune response to the infected cells [3].

Research efforts are in progress to extend to other non-biological objects such as fullerenes, carbon nanotubes (CNTs, single-walled or multi-walled) and render them biocompatible by the modification either by attachment (e.g. PEG) to an NP surface or by coating, or PEGylation. Nanocontainers are altered to drive the targeting purpose, by molecular groups that identify receptors on the surface of target cells, such as folic acid, antibodies. Other nanomaterial combinations can be nano-diamonds (NDs), graphene [4–6] and inorganic materials [7–9] like mesoporous silica NPs (MSNPs), superparamagnetic iron oxide NPs (SPIONs), quantum dots (QDs), plasmonic NPs, gold nanoclusters (GNCS), upconverting NPs (UCNPs), etc [10].

Nanocontainers where targeting molecules directly attached to the individual drug are developed without the need of any carrier. Such examples include, hybrid molecules (consisting of antibody to cell surface ferritin receptor and biotin binding

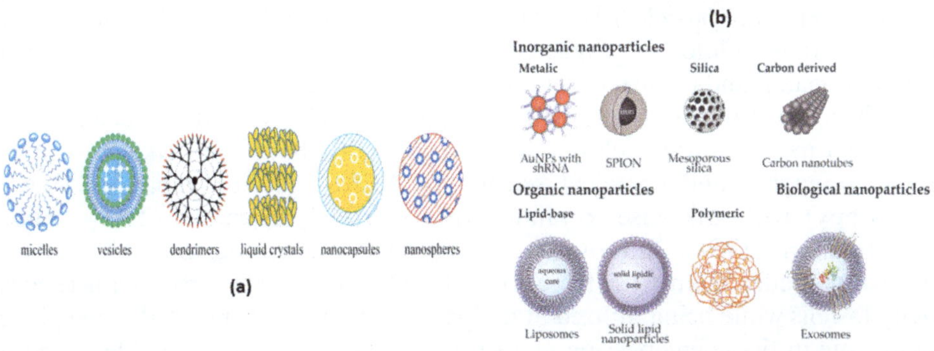

Figure 6.1. (a) and (b) nanocarriers or vectors for various modes of drug delivery for potential nano-medicinal applications and different classes of NPs utilized in biomedical applications.(a) Copyright 2017; adapted from [2] and, an open access article distributed under creative commons Attribution license (CC BY 3.0). (b) Adapted from [10] copyright 2020, an open access article distributed under creative commons Attribution license (CC BY 4.0).

protein, avidin) made by genetic engineering techniques, e.g. by chemical biotinylation of pharmaceutical ingredients or modification by biotin to ensure their delivery and strong binding to avidin. This ensures the transport of drugs to the cells, especially to central nervous system (CNS) cells through the endothelium of brain capillaries via active transport [11]. Due to the usual barrier function of some organs (e.g. spleen, liver, lungs) nanocontainers loaded with drugs can be accumulated in large amounts in these organs without the need of specific targeting. Similarly, accumulation of drug loaded nanocontainers can occur in tumors due to increased permeability of tumor microvessels, that allow bigger molecules and particles to pass easily from the blood to the extracellular space and in the extravascular tissues. Nevertheless, there is not much or low difference between the tumor tissue and normal tissue in terms of accumulating therapeutic agents, which creates difficulty in targeting tumor specific agents and requires them to be effective agents [12].

6.2 Types of nanoparticles

6.2.1 Gold, silver and other nanoparticles

Inorganic NPs, owing to their unique characteristics either alone or in combination with other materials, e.g. as composites, have contributed enormously towards biomedical applications because of their classical properties like large surface area, offering high local or surface concentrations, requiring low concentration of active material. In particular, NPs studied as therapeutic agents belong to the class of metals silver (Ag) gold (Au) and platinum (Pt) and oxides of metals, zinc (Zn) and cerium, etc [13, 14]. The characteristics like distinct size, shape, surface chemistry and very low impurities make them an ideal choice with advantageous results while interpreting and predicting their unusual properties towards optical, magnetic and electronic behavior [13] as well as catalytic behavior contributing to enhanced surface properties when existing in nanoscale size or due to their physical properties (e.g. platinum NPs) [15] or surface catalytic capabilities. Similarly, silver from AgNPs (silver nanoparticles) [16] or AgNP composites [17] contribute to antimicrobial activity. Gold NPs triggered a breakthrough as theranostic tools to lead extensive research and clinical developments for evidence-based approaches [18, 19] due to their usage in both therapy and diagnostics. The optical characteristics of AuNPs that include surface plasmon resonance (SPR) have been taken advantage of for bioimaging and chemical sensing by SERS (surface enhanced Raman spectroscopy) [20]. Likewise, ceramic NP oxides of zirconium (ZrO_2), silicon (SiO_2), titanium (TiO_2), and aluminum (Al_2O_3) that are biocompatible, are also prepared to render them with the chemical and physical properties with reduced toxicity to cells while being utilized in biological systems. Ceramic NPs have played a major role in tissue engineering and regeneration due to their tunable morphology, mesostructured existence and convenient functionalization [21, 22] large pore capacity (loading and sustained release of (hydrophobic) drugs or cargo) and surface functional (hydrophilic or bioactive) groups. In the same manner magnetic NPs (Fe_3O_4/magnetite and γ-Fe_2O_3) due their surface (or functionalized with biocompatible polymers)–antibody conjugation capability, and being target specific with externally controlled magnetic field, can also achieve separation of cells from biological samples or fluids. In addition, SPIONs, a kind of NP with remarkable magnetic properties at low size (average diameter ≈ 10 nm) are small enough to limit themselves to single domain state for efficient utility in drug delivery [23, 24]. The aforementioned basic features of SPIONs like morphological, crystalline and magnetic characteristics offer potential diversity towards targeting the drugs and ligands to facilitate their study by fluorescence and conjugation [25]. For instance, targeted drug delivery aimed at the possibility of locating and guiding magnetic NPs conjugated with drugs, ligands or genes can be visualized by magnetic resonance imaging (MRI) without affecting the healthy organs. Furthermore, local heating of these NPs by a high-frequency magnetic field helps to release the encapsulated drugs or to induce hyperthermia (to treat tumors) and also to aid in repairing damaged tissue [26–28].

6.2.2 Quantum dots (or carbon materials)

The properties of quantum dots (QDs), also termed 'semiconductor crystals in nanometer range', depend primarily on particle size and luminescence nature displaying photochemical and photophysical phenomena. The investigation of QDs started in 1982, and since then with quantum confinement, the size-dependent, small (that range from diameter in 2–10 mm) particles that are semiconducting in nature, with optical and electrical features have been extensively studied. The characteristic QDs are composed of an inner core made of an inorganic element (e.g. cadmium, mercury) and outer wide-gap semiconducting covering (e.g. zinc oxide). On excitation with characteristic ultraviolet light, QDs fluoresce by electronic excitation, and produce built-in fluorescence emission spectra from 400 to 2000 nm, a wavelength range that enables them to be utilized both for imaging and treatment. They are used as cellular labels for *in vivo* and *in vitro* fluorophores, and for imaging; and in nanobiosensors to track in the long term, image sensitive deep tissue, i.e. as contrast agents or as photodynamic agents to be guided by light; bio-barcoding, as NP mediated drug delivery tools [29–33]. However, their toxicity is an issue due to the presence of small amounts of heavy metal impurities and this restricts the human (internal) applications [34].

6.2.3 Other nanohybrid materials

Liposomes, 'lipos' meaning fat and 'soma' meaning body, are used because of their primary composition as phospholipid [35]. Primarily, liposomes are regarded as spherical vesicles with at least one lipid bilayer. They are composed of phospholipids, phosphatidylcholine or natural lipids that are compatible biologically and with lipid bilayer structure such as egg phosphatidyl ethanolamine, and thus can disrupt biological membranes to utilize them as a drug delivery carrier for administering nutrients, pharmaceutical ingredients/drugs or lipid NPs, e.g. as vaccines based on mRNA and DNA.

Since the liposomal structure (as shown in figure 6.1) is built up with an aqueous core and outer phospholipid bilayer, they can function by encapsulating or incorporating antimicrobial or immunomodulatory drugs that are both hydrophilic as well as hydrophobic in nature [36, 37], respectively. Properties like increased solubility, improved permeability along the biological membranes and consequent release of the encapsulants into the desired location [38] and no or minimum toxicity with side effects along with improved pharmacokinetics, targeted delivery to the infection site increasing the efficacy and efficiency of drugs, all make liposomes preferable nano-delivery carriers. Liposomes exist as multilamellar or small unilamellar vesicles or large or cochleate vesicles. Due to their unique structures, compositions, amphiphilic nature with distinct sizes, they are considered as imaging and therapeutics tools to diagnose and facilitate disease treatments [39–42]. Due to the inclusion of synthetic polymers, e, g, poly(ethylene glycol), PEG, in liposome compositions, long circulating sterically stabilized or stealth liposomes [43–45] can be prepared, and, further, a liposomal carrier surface functionalized with PEG can help extend the time of blood circulation along with reduction in system uptake by mononuclear phagocytes (i.e. stealth liposomes). This technique has helped in designing formulations with encapsulated active molecules having improved efficiency and activity towards the target. For example, PEG-based stealth liposomes have been employed actively targeted with monoclonal antibodies or ligands and subsequently the PEG coating helped distribution of the drug by prolonging the duration of its circulation [46, 47], but the liposomes remain inactive towards the mononuclear phagocytes and plasma proteins. However, the drawback lies in reduced encapsulation potency and shelf life due to the rapid leakage of active constituents or pharmaceuticals that are water soluble in proximity of blood ingredients.

Polymeric micelles (PMs) are formed into nanoscopic aggregations by the self-assembly of single chain amphiphilic molecules or block copolymers [48]. The versatility of core–shell structure with interior core of hydrophobic segments/tail with the ability to solubilize lipophilic substance and an outer hydrophilic head or corona, behave in stabilizing large layers built among hydrophobic core and the external aqueous environment (illustrated in figure 6.1) [49] and together make PMs a unique colloidal delivery system. The hydrophobic core encapsulates the drugs (that are hydrophobic in nature), proteins, or genetic materials, whereas hydrophilic copolymer block (exterior micellar covering) saves encapsulated content (e.g. drug) from outside the aqueous environment, and from the reticular endothelial system (RES) [50]. The variation in the nature of core block and its chemical structure of PM offers unique features to facilitate encapsulation of drugs, stability of micelles, and controlled drug release or delivery systems from the micro-reservoir. However, some of the drawbacks like toxicity, loss in shelf-life and biodegradability are due to the existence of covalent crosslinking in copolymers [51].

Dendrimers are another unique nanomaterial that display superior control on synthetic conditions of nanofabrication properties, such as shape, size, function and core, with inner void space. A number of terminal units or tree-like models are formed on the outer surfaces of dendrimers known to be dendritic branches [52]. Their host–guest chemistry fits the functions of efficient drug carriers, such as rapid cell entry, reduced uptake of macrophages, designating action at the site, evading the biological obstacle through transcytosis, as compared to other potential NPs/

liposomes. The first group of dendrimers that are commercialized and well-studied belongs to the class of Tomalia-type poly (amidoamine) (PAMAM) Starburst series. PAMAM dendrimers are functionalized with either amine or carboxylic groups on their periphery with a fixed chemistry to promote chemical transformations and increased solubility. Depending on the route of administration, drug bioavailability is enhanced by encapsulating and solubilizing feebly water-soluble drugs in the interior hydrophobic cavities of dendrimers [53, 54]. The physical and chemical properties of peripheral groups on dendrimers influence their loading and drug releasing capability.

Polymeric nanomaterials have been applied for the potential systems in medical applications, as an example gene therapy, an advanced treatment used to tackle various disorders in modern times. Gene therapy involved with delivery of genes in the living system is associated with barriers like efficiency of the delivery vectors or media to the target site. Non-viral vector delivery systems have characteristics such as low toxicity, effective in targeted delivery, stable in the long term, nonexistent immunogenicity and comparatively less cost, making them an ideal choice as gene delivery systems. Polymeric nanomaterials have come a long way; in 1987 Felgner *et al* applied cationic lipid polymer, non-viral gene delivery systems to the most recent US FDA (Food and Drug Administration) approved RNAi nanoparticle therapeutics that deliver the drug directly to the liver via an infusion, and thus disease-causing proteins [55] production was prevented by the body. The attempts are being made in the direction of resolving the issues of gene delivery, and safety aspects of viral vectors. Even though they are efficient, they need robust and significant attention for their safe delivery to disease systems.

Cationic lipid-based systems with negatively charged phosphate groups (as in nucleic acids) by electrostatic forces to form NPs or lipoplexes (non-viral, synthetic lipid carriers of DNA) are one of the primary polymeric systems utilized for non-viral gene delivery. These lipoplexes offer a variety of favorable factors for gene delivery, e.g. ease of synthesis to derive flexible properties, or conjugation of polymer with genetic material, and physiological pH among other properties. Some of them are synthetic polymers, i.e. poly(l-lysine), poly(l-ornithine), linear and branched polyethyleneimine, diethyl aminoethyl-dextran, poly(amidoamine) dendrimers, and poly(dimethyl aminoethyl methacrylate) and others naturally derived, for example, chitosan, dextran, and gelatin and also the combinations of both natural and synthetic, to achieve bio-reducibility. The advantage of tailoring the properties by tuning the combination to form biodegradable polymer systems has provided the capabilities of preventing toxicity and ease of elimination from the body without accumulation after repeated administration and targeted delivery [56].

Some of the polymeric nanoparticles showing reduced toxicity and highly efficient transfection, are produced from the class of diene-based polymers that are amine-functionalized, e.g. poly [2-(*N*,*N*-diethylaminomethyl)-1,3-butadiene] [57]. To direct the gene delivery to the affected tumor cells, often polymeric systems are functionalized with tumor targeting peptides, as illustrated in the case of human cancer cells, where peptide targeting glucose regulated antigens (or protein-78 kDa) is designed by a polymeric system made of linear, dendritic hybrid polymers [58] to deliver plasmid deoxyribonucleic acid (pDNA).

Polymers alone or in combinations (i.e. poly-lactic-acid (PLA), poly-d-l-glycolide (PLG), poly-d-l-lactide-co-glycolide (PLGA), and poly-cyanoacrylate (PCA)) have been studied to formulate PNPs [59] that are biodegradable. The extent of biodegradability in these PNPs, is influenced by factors such as monomer content, polydispersity index (PDI), molecular weight or the nature/type of cargo that is encapsulated in these polymers. PLGA NPs have been utilized as implantable materials to treat brain tumors [60] and others such as PLA, due to ease of its acid hydrolysis into lactic acid and then glucose with low risk of accumulation and favorable drug delivery entity to complex sites (hair follicles and sebaceous glands) [61], or base hydrolyzed PCA slow degradation rate (as compared to polylactides) beneficial for implanted devices for long term function [62].

Other characteristics include their unique ability to be functionalized by solubilization in a variety of solvents, to facilitate chemical modifications [63, 64], stability at high temperature, sonication or robust synthetic conditions required for functionalization of hard NPs, for example by polyethylene glycol or PEGylated NPs [65]. Similarly, the combination of a HA nanocomposite with PEI-g-chitosan oligosaccharide, and siRNA has been reported to treat endometriosis by targeting gene therapy. The effective delivery of therapeutic gene has been achieved in CD44 cells using this formulation, and significant reduction of clinical clues in tissues towards endometriosis was found along with favored biocompatibility in reproductive organs [66].

Another such combination that utilizes different bonds or chemical linkages in the NPs, is the case of hollow mesoporous silica NPs that are fist coated with cyclodextrins (CDs), conjugated with PEG by a linking moiety adamantine to mimic the natural environment of tumor having a change in pH and linkages that are cleavable [67]. PNPs are also subjected to extensive research and potential for large scale industrial production and employed/designed, sophisticated and precision nanosystems like automated Nanoassemblr® platforms [68]. These are aimed to modify the existing methods to generate non-spherical, or shape specific nanobiomaterials utilizing a costly top-down method copying the shape shown by the photolithographic mask, known as particle replication in a non-wetting template or PRINT [69]. Other simple, industrial scalable methods without affecting core NP properties may be single-step nanoprecipitation, that involves dilute solutions of polymers that result in less than 500 ppm solid content or multi-step, and nanoemulsion techniques that could facilitate the encapsulation of protein, nucleic acids or peptides to equip them with mucous penetrating abilities and enable their use in targeted respiratory treatments [70, 71].

The primary strategies to generate PNPs are dependent upon their efficiency to entrap moieties (water soluble or insoluble), size, or surface chemistry of the particles and NP/polymer complexes, e.g. polyplexes. The two approaches are: first, the top down [72–75] breaking polymers into sized particles (by solvent evaporation, salting-out dialysis, nanoprecipitation, and sophisticated supercritical fluid technology for high purity (rapid expansion of supercritical solution, RESS or rapid expansion of supercritical solution into liquid solvent, RESOLV), alone or in combination used for material systems such as PLA, without or with colloidal stabilizers like polyvinyl pyrrolidine, PVP or hydroxyethyl cellulose, HEC and Poly (perfluoropolyetherdiamide) and poly(heptadeca-fluorodecylacrylate) (PHDFDA) NPs); or bottom up strategy (as in emulsion polymerization) where the polymers, e.g. PMMA, PECA, and PBCA NPs, are produced by means of surfactant-based dispersion into solvents (cyclohexane, n-pentane, or toluene) as in the continuous organic phase [76]. With the recombinant DNA method, utilizing multiple functionality approaches, (e.g. as in amino based polymers, produced by *E. coli*, specific composition and function that depends on the amino acid sequence) in contrast to synthetic biomaterials, a single biopolymer can display multiple functionalities simply by protein expression changing [77, 78].

6.3 Bionanomaterials application in nanomedicine

The applications of nanotechnology have branched out among various disciplines with innovative and collaborative research efforts of chemists, biotechnologists and material scientists for biomedical applications such as delivery of genes, small molecules, cell imaging and designing the scaffolds for tissue engineering. Innovative medical technologies involving nanomaterials, as 'nanomedicines' are utilized for curing ailments, repairing damaged tissues, with therapeutic and imaging interventions that direct clinical and surgical practices. Henceforth, these advances will have a promising impact on the wide range of fields in medical diagnostics, drug development and clinical benefits [79].

Some of the significant features of bionanomaterials used for biomedical applications:

- ✓ The drugs associated with NPs do not adsorb easily (to plasma protein) and/or are protected from loss by circulating nucleases due to degradation.
- ✓ Nanomaterials increase the bioavailability of active agents at the target site as they escape reticuloendothelial system (RES).
- ✓ Drugs conjugated with NPs, offer several advantages—considerable reduction in clearing the drug from organs, and enable the drug to prevail in the proximity of target tissues for longer, as well as better *in vivo* stability and biodistribution, enhanced solubility of weakly soluble (in water) drugs, efficient drug delivery to the targeted site, release of drug in significant amounts to maintain efficiency.
- ✓ In the case of combination therapy, favoring either the macromolecular drug delivery or two or more drugs co-delivery to the action sites within a cell, or combining imaging modes with therapeutic agents can provide the capability of visualizing the sites of drug delivery.
- ✓ Additionally, the advantages in extension of half-life of an intended drug, increasing a hydrophobic drug's solubility, least potential for eliciting immune response (or immunogenicity) and toxicity towards the cells (or cytotoxicity), and/or stimuli-triggered uninterrupted delivery of drugs are also offered.

- ✓ Reduced toxic side effects as well as reduced frequency of administration is also possible due to the formation of drug–nanoparticle complexes.
- ✓ Next generation, smart drug delivery systems in the form of drug–nanoparticle complexes are in action for novel tissue/organ-specific therapies.

The following case studies have demonstrated the design of biopolymers to achieve endosomal escape. For example, 249AL, reported by Aris *et al*, is an engineered gene delivery system composed of oligomer of cationic lysine, K10 conjugated with ß-galactosidase-derived protein presenting a cell attachment peptide, RGD or arginylglycylaspartic acid. Here, condensation of plasmid DNA (pDNA) is supported by K10 and the interaction of RGD is with the αVβ3 integrin existing on the cell membrane [80]. The efficiency of the system was determined by complexing 249AL with pDNA encoding a luciferase reporter gene and transfecting $CaCO_2$ cells. The efficiency of the system and target specificity of 249AL is expressed by the percentage of transfected cells and total gene expression. As compared to commercial transfecting agents, the efficiency of 249AL was found to be less, due to inability of 249AL to escape the endosome [81]. In the same way, a biopolymer composed of cationic oligomer block, VGK8G, conjugated with elastin-like polymer, (thermoresponsive) with 60 repeats of Val–Pro–Gly–Xaa–Gly (VPGXG) has been reported by Furgeson *et al* as a recombinant biopolymer to be used in gene delivery [81, 82] and this biopolymer, as with the case of 249AL could not escape the endosome. Other groups have advanced the research efforts to overcome all these challenges to condense pDNA into NPs to induce significant proliferation of cells [1, 83–85].

6.3.1 Bioimaging

Nanoparticles intended for delivery of active agents or drugs have the unique ability to enter tumors by crossing the biological barriers through their localized and vasculature leak in the microenvironment of tumors and then are retained owing to poor lymphatic drainage. Thus, passive targeting is effected, also called enhanced permeation and retention (EPR) effect [86–88]. There is an ongoing debate over the effectiveness of active targeting (i.e. ligand/receptor mediated targeting) and passive targeting; in either case, the carrier has to be delivered to the intended site, before it binds to the receptors on the cell surface or is retained by any other effects [89, 90]. NPs aimed at nanomedicinal applications, need to be assessed for their efficacy and safe use in biological systems and that can be done by tissue imaging, carrier particle tracking after the drug is delivered, validating NPs performance once they are required and administered in the body. Similarly, elimination of particles is tracked or cleared via potential renal or hepatobiliary conditions. The imaging modalities provide the idea, whether they are eliminated or not. It is not clear whether the NPs degrade and are removed via the renal route, as they are not able to get filtered through the slits of the kidney [91, 92] and are believed to concentrate in unintended cells or organs. Thus a dynamic *in vivo* mechanism of NPs requires a better knowledge of nano/bio/pharmacokinetics. In view of the above conclusions, key areas of nanomedicine are focused on the imaging of functional and anatomical aspects to utilize nanomaterials utilized as contrast agents to help visualize deep structures of the human body and support clinical personnel in demarcating the healthy tissues from diseased and lead the way to deciding suitable treatment options. Engineering the nanoparticles can equip them with various contrast properties to be utilized for common imaging techniques and modalities such as: fluorescence imaging; photoacoustic imaging; magnetic resonance imaging (MRI); computed tomography (CT); imaging of radioactivity, like positron emission tomography (PET) or single-photon emission computed tomography (SPECT). The crucial aspects to utilize the above techniques depend on the use of advanced materials, ability to engineer the NPs to act locally (or in specific tissue sites) and effectively to arrive at high quality contrast images.

6.3.2 Antibacterial activity and wound healing

The propagation of antibiotic (or multi-drug) resistant bacteria and biofilm formation due to indirect transmission of contaminated surfaces is considered a major global concern. The common surfaces that include knobs, frames, etc. made of materials, i.e. steel, aluminum in the hospital environment pose limited or low antimicrobial protection and hence antibacterial coating materials that control antibiotic resistance bacteria have prime importance. Due to the increase in the occurrence of multi drug resistant bacteria, not adhering to the present treatment methods, it is imperative to explore the new material combinations, especially nanomaterial composites. The motivation is to achieve controlled or sustained release, improve patient confidence and adherence to the treatment and supervision and reduce the toxic side effects, thus increasing safe applications.

Antimicrobial dressings have been utilized to treat the infection after a standard treatment of wound [93, 94]. The untreated wound will result in chronic or acute wounds, especially in patients with disorders (e.g. diabetic foot ulcers) or deficiency in the immune system. In the case of normal or intact skin, the balance of bacterial colonization is persistent. This balance is endangered by wounds that trigger infection, and prevalence of bacterial species such as *Staphylococcus aureus* poses a risk factor for the recurrence of infection, subsequently leading to chronic wounds, which are majority contributors in clinical cases. Research efforts in wound care management are aimed at continuous development of novel technologies [95]. The combination of nanomaterials with biomaterials has made potential agents for antimicrobial activity in controlling infection due to wounds. Nanomedicinal materials and/or biomaterials are believed to mimic the skin's extracellular matrix in the form of nanofibers, films and hydrogels made of polymeric or non-polymeric combinations, and efficient strategies are adopted to incorporate and deliver bioactivity to enhance the healing characteristics and finally to arrive at smart, ideal wound dressings.

In this direction, one of the authors has investigated [96] polyvinyl alcohol-based silver nanocomposite (PVA-MFR/AgNP) films, sprays and dressings (as shown in figures 6.2 and 6.3), and reported elsewhere [97] antimicrobial activity *in vitro* towards the microorganisms responsible for diabetic foot ulcers. The antimicrobial

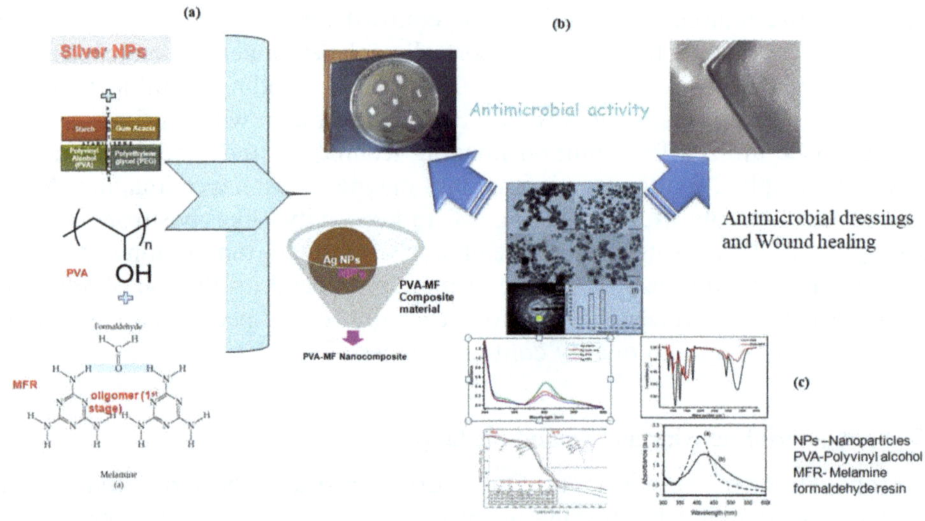

Figure 6.2. Investigation into PVA-based composites and silver nanocomposites: (a) scheme depicting the preparation of composite and nanocomposites, (b) scanning electron micrograph (SEM) of AgNPs (bare and starch stabilized), antimicrobial activity of films (activity studies presented in figure 3), and (c) characterization (UV visible, FTIR and TGA) studies of composites and nanocomposites (AgNPs). Copyright 2015, adapted with permission from [95, 96].

composites were cast into films, also soaked to form foams, and coated on Whatman paper. Antimicrobial efficacy of such prepared dressing materials was tested against the samples collected from the case studies and repeated over a period of time. The composites are reported to be stable and do not lose their antimicrobial activity with time. PVA and multiwalled CNTs (MWCNTs) scaffolds prepared by conjugation with glucose oxidase are reported for wound healing [98] in the literature. Recently, a few case studies were reported to check the potency of topical administration of AgNPs (1.8 mg mL^{-1} of metallic silver) along with conventional antibiotics employed for the treatment of diabetic foot ulcers of Wagner classification degrees II and III and other chronic ulcers [98].

6.3.3 Miscellaneous applications—special emphasis on cancer nanotherapeutics

Potential nanomedicinal research is progressing in the direction of cancer nanotherapeutics, which are the need of the hour. The World Health Organization (WHO), accounted 9.6 million deaths in 2018 to cancer, which is the second leading cause of death worldwide. The challenges in complexity and unpredictability of incidence of tumors has triggered global efforts focused on prevention, early-stage diagnosis, consultation, screening and treatments.

The key factors for tumor growth are believed to be instability in tumor cells genomics and proinflammatory environment, along with major and common characteristics of tumor cells leading to continuous proliferative signaling, evasion of growth suppressors, cell death resistance, deregulation in cellular energetics, promotion of angiogenesis, invasion and metastasis activation and evading immune

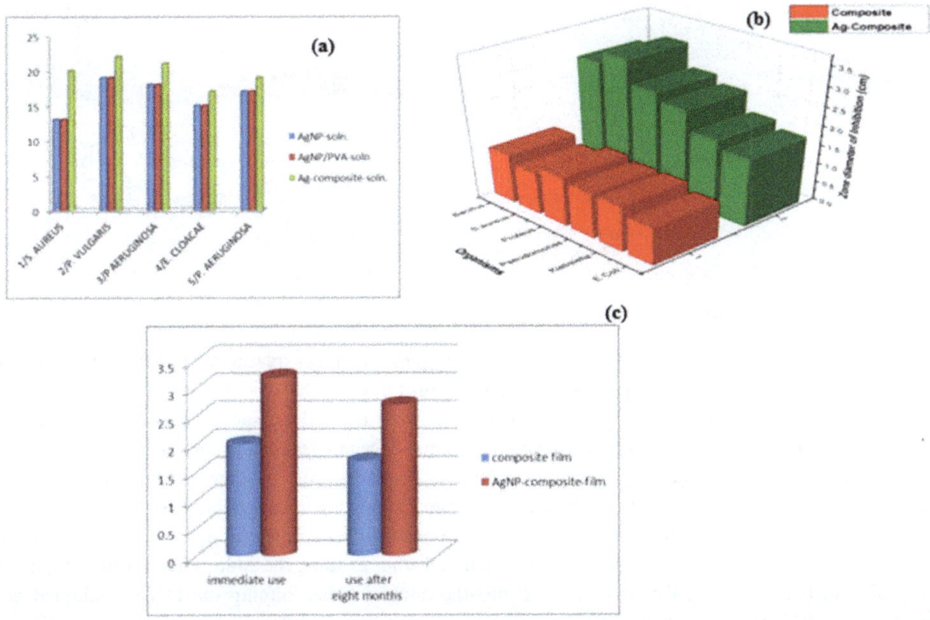

Figure 6.3. Studies on antimicrobial activity of AgNPs, Ag-PVA, PVA-MFR-AgNP by measuring the zone of inhibition: (a) susceptibility of microorganisms from foot infections of different diabetic patients showing highest efficacy in PVA-MFR-AgNPs in solution form, (b) respective solutions of sample (a) are cast into films, composite (PVA-MFR, red) and (Ag-PVA-MFR, green), and (c) *Pseudomonas aeruginosa* demonstrating the stability and antimicrobial efficacy of composite films even after eight months. Copyright 2015, adapted with permission from [96].

system destruction [99–102]. Figure 6.4(a) depicts the major strategies for cancer treatment by non-viral gene therapies and figure 6.4(b) displays the pictorial representation of systemic barriers required to be overcome by nanoparticles to arrive at effective gene delivery in the treatment of cancer [10]. Not only viral-based gene delivery, but also non-immunogenic and biocompatible NPs have raised success and are encouraged to show some clinical use. Even though novel nanomedicine strategies are believed to be useful prerequisite studies for *in vitro* and as proof-of-concept, a quick progression to *in vivo* testing is encouraging and some of them have displayed potential clinical utility. A number of clinical trials proposed recently using nanovectors for cancer treatment provide significant and promising gene delivery schemes and have employed lipid-based NPs and exosomes, owing to their reduced immunogenicity and ease in cell membrane penetration. Undeniably, clinical studies are in progress [103–107] that stress the importance of miRNA- and siRNA-based therapeutics in improving nanomedicine for treating cancer. However, the effective utilization of nanomedicine in the clinic is limited by poor study design, and would require more thoughtful investigations with sound knowledge in characterization of NPs and their biological effect. Moreover, the heterogeneity and complexity of tumors in the tumor microenvironment (TME) are still

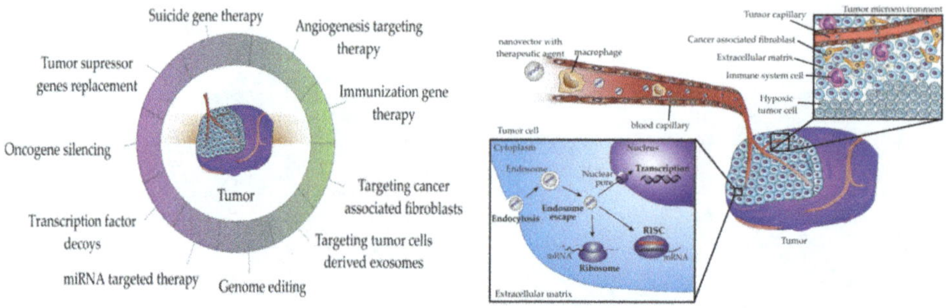

(a) (b)

Figure 6.4. (a) Major strategies used in non-viral gene therapies for cancer treatment. Therapies targeting the tumor microenvironment (in green), that include angiogenesis targeting therapy, immunization gene therapy, targeting cancer associated fibroblasts and targeting tumor cells derived exosomes, also use the molecular strategies as described (in purple), such as genes replacement, gene silencing, transcription factor decoys, miRNA targeted therapy and genome editing. (b) Barriers that NPs cross to effect potent gene delivery in cancer treatment. Passive targeting by NPs, due to accumulation in tumors to improve permeability and retention effect. NPs also cross barriers to infiltrate tumor areas with less oxygen (or hypoxia) and dense ECM. In the tumor cells, internalization of NPs or endocytosed and while evading the endosomes during cytoplasmic delivery of load (while aiming RNA) or ported into the nucleus (when aiming the DNA). Adapted with permission from [10]; copyright 2020, an open access article distributed under creative commons Attribution license (CC BY 4.0).

posing limitations and thus an effective treatment focusing on gene therapy, and the formulation of novel strategies using combination of anti-tumor therapies are required.

6.4 Current challenges and future directions

The chapter aimed to briefly summarize the fundamental nanotechnology methodologies and a number of (but not all) distinctive nanomaterials utilized for potential applications in the biomedical field. A quick mention of conventional therapies and innovative strategies in cancer research has also been introduced in the miscellaneous applications.

Although novel methods of NP synthesis have been introduced from time to time, the eco-friendly, sustainable and green methods utilizing plants and microorganisms and recent biopharmaceuticals have attracted much attention as preferred and extensively applied technologies while scaling up and translating into industrial or commercial applications [108]. As stated in a number of reviews [109], a nanomedicine product after therapeutic optimization is further refined with various stages, scaling up approaches (based on precursors or specific application), and approvals before reaching the final market release [109]. Even though enormous exchange of information with successful attempts and approvals is used while nurturing interdisciplinary academic research to clinical scenarios (as in the case of nanodrugs), industrial scale-up is still limited by the demand of large-scale funding, extreme precision, along with proven efficacy and safety [110, 111].

Safety and stability of (non-viral) nanocarriers are some of the primary challenges to be considered even while engineering the bio/nanomaterials for nanomedicine. Other challenges include immunogenicity, systemic toxicity, designing membranes mimicking the biological scenarios and tumor microenvironments, along with significant efforts to reduce accumulation in off-targets and trafficking, and also to encourage behavior only by appropriate stimulus response. The various modalities depend on the key points such as identifying the precise target for efficacy, tissue for exposure, safety of the model or patient to be studied and translating the benchtop research to a potential clinical or commercial setting without much modification. Most of these key points have been addressed by utilizing multifunctional materials that could facilitate monitoring the effect in real time, i.e. imaging, diagnostics and treatment, either by release control at the appropriate target or hand-in-glove strategy for therapy. Further, these are all possible by dynamic functionalization, complex chemical reactions with designed process parameters that enable tracking the elaborate metabolic (or degradation) products and nonetheless all amalgamate to increased costs, development times, and regulatory hurdles making expensive final market output. However, each new technology comes with its own value, and nanomedicine has allowed prevention, initial identification for detecting and managing the disease (e.g. preliminary malignancies in cancer), improved diagnostic precision leading to improved therapy and reduced demand for hospitalization and paving the way to full recovery emerging into cost effective treatments in future medicine.

Acknowledgements

One of the authors, KM acknowledges the support of her supervisor, Sumedh P Surwade, CEO and Founder, SAS Nanotechnologies LLC for encouraging work towards polymer nanocomposite self-healing materials. VSP acknowledges the support of Young Talent Fellowship (File number: 88887.468130/2019–00 funding by CAPES-PRINT Program—Call no. 41/2017), (PRINT-Programa Institucional De Internacionalizaa˜o), Brazil.

References

[1] Rajesh S, James W and Lillard Jr 2009 Nanoparticle-based targeted drug delivery *Exp. Mol. Pathol. [Internet]* **86** 215–23

[2] Fu D, Aman W, Ullah I, Qureshi O S, Mustapha O, Shafique S and Zeb A 2017 Effective use of nanocarriers as drug delivery systems for the treatment of selected tumors *Int. J. Nanomed.* **12** 7291–309

[3] Dudek T and Knipe D M 2006 Replication-defective viruses as vaccines and vaccine vectors *Virology* **344** 230–9

[4] Yu S J, Kang M W, Chang H C, Chen K M and Yu Y C 2005 Bright fluorescent nanodiamonds: no photobleaching and low cytotoxicity *J. Am. Chem. Soc.* **127** 17604–5

[5] Baughman R H, Zakhidov A A and de Heer W A 2002 Carbon nanotubes—the route toward applications *Science* **297** 787–92

[6] Nurunnabi M, Khatun Z, Reeck G R, Lee D Y and Lee Y 2014 Photoluminescent graphene nanoparticles for cancer phototherapy and imaging *ACS Appl. Mater. Interfaces* **6** 12413–21

[7] Colombo M, Carregal-Romero S, Gutierrez C M F, Morales L, Böhm M P, Heverhagen I B, Prosperi J T and Parak W J 2012 Biological applications of magnetic nanoparticles *Chem. Soc. Rev.* **41** 4306–34

[8] Parak W J, Pellegrino T and Plank C 2005 Labelling of cells with quantum dots *Nanotechnology* **16** R9–25

[9] Sperling R A, Rivera Gil P, Zhang F, Zanella M and Parak W J 2008 Biological applications of gold nanoparticles *Chem. Soc. Rev.* **37** 1896–908

[10] Roma-Rodrigues C, Rivas-García L, Baptista P V and Fernandes A R 2020 Gene therapy in cancer treatment: why go nano? *Pharmaceutics* **12** 233

[11] Kaparissides C, Alexandridou S, Kotti K and Chaitidou S 2006 Recent advances in novel drug delivery systems *J. Nanotechnol.* (Online) Available from: www.azonano.com/Details.asp?ArticleID=1538 DOI: 10.2240/azojono0111

[12] Beatriz Pelaz *et al* 2017 Diverse applications of nanomedicine *ACS Nano* **11** 2313–81

[13] Daniel M-C and Didier Astruc D 2004 Gold nanoparticles: assembly, supramolecular chemistry, quantum-size-related properties, and applications toward biology, catalysis, and nanotechnology *Chem. Rev.* **104** 293–346

[14] Singh K R, Nayak V, Sarkar T and Singh R P 2020 Cerium oxide nanoparticles: properties, biosynthesis and biomedical application *RSC Adv. [Internet]* **10** 27194–214

[15] Dongguo Li C W, Dusan Tripkovic S S, Nenad M M and Vojislav R S 2012 Surfactant removal for colloidal nanoparticles from solution synthesis: the effect on catalytic performance *ACS Catal.* **2** 1358–62

[16] Escárcega-González C E *et al* 2018 *In vivo* antimicrobial activity of silver nanoparticles produced via a green chemistry synthesis using Acacia rigidula as a reducing and capping agent *Int. J. Nanomed.* **13** 2349–63

[17] Kakkar R, Sherly E D, Madgula K, Devi D K and Sreedhar B 2012 Synergetic effect of sodium citrate and starch in the synthesis of silver nanoparticles *J. Appl. Polym. Sci.* **126** E154–61

[18] Dreaden E C, Alaaldin M, Alkilany X H, Murphy C J and El-Sayed M A 2012 The golden age: gold nanoparticles for biomedicine *Chem. Soc. Rev.* **41** 2740–79

[19] Riley R S and Day E S 2017 Gold nanoparticle-mediated photothermal therapy: applications and opportunities for multimodal cancer treatment *Wiley Interdiscip. Rev. Nanomed. Nanobiotechnol.* **9** e1449

[20] Soliman M G, Pelaz B, Parak W J and del Pino P 2015 Phase transfer and polymer coating methods toward improving the stability of metallic nanoparticles for biological applications *Chem. Mater.* **27** 990–7

[21] Popat A, Hartono S B, Stahr F, Qiao L J and Qing S Z M 2011 Mesoporous silica nanoparticles for bioadsorption, enzyme immobilization, and delivery carriers *Nanoscale* **3** 2801–18

[22] Mai W X and Meng H 2013 Mesoporous silica nanoparticles: a multifunctional nano-therapeutic systems *Integr. Biol. (Chamb.)* **5** 19–28

[23] Hadjipanayis C G, Machaidze R K, Wang M, Schuetter L and Chen A J H 2010 EGFR v III antibody-conjugated iron oxide nanoparticles for magnetic resonance imaging-guided convection-enhanced delivery and targeted therapy of glioblastoma *Cancer Res.* **70** 6303–12

[24] Smith J E, Sapsford K E, Tan W and Ligler F S 2011 Optimization of antibody conjugated magnetic nanoparticles for target preconcentration and immunoassays *Anal. Biochem.* **410** 124–32

[25] Patil U S, Adireddy S, Jaiswal A, Mandava S, Lee B R and Douglas B 2015 *In vitro/in vivo* toxicity evaluation and quantification of iron oxide nanoparticles *Int. J. Mol. Sci.* **16** 24417–50

[26] Wang W, Xu Y, Wang D I and LI Z 2009 Recyclable nanobiocatalyst for enantioselective sulfoxidation: Facile fabrication and high performance of chloroperoxidase-coated magnetic nanoparticles with iron oxide core and polymer shell *J. Am. Chem. Soc.* **131** 12892–3

[27] Cherukuri P, Glazer E S and Curley S A 2010 Targeted hyperthermia using metal nanoparticles *Adv. Drug Delivery Rev.* **62** 339–45

[28] Kai W, Xiaojun X, Ximing P, Zhenqing H and Qiqing Z 2011 Cytotoxic effects and the mechanism of three types of magnetic nanoparticles on human hepatoma BEL-7402 cells *Nanoscale Res. Lett.* **6** 480

[29] Petryayeva E, Medintz I L and ALgar W R 2013 Quantum dots in bioanalysis: a review of applications across various platforms for fluorescence spectroscopy and imaging *Appl. Spectrose* **67** 215–52

[30] Rosenthal S J, Chang J C, Kovtun O, McBride J R and Tomlinaon I D 2011 Biocompatible quantum dots for biological applications *Chem. Biol.* **18** 10–24

[31] Algar W R and Krull U J 2010 New opportunities in multiplexed optical bioanalyses using quantum dots and donor-acceptor interactions *Anal. Bional. Chem.* **398** 2439–49

[32] Walters R, Kraig R P, Meintz I L, Delehanty J B, Steart M H and Susumu K 2012 Nanoparticle targeting to neurons in a rat hippocampal slice culture model *ASN Neuro* **4** e00099

[33] Spillmann C M and Ancona M G 2013 Achieving effective terminal exciton delivery in quantum dot antenna-sensitized multistep DNA photonic wires *ACS Nano* **7** 7101–18

[34] Derfus A M, Chan W C W and Bhatia S N 2004 Probing the cytotoxicity of semiconductor quantum dots *Nano Lett.* **4** 11–8

[35] Melis Çağdaş A D S and Buca S 2014 Liposomes as potential drug carrier systems for drug delivery *Application of Nanotechnology in Drug Delivery* (Rijeka: InTech) ch 1 pp 1–51

[36] Sosnik A, Carcaboso A M, Romina A L, Glisoni J, Moretton M A and Chiappetta D A 2010 New old challenges in tuberculosis: potentially effective nanotechnologies in drug delivery *Adv. Drug Del. Rev.* **62** 547–49

[37] Tagawa T and Liposome U M 2007 *Google Patents US* 200770248541

[38] Yang D, Pornapattananangkul D, Nakatsuji T and Chan M 2009 The antimicrobial activity of liposomal lauric acids against propionibacterium acnes *Biomaterials* **30** 6035–40

[39] Vasir J K and Labhasetwar V 2007 Biodegradable nanoparticles for cytosolic delivery of therapeutics *Adv. Drug Deliv. Rev.* **59** 718–28

[40] Torchilin V P 2008 Antibody-modified liposomes for cancer chemotherapy *Exp. Opin. Drug Deliv.* **5** 1003–25

[41] Zylberberg C and Matosevic S 2016 Pharmaceutical liposomal drug delivery: a review of new delivery systems and a look at the regulatory landscape *Drug Deliv.* **23** 3319–29

[42] Lou J and Best M D 2020 A general approach to enzyme-responsive liposomes *Chem.—A Eur. J.* **26** 8597–607

[43] Immordino M L, Dosio F and Cattel L 2006 Stealth liposomes: review of the basic science, rationale, and clinical applications, existing and potential *Int. J. Nanomed.* **1** 297–315

[44] Nag O K and Awasthi V 2013 Surface engineering of liposomes for stealth behavior *Pharmaceutics* **5** 542–69
[45] Leaf H 1992 Stealth liposomes, ninja liposomes, or cryptosomes: are they really sterically stabilized liposomes? *J. Liposome Res.* **2** 451–4
[46] Ferrari M 2005 Cancer nanotechnology: opportunities and challenges *Nat. Rev. Cancer* **5** 161–71
[47] Fassas A and Anagnostopoulos A 2005 The use of liposomal daunorubicin (DaunoXome) in acute myeloid leukemia *Lymphoma* **46** 795–802
[48] Moom S A, Mima K and Dusan L 2013 Polymeric micelles for multidrug delivery and combination therapy *Chem. Eur. J.* **19** 12586–601
[49] Aliabadi H M and Lavasanifar A 2006 Polymeric micelles for drug delivery *Exp. Opin. Drug Deliv.* **3** 139–62
[50] Bronich T K, Kobanov V A, Kobanov A V and Esenberg A 1997 Soluble complexes from poly (ethylene oxide)-block-olymethacrylate anions and *N*-alkylpyramdinium cations *Macromolecules* **30** 3519–25
[51] Yuichi O 2013 Polymeric micelles stabilized by electrostatic interactions for drug delivery *Tailored Polymer Architectures for Pharmaceutical and Biomedical Applications (ACS Symposium Series)* (Washington, DC: American Chemical Society) p 1135
[52] Menjoge A R, Kannan R M and Tomalia D A 2010 Dendrimer-based drug and imaging conjugates: design considerations for nanomedical applications *Drug Disc. Today* **15** 171–85
[53] D'Emanuele A and Attwood D 2005 Dendrimer-drug interaction *Ad. Drug Deliv. Rev.* **57** 2147–62
[54] Jain N K and Gupta U 2008 Application of dendrimer-drug complexation in the enhancement of drug solubility and bioavailability *Expert Opin. Drug Metab. Toxicol.* **8** 1035–52
[55] Alnylam Pharmaceuticals Inc. 2019 Alnylam Announces First-Ever FDA Approval of an RNAi Therapeutic, ONPATTRO™ (patisiran) for the Treatment of the Polyneuropathy of Hereditary Transthyretin-Mediated Amyloidosis in Adults. Available online: http://investors.alnylam.com/news-releases/news-release-details/alnylam-announces-first-ever-fda-approval-rnai-therapeutic (Accessed on 23 April)
[56] Bolhassani A, Javanzad S, Saleh T, Hashemi M, Aghasadeghi M and Sadat S 2014 Polymeric nanoparticles potent vectors for vaccine delivery targeting cancer and infectious diseases *Hum. Vaccin. Immunother* **10** 321–32
[57] Yang Y, Lee J, Cho M and Sheares V 2006 Synthesis of amine-functionalized diene-based polymers as novel gene delivery vectors *Macromolecules* **39** 8625–31
[58] Wood K, Azarin S, Arap W, Pasqualini R, Langer R and Hammond P 2008 Tumor-targeted gene delivery using molecularly engineered hybrid polymers functionalized with a tumor-homing peptide *Bioconjug. Chem.* **19** 403–5
[59] Mahapatro A and Singh D 2011 Biodegradable nanoparticles are excellent vehicle for site directed in-vivo delivery of drugs and vaccines *J. Nanobiotechnol.* **9** 55
[60] Brem H and Gabikian P 2001 Biodegradable polymer implants to treat brain tumors *J. Control. Release* **74** 63–7
[61] Rancan F, Papakostas D, Hadam S, Hackbarth S, Delair T, Primard C, Verrier B, Sterry W, Blume-Peytavi U and Vogt A 2009 Investigation of polylactic acid (PLA) nanoparticles as drug delivery systems for local dermatotherapy *Pharm. Res.* **26** 2027–36

[62] Han M, Kim S and Liu S 2008 Synthesis and degradation behavior of poly(ethyl cyanoacrylate) *Polym. Degrad. Stab.* **93** 1243–51

[63] Zubris K, Khullar O, Griset A, Gibbs-Strauss S, Frangioni J, Colson Y and Grinstaff M 2010 Ease of synthesis, controllable sizes, and *in vivo* large animal lymph migration of polymeric nanoparticles *Chem. Med. Chem.* **5** 1435–8

[64] Watkins R, Wu L, Zhang C, Davis R and Xu B 2015 Natural product-based nanomedicine: recent advances and issues *Int. J. Nanomed.* **10** 6055–74

[65] Fang Y P, Wu P C, Huang Y B, Tzeng C C, Chen Y H, Hung Y H, Tsai M J and Tsai Y H 2012 Modification of polyethylene glycol onto solid lipid nanoparticles encapsulating a novel chemotherapeutic agent (PK-L4) to enhance solubility for injection delivery *Int. J. Nanomed.* **7** 4995–5005

[66] Zhao M *et al* 2016 Hyaluronic acid reagent functional chitosan-PEI conjugate with AQP2-siRNA suppressed endometriotic lesion formation *Int. J. Nanomed.* **11** 1323–36

[67] Liu J, Luo Z, Zhang J, Luo T, Zhou J, Zhao X and Cai K 2016 Hollow mesoporous silica nanoparticles facilitated drug delivery via cascade pH stimuli in tumor microenvironment for tumor therapy *Biomaterials* **83** 51–65

[68] Florez L, Herrmann C, Cramer J M, Hauser C P, Koynov K, Landfester K, Crespy D and Mailänder V 2012 How shape influences uptake: interactions of anisotropic polymer nanoparticles and human mesenchymal stem cells *Small* **8** 2222–30

[69] Rolland J P, Maynor B W, Euliss L E, Exner A E, Denison G M and DeSimone J M 2005 Direct fabrication and harvesting of monodisperse, shape-specific nanobiomaterials *J. Am. Chem. Soc.* **127** 10096–100

[70] Behrendt J, Guzman J, Purdie L, Willcock H, Morrison J, Foster A, O'Reilly R, McCairn M and Turner M 2016 Scalable synthesis of multicolour conjugated polymer nanoparticles via Suzuki-Miyaura polymerisation in a miniemulsion and application in bioimaging *React. Funct. Polym.* **107** 69–77

[71] Xu Q, Boylan N J, Cai S, Miao B, Patel H and Hanes J 2013 Scalable method to produce biodegradable nanoparticles that rapidly penetrate human mucus *J. Control. Release* **170** 279–86

[72] Zambaux M F, Bonneaux F, Gref R, Maincent P, Dellacherie E, Alonso M J, Labrude P and Vigneron C 1998 Influence of experimental parameters on the characteristics of poly (lactic acid) nanoparticles prepared by a double emulsion method *J. Control. Release* **50** 31–40

[73] Zhang Z, Grijpma D W and Feijen J 2006 Poly (trimethylene carbonate) and monomethoxy poly(ethylene glycol)-block-poly(trimethylene carbonate) nanoparticles for the controlled release of dexamethasone *J. Control. Release* **111** 263–70

[74] Fattahi A, Karimi-Sabet J, Keshavarz A, Golzary A, Rafiee-Tehrani M and Farid A 2012 Dorkoosh. Preparation and characterization of raloxifene nanoparticles using rapid expansion of supercritical solution (RESS) *J. Supercrit. Fluids* **63** 169–79

[75] Meziani M, Pathak P, Hurezeanu R, Thies M, Enick R and Sun Y 2004 Supercritical-fluid processing technique for nanoscale polymer particles *Angew. Chem. Int. Ed.* **43** 704–7

[76] Reis C P, Neufeld R J, Ribeiro A J and Veiga F 2006 Nanoencapsulation I. Methods for preparation of drug-loaded polymeric nanoparticles *Nanomedicine* **2** 8–21

[77] Canine B and Hatefi A 2010 Development of recombinant cationic polymers for gene therapy research *Adv. Drug Deliv. Rev.* **62** 1524–9

[78] Ghoderao P, Sanghavi S, Bhave T and Kulkarni A A 2019 Drug-coated nanoparticles: the magic bullets for threatening diseases, with special reference to tuberculosis *Materials for Biomedical Engineering: Nanomaterials-Based Drug Delivery* (Amsterdam: Elsevier) 41–84

[79] Salata O V 2004 Applications of nanoparticles in biology and medicine *J. Nanobiotechnol.* **2** 3

[80] Thanki K, Zeng X and Foged C 2019 Preparation, characterization, and *in vitro* evaluation of lipidoid-polymer hybrid nanoparticles for siRNA delivery to the cytosol *Methods Mol. Biol.* **1943** 141–52

[81] Gessner I, Yu X, Jungst C, Klimpel A, Wang L, Fischer T, Neundorf I, Schauss A C, Odenthal M and Mathur S 2019 Selective capture and purification of microRNAs and intracellular proteins through antisense-vectorized magnetic nanobeads *Sci Rep.* **9** 2069

[82] Syed S N, Frank A C, Raue R and Brune B 2019 MicroRNA-A tumor trojan horse for tumor-associated macrophages *Cells* **8** 1482

[83] Chen X *et al* 2019 Identifying and targeting angiogenesis-related microRNAs in ovarian cancer *Oncogene* **38** 6095–108

[84] Lo A *et al* 2015 Tumor-promoting desmoplasia is disrupted by depleting FAP-expressing stromal cells *Cancer Res.* **75** 2800–10

[85] Wang L C *et al* 2014 Targeting fibroblast activation protein in tumor stroma with chimeric antigen receptor T cells can inhibit tumor growth and augment host immunity without severe toxicity *Canc. Immunol. Res.* **2** 154–66

[86] Zhang Q *et al* 2012 Mechanical properties and biomineralization of multifunctional nanodiamond-PLLA composites for bone tissue engineering *Biomaterials* **33** 5067–75

[87] Altinoğlu E I, Russin T J, Kaiser J M, Barth B M, Eklund P C, Kester M and Adair J H 2008 Near-infrared emitting fluorophore-doped calcium phosphate nanoparticles for *in vivo* imaging of human breast cancer *ACS Nano* **2** 2075–84

[88] Matsumura Y and Maeda H 1986 A new concept for macromolecular therapeutics in cancer chemotherapy: mechanism of tumoritropic accumulation of proteins and the antitumor agent smancs *Cancer Res.* **46** 6387–92

[89] Wilhelm S *et al* 2016 Analysis of nanoparticle delivery to tumors *Nat. Rev. Mater.* **1** 16014

[90] Kolosnjaj-Tabi J *et al* 2015 The one year fate of iron oxide coated gold nanoparticles in mice *ACS Nano* **9** 7925–39

[91] Chou L Y, Zagorovsky K and Chan W C 2014 DNA assembly of nanoparticle superstructures for controlled biological delivery and elimination *Nat. Nanotechnol.* **9** 148–55

[92] Kreyling W G *et al* 2015 *In vivo* integrity of polymer-coated gold nanoparticles *Nat. Nanotechnol.* **10** 619–23

[93] Dreifke M B, Jayasuriya A A and Jayasuriya A C 2015 Current wound healing procedures and potential care *Mater. Sci. Eng.* C **48** 651–62

[94] Suarato G, Bertorelli R and Athanassiou A 2018 Borrowing from nature: biopolymers and biocomposites as smart wound care materials *Front. Bioeng. Biotechnol.* **6** 137

[95] Kakkar R, Madgula K, Saritha Nehru Y V, Shailaja R M and Sreedhar B 2014 Polyvinyl alcohol-melamine formaldehyde resin composite and nanocomposites with Ag, TiO_2, ZnO nanoparticles as antimicrobial films *Coat. Sprays* **3** 1088–97

[96] Rita Kakkar K M, Saritha Nehru Y V and Kakkar J 2015 Films and coatings of silver nano composites for wound dressings in diabetic foot disease *Eur. Chem. Bull. Section C—Chem. Biol. Sci.* **4** 98–105

[97] Santos J C C, Mansur A A, Ciminell V S and Mansur H S 2014 Nanocomposites of poly (vinyl alcohol)/functionalized-multiwall carbon nanotubes conjugated with glucose oxidase for potential application as scaffolds in skin wound healing *Int. J. Polym. Mater. Polym. Biomater* **63** 185–96

[98] Almonaci Hernández C A *et al* 2017 Silver nanoparticles for the rapid healing of diabetic foot ulcers *Int. J. Med. Nano. Res.* **4** 019

[99] Kapadia C H, Luo B, Dang M N, Irvin-Choy N ' D, Valcourt D M and Day E S 2020 Polymer nanocarriers for microRNA delivery *J. Appl. Polym. Sci.* **137** 48651

[100] Zhu J-Y *et al* 2016 Preferential cancer cell self-recognition and tumor self-targeting by coating nanoparticles with homotypic cancer cell membranes *Nano Lett.* **16** 5895–901

[101] Kapadia C H, Perry J L, Tian S, Christopher Lufta J and DeSimone J M 2015 Nanoparticulate immunotherapy for cancer *J. Control Rel.* **21910** 167–80

[102] Valcourt D M, Kapadia C H, Scully M A, Dang M N and Day E S 2020 Best practices for preclinical *in vivo* testing of cancer nanomedicines *Adv. Healthcare Mater.* **9** 2000110

[103] Lu C *et al* 2012 Phase I clinical trial of systemically administered tusc2(fus1)-nanoparticles mediating functional gene transfer in humans *PLoS One* **7** e34833

[104] Schultheis B *et al* 2014 First-in-human phase I study of the liposomal RNA interference therapeutic atu027 in patients with advanced solid tumors *J. Clin. Oncol.* **32** 4141–8

[105] El Dika I *et al* 2019 An open-label, multicenter, phase I, dose escalation study with phase II expansion cohort to determine the safety, pharmacokinetics, and preliminary antitumor activity of intravenous TKM-080301 in subjects with advanced hepatocellular carcinoma *Oncologist* Available from: https://doi.org/10.1634/theoncologist.2018-0838

[106] Clinical trials. gov. Available online: http://clinicaltrials.gov (accessed on 28 December 2019)

[107] Burris H A *et al* 2019 A phase I multicenter study to assess the safety, tolerability, and immunogenicity of mRNA-4157 alone in patients with resected solid tumors and in combination with pembrolizumab in patients with unresectable solid tumors *J. Clin. Oncol.* **37** 2523

[108] Saleh N and Yousaf Z 2018 Tools and techniques for the optimized synthesis, reproducibility and scale up of desired nanoparticles from plant derived material and their role in pharmaceutical properties *Nanoscale Fabrication, Optimization, Scale-Up and Biological Aspects of Pharmaceutical Nanotechnology* ed A M Grumezescu (Amsterdam: Elsevier) pp 86–131

[109] Paliwal R, Jayachandra Babu R and Palakurthi S 2014 Nanomedicine scale-up technologies: feasibilities and challenges *AAPS Pharm. Sci. Tech.* **15** 1527–34

[110] Ventola C L 2017 Progress in nanomedicine: approved and investigational nanodrugs *P. T* **42** 742–55 PMID: 29234213; PMCID: PMC5720487

[111] Van der Meel R *et al* 2019 Smart cancer nanomedicine *Nat. Nanotechnol.* **14** 1007–17

IOP Publishing

Bionanomaterials
Fundamentals and biomedical applications
Ravindra Pratap Singh and Kshitij RB Singh

Chapter 7

Bionanomaterials utility for therapeutic applications

Sadhucharan Mallick, Ajay Shankar and Bhavabhuti Prasad

Bionanomaterials (BNMs) are nanotechnology-empowered biomaterials. Nowadays, the growth of BNMs has moved further than the finding of entirely novel materials and compositions. Advances in nanotechnology have enabled the design of functional nanostructured biological materials, i.e. bionanomaterials engineered biological entities (e.g. liposomes, proteins, enzymes, nucleic acids, oligonucleotides, receptor, antibodies, and macromolecules of peptides, polysaccharides, biological cofactors, organelles, cell, tissue, microorganism, and ligands). Biomolecules have been conjugated with nanoscale materials like metal nanoparticles (NPs), nanowires, nanofibers, nanotubes, hydrogel, graphene, etc. The present chapter mainly describes bionanomaterial's possible biomedical domain activity, which makes it a possible theragnostic and therapeutic agent.

7.1 Introduction

Nanomaterials' interactions with proteins, cell membranes, cells, DNA, organelles, and biofluids have profound remains in the origin of nanomaterial bio-activity and therapeutic applications. BNMs are new hybrid materials that are composed partly or entirely of biological molecules such as proteins, peptides, enzymes, antibodies, deoxyribonucleic acid (DNA), ribonucleic acid (RNA), oligonucleotides, lipid, polysaccharide, viruses, cells, etc, and resulting materials having nanoscale-dimensions, i.e. nanocellulose, lignin NPs, lipid-based NPs (about 100 nm in dimension) influenza virus NPs, human immunoglobulin G (IgG) ligands, and human IgG coated NPs, NP–DNA materials, lipid-based nano emulsified drug delivery systems, metal NPs-enzyme biohybrids figures 7.1(a) and (b) [1]. Nature, as the most well-known bioengineer, applies smooth procedures for the development of robust and well-designed bionanomaterials, for example, metalloenzymes, three-dimensional protein, and lipid nano scaffolds. The formation of hybrid bionanomaterials is

doi:10.1088/978-0-7503-3767-0ch7

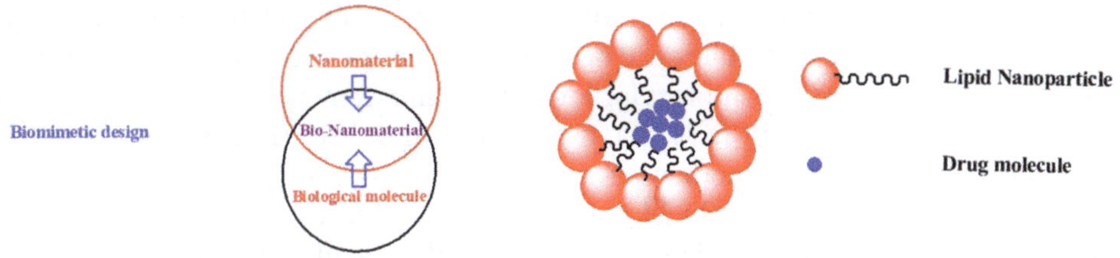

Figure 7.1. (a) Schematic diagram of BNMs. (b) Schematic diagram of drug encapsulated lipid BNMs.

primarily performed following two methodologies: biomolecular self-assembly and bioconjugation techniques (peptide-gold NP bioconjugate, lipid drug conjugates, anti-epidermal growth factor receptor (EGFR) antibody conjugated gold NPs). Self-assembly is a simple but effective bottom-up technique for formulating well-designed BNMs with orderly structures comprising DNA, proteins, peptides, viruses, enzymes, and their novel functions.

Impressive research has been devoted to advancing the field of bionanomaterials for a bunch of biomedical applications, including combating bone cancers. Several researchers have integrated biosystems into nanoscale materials as a vital and new task in recent years. These include quantum dots (QDs) made of semiconductors with size-dependent photoluminescence and various carbon forms such as single-walled, multi-walled carbon nanotubes, and graphene. They impart ballistic transport properties. Also, the large surface area of nanomaterials facilitates functionalization with biopolymers, ligands, including small molecules, DNA or RNA strands, aptamers or antibodies, oligonucleotides, proteins, peptides, drugs or for achieving the target-specific activity, selectivity, and sensitivity for their several applications in drug delivery, therapeutics and theranostics. In recent times QDs conjugated with biomolecules have been used for long-term multicolor bioimaging. These functional BNMs are highly beneficial for diverse biomedical applications, i.e. biosensing, bioimaging, bioanalysis, biocatalysis, drug delivery, and diagnostic and therapeutic uses in healthcare [1–9]. The established bioconjugation (quantum dot-antibody, Tat peptide-conjugated quantum dots) approaches have improved the stability, solubility, biocompatibility, and interfacial activity of classic inorganic NPs and quantum dots [5–17]. These nanoprobe BNMs have quite distinct properties and functions compared to their inorganic or organic counterparts. In an organic NP, carbon plays an important role, i.e. fullerenes, carbon dots, carbon nanotubes, carbon nanofibers, graphene nanosheets are the renowned members. In an inorganic NP, they comprise inorganic metals like Fe, Ni, Zn, Cr, coinage metals (Cu, Ag, and Au), silica, etc [18, 19].

Biomolecular engineering can be utilized to control biological molecules deliberately; a few prominent examples are proteins, lipids, nucleic acids, peptides, in the background of the relationships amongst their structures, purposes, properties, and their application to various areas such as emerging biomaterials, medical diagnostics, bioimaging, therapeutics, and biosensing. Nanoscience and nanotechnology are frequently used to fabricate and modulate nanomaterials' shapes, dimensions, properties, and utility. There are significant influences among biomolecular engineering and nanotechnology. They are both focused on the behavior and structure of materials on the nanoscale or molecular level. So, nanoscience, nanotechnology, and the biomolecular engineering fields have created and developed novel bionanomaterials. Based on this, nanobiodevices and nanobiosystems have been developed. Nanotechnology in the field of BNM development has gained great attention during the last 20 years. Two approaches have been used to synthesize BNMs: first, the bottom-up approach; and second, the top-down approach. Some BNM preparation goes from the top down, such as microfluidics to nanofluidic biochips, viz., lab-on-a-chip. Here, the continuous-flow-based separation and the individual or collective detection of such macromolecules, e.g. proteins and DNA, microfluidic-based biosensors; nucleic acid and protein sensors; solid-state nanopore sensors for DNA sequencing, and cancer biomarker [1–3]. Microorganisms, plant- and animal-based products, have been used to synthesize BNMs, which can be either intracellular or extracellular in their mode of working. For example, siliceous (silica-based) material may include other substances (e.g. pectin, lignin, and other chemicals), including sillafins and polyamines, and magnetic NPs have been synthesized from magneto-bacteria [20]. BNMs have also been synthesized by bioreduction method where reduction is due to reducing sugar, protein, enzyme, polysaccharide, etc. BNMs play a significant role in agriculture, biology, medicine, pollution control, drug delivery, biomimetics, and their use decreases the risk of various toxic chemicals in the environment [21, 22]. Pavlovic *et al* formulated functional BNMs (Mg/Al-CO_3-LDH-SOD) that showed excellent activity in the decomposition of superoxide radicals [23]. They immobilized superoxide dismutase (SOD) enzyme with the help of heparin coating on solid support layered double hydroxide (LDH) Mg/Al-CO_3-LDH. The unique and novel features and functions of BNMs such as low volume-to-surface ratio, greater solubility, nano size, and multifunctionality such as being natural, renewable, biodegradable, biocompatible, and safe are amply utilized for biomedical applications. The engineered BNMs are most useful in imaging/sensing, and immunomodulation also can be used as a vector to carry drugs. These BNMs are already finding many non-biotic applications for the harvesting of energy in solar cells, enhanced data storage capacity, optical display, and chemical catalysis and remediation purposes. The metal NP has tremendous features but has some limits such as toxicity or other side effects; to overcome these borders BNMs have been developed. In general, BNMs have extraordinary features like low toxicity, biocompatibility, enhanced eco-friendliness, etc. BNMs have already been used in novel therapies, such as targeted drug delivery, cell imaging, for various diagnostics purposes, tissue engineering, and wound dressing purposes [21, 22]. DNA is naturally water-soluble and biocompatible. As the dimensions of DNA are characteristically on the nanoscale, their self-assembly provides an opportunity for a programmable bottom-up approach to produce complicated structures from nanosized components. DNA has recently demonstrated itself to be an adaptable construction unit for the programmable formation of such objects, including two-dimensional crystals, nanotubes, and three-dimensional wireframe nanopolyhedra with precisely measured sizes extending from 10 to 100 nm.

Moreover, DNA has recently appeared as an encouraging material for constructing DNA nanostructures with capable applications in bionanotechnology and biomedicine. DNA nanostructures are also water-soluble and possess excellent biocompatibility, eco-friendliness, high tissue infiltration efficacy, and adequate stability in biological fluids, enabling their *in vitro* and *in vivo* applications. Molecular self-assembly of biomolecules with diverse structures such as NPs, nanorods, nanotubes, etc, is a constant inspiration for researchers in biomedical and biological applications.

Characterization is required to establish understanding and control of BNM synthesis and applications. Essential physicochemical properties and their characterization has usually completed the preparation of BNMs afterward. The constraints desirable to estimate BNMs include hydrodynamic dimension, zeta-potential (ζ) measurements, the extent of crystallinity, release of the drug, efficiency of entrapment (% EE), and morphology of the surface. Numerous nanoscience instruments have been used to characterize BNMs like UV–visible spectroscopy, dynamic light scattering (DLS), powder x-ray diffraction (XRD), energy dispersed x-ray spectroscopy, Fourier transform infrared spectroscopy (FTIR), scanning electron microscopy (SEM), transmission electron microscopy (TEM), field emission scanning electron microscopy (FESEM), atomic force microscopy (AFM), atomic absorption spectroscopy (AAS), x-ray photoelectron spectroscopy (XPS), fluorescence microscopy, atomic force microscopy (AFM), etc. The main objective of this chapter is to discuss biomedical and pharmaceutical use of BNMs that comprise inorganic NPs such as Cu, Ag, and Au, and their alloy NPs, core–shell NPs, mesoporous silica, titania, magnetic NPs, carbon nanotubes, carbon dots (C-dots), graphene and graphene oxide as well as organic functional BNMs such as cellulose, starch, chitosan, functional chitosan, dendrimer, lipid-based and protein-based NPs. During the past few years, BNMs have been developed for applications in fields such as delivery vehicle (drug, genes, and siRNA), diagnostic or therapeutic agents, bioelectronics, biosensing, bioimaging, biocatalysis, biological actuators, and tissue engineering and regenerative medicine, and many other clinical applications because of their outstanding physicochemical characteristics. Hence, this chapter elaborates properties of polysaccharide, lipid, protein, nucleic acid, DNA, peptide nucleic acids based BNMs, and their potential use as pharmaceutical nanocarriers, targeted drug delivery vehicles as well as diagnostics tools, imaging and anticancer agents.

7.2 Advantages of bionanomaterials

The influence of nanoscience and nanotechnology for theranostic use has been growing exponentially in the previous few decades. NPs, in addition to nanostructured materials made of hydrophobic engineered polymeric materials, metals, or inorganic materials, are generally not blood compatible. NPs injected inside the body may incite a clotting response and trigger the complement cascade; subsequently, they may be familiarized by phagocytes and macrophages and understand them as unusable or hazardous. On the other hand, biomolecules present in biological sources can reduce metallic ions to metal NPs and form stable and biocompatible bionanomaterials [9, 10]. The surface modification of NPs with biological molecules and polymers, i.e. homopolysaccharides, heteropolysaccharides, proteins, polypeptides, enzymes, antibodies, DNA, RNA, lipid, viruses, and cells, etc have been developed by several scientists [21, 22]. This type of external surface modification exhibits increased intrinsic anti-complement and anti-coagulant properties, along with other biological activities. Generally, BNMs are considered safe. This is because they originated from plant and animal resources and the gentle nature of their larger forms. There are several published results so far on safety. They have shown that BNMs are usually less noxious to humans and the environment. Engineered BNMs and biopolymeric nanomaterials with superb biodegradability and biocompatibility are regarded as one of the best vehicles for the delivery of drug systems in numerous medicinal applications.

Functionally incorporating DNA and other nucleic acids with nanomaterials, i.e. quantum dots or NPs made from Cu, Ag, Au metals and their metal oxides, polymeric NPs, and carbon allotropes in all their different forms have produced an enriched type of hybrid BNMs which, in many cases, display unique or augmented optical, physical, magnetic, and electrochemical features owing to the synergistic action of both components. These competencies are enticing greater consideration, in turn, from several research groups in the exploration of new nano-level tools for diversified uses that comprise targeted imaging, cellular delivery, labeling, biosensing, therapeutics, diagnostics, theranostics, biocomputing, and bioelectronics, to name just a few among several others (figure 7.2). Beyond this, synthetic polymer-based only and viral or proteinaceous nanomaterials are similarly useful in the same role since they can provide a defined and biocompatible transport and targeting capability.

7.3 Utility of polysaccharide-based bionanomaterial

Carbohydrate-based polymers are easily available in nature and show an exceptional role in therapeutic applications in various human diseases. Numerous natural polymers, such as gum acacia, silk, sodium alginate, chitosan, albumin, and gelatin,

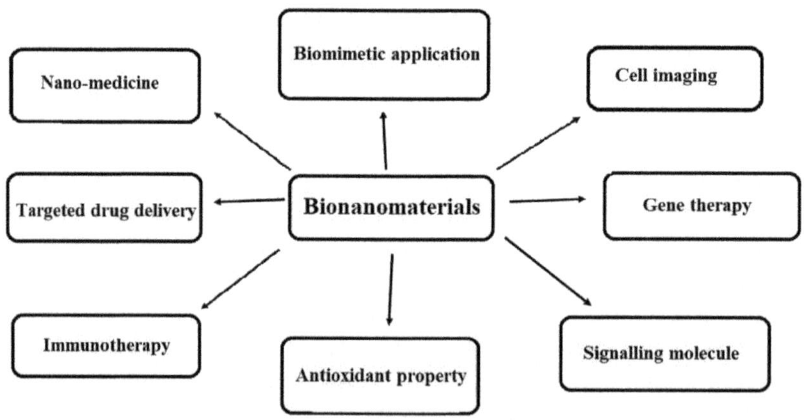

Figure 7.2. BNMs employed for numerous biomedical applications.

plant dietary fiber, which is generally composed of cellulose, hemicellulose, and lignin, are widely abundant. The main advantage comes from their eco-friendly, renewable, and physiologically benign nature to humans. The different structures and inherent functional groups in polysaccharides like hydroxyl, carboxyl, and amine groups show various chemical transformations. These transformations can make these molecules more effective in biomedical and pharmaceutical applications. The application of carbohydrates and natural polysaccharides combined with nanotechnology in tissue engineering and medicine are the new and potential research areas developing novel biomaterials for biosensing, bioimaging, diagnostic, and drug delivery systems. NPs with a biological polymer like protein, polysaccharide, collagen, chitosan have been recently used with various morphologies in biomedical applications and stem cell differentiation [21–27]. These polymeric nanomaterials are used as carriers for targeted drug delivery as these polymeric nanocarriers release drugs at controlled rates over long periods. Also, they have been used as polymeric nanocarriers with a smart and multifunctional drug as a neuroprotector, which helps to avoid acute ischemic stroke [28, 29]. Recent research provides the information that led to the development of polysaccharide-based NPs, which are highly effective for basic structure for controlled release of the therapeutic agent, especially for a vehicle for tumor targeting and several other biomedical applications [21–23]. They have many advantages, like avoiding drug degradation and improving the pharmacokinetic profile and its onsite specificity. The hydrophilic functional group in polysaccharides shows bio-adhesion property with biological tissue and results in valuable materials for improving the therapeutic agent's bioavailability, particularly in the mucosal oral drug delivery system [13, 14]. The remarkable absorption capacity, biodegradability, and non-toxicity of lignin NPs have possible applications in the environmental aspects and biomedical fields such as strong underwater antifouling materials, tissue engineering, regeneration, and artificial muscles [13, 14]. Among numerous NPs, coinage metals, i.e. Cu, Ag, and Au, have attractive optical properties and chemical and biological properties [24–27]. The coinage monometallic NPs and their bimetallic NPs, i.e. alloy NPs and layered (core–shell) NPs fabricated with chitosan, provide special opportunities owing to their remarkable antibacterial, antifungal and anticancer applications at relatively low concentrations [24–27]. Our recent studies have confirmed that antimicrobial formulations consisting of chitosan metal NPs of Ag, Cu, hybrid, and core–shell (e.g. Cu@Ag NPs) might be effective bactericidal nanocomposites [24–27]. Further, following the same approach, it has been found that core–shell NPs with magnetic core (e.g. mixed iron oxides, metallic Fe, Co) and non-magnetic shell (e.g. Au, Ag) are conjugated with a biomolecule, which is also helpful in these biomedical applications. Magnetic NPs are favored primarily because of their superparamagnetic property, which is controllable by an external magnetic field [30, 31]. These unique magnetic materials functionalized with proteins and polysaccharides offer various applications in enhanced mode, e.g. tissue engineering [32], ferroelastomers for artificial muscles [33], bioseparation of proteins [34], and so on. The additional opportunity via an external magnetic field to tune the mobility, spatial distribution and on-spot heat generation in biological systems enhances their applicability.

In 2003 Pan *et al* reported the synthesis of insulin- loaded bioadhesive chitosan nanoparticles (CS-NPs) by ionotropic gelation of CS with tripolyphosphate anions [35]; they had explored insulin attached CS-NPs, which exhibited a positive charge and fast release kinetics *in vitro*. They had also shown that insulin-loaded CS-NP BNMs might release active insulin form *in vivo* and increase the intestinal absorption of insulin to a greater amount than an insulin–chitosan solution. They had measured the comparative pharmacological bioavailability of insulin by monitoring the plasma glucose level of alloxan-induced diabetic mice after oral administration of various doses of insulin-loaded CS-NPs [35]. The effect of CS-NPs to increase the intestinal absorption of insulin was investigated by determining the decrease of the plasma glucose levels following oral administration, and the comparative pharmacological availability was calculated [35].

7.4 Lipid-based bionanomaterial as pharmaceutical carriers

Liposomes are important nano-sized (naturally 50–100 nm) biological molecules which are closed spherical vesicles made of the membranous phospholipid bilayer and aqueous central core, first described by Torchilin in 1964 [36, 37]. The liposome is hydrophobic or amphiphilic small molecules that have been able to encapsulate the drug (doxorubicin, docetaxel, doxorubicinol, paclitaxel) in the lipid bilayer, genes, and siRNA into the aqueous core [36–47]. One of the key benefits is that liposome can be easily produced in the laboratory and used in a broad-spectrum drug delivery system. Lipid-based nanomaterial and polymeric lipid hybrid nanomaterial with long-term stability show a tremendous property of drug delivery into the tumor cells. It will be supportive for therapeutics application and theranostics applications in the cancer research field [36–49]. Among the colloidal drug carriers, nanolipid dispersions such as liposomes, deformable liposomes, solid lipid NPs, niosomes (nonionic surfactant vesicle composed of cholesterol and alkyl or dialkyl polyglycerol ether group), virosomes (non-replicating artificial viruses), and ethosomes (phospholipid-based noninvasive soft vesicles) can deliver drugs to target locations [38]. Nanostructured lipid carriers and solid lipid NPs (SLNs) are stable and non-biotoxic; they are subsequently biodegradable compared to polymeric NPs [36, 37]. Liposome-based BNMs are extensively used as a drug, nucleic acids, proteins, enzymes, vaccines, or other entities in the diagnosis carriers for their inherent characteristic properties such as biocompatibility, self-assembly capabilities, low toxicity, and controlled pharmacokinetic profile, and capacity to cross the blood–brain barrier, although challenging tasks exist in the control of their surface properties, particle size, and their targeting ability. More than a dozen U.S. Food and Drug Administration (FDA) and European Medicines Evaluation Agency (EMA)-approved liposomal drugs have been in clinical trials from 1995 to the present, and among these, Doxil has the most widespread clinical practice. The greatest advantage is protecting entrapped drugs from degradation, prolonging drug circulation time, oral bioavailability, biodegradability, biocompatibility, focusing on when they are defined as nanostructured lipid carriers, solid lipid NP, lipospheres, and self/micro/nano emulsified drugs delivery framework, as shown in figures 7.3 and 7.4.

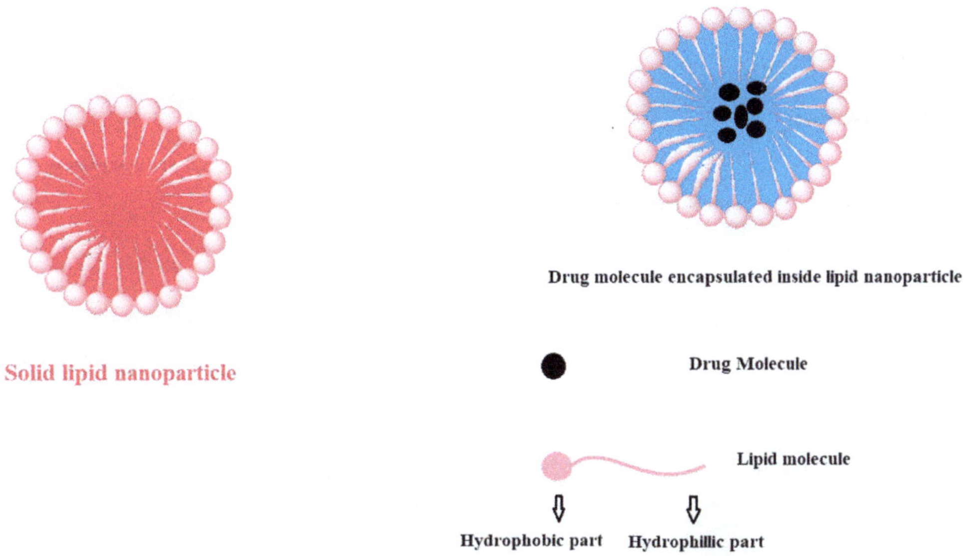

Figure 7.3. Schematic representation of solid lipid NP and drug encapsulated lipid NP.

The concept of a liposomal drug delivery system has revolutionized the pharmaceutical field. Liposomes are easy to synthesize, have greater biocompatibility, and can be loaded with diagnostic agents, DNA, and a wide diversity of drugs [36–47]. Physiologically suitable liposomes' *in vivo* properties are easy to control. Many liposomal drugs are presently in progress, and some of them are now approved for clinical use. The use of liposomes (lipid spherules) was an enzyme (amyloglucosidase with iodinated albumin) carrier in enzyme replacement therapy first reported by Gregoriadis *et al* in 1971 [39, 40]. Liposomes can capture hydrophobic drugs in the lipid bilayer and genes, hydrophilic drugs, and siRNA into the water-based core. Stealth or sterically stabilized liposomes capable of circulating with very long half-lives have facilitated innovative cancer drug delivery studies. In recent years, several scientists had established the careful delivery of anticancer agent doxorubicin in polyethylene glycol (PEG) liposomes for action on solid tumors of humans with breast-carcinoma metastases, which have resulted in successful improvements in life saving [43, 44]. Due to its analogous tumor-targeted effectiveness and promising safety profile, scientists found that pegylated liposomal doxorubicin might be a useful substitute to traditional doxorubicin and other agents normally used in the handling of breast cancer [43, 44]. Ahmad *et al* had developed a liposomal (lipid-DNA complex) formulation for delivering anticancer drug estrogenic derivative (ESC8) in well-established synthetic ligand dexamethasone (Dex)-to form an ESC8-entrapped liposome named DXE lipoplex [44]. This DXE liposome is tumor-selective in its anticancer action with an advantageous pharmacokinetic and tumor regressing profile that might sensitize and destroy highly aggressive and drug-resistive mice bearing breast cancer ANV-1 cells [44]. Sun *et al* had synthesized biocompatible and decomposable quercetin (3,3′,4′,5′,7-pentahydroxyflavone) encapsulated nanostructured lipid carriers (Q-NLCs) using soy lecithin, glyceryl

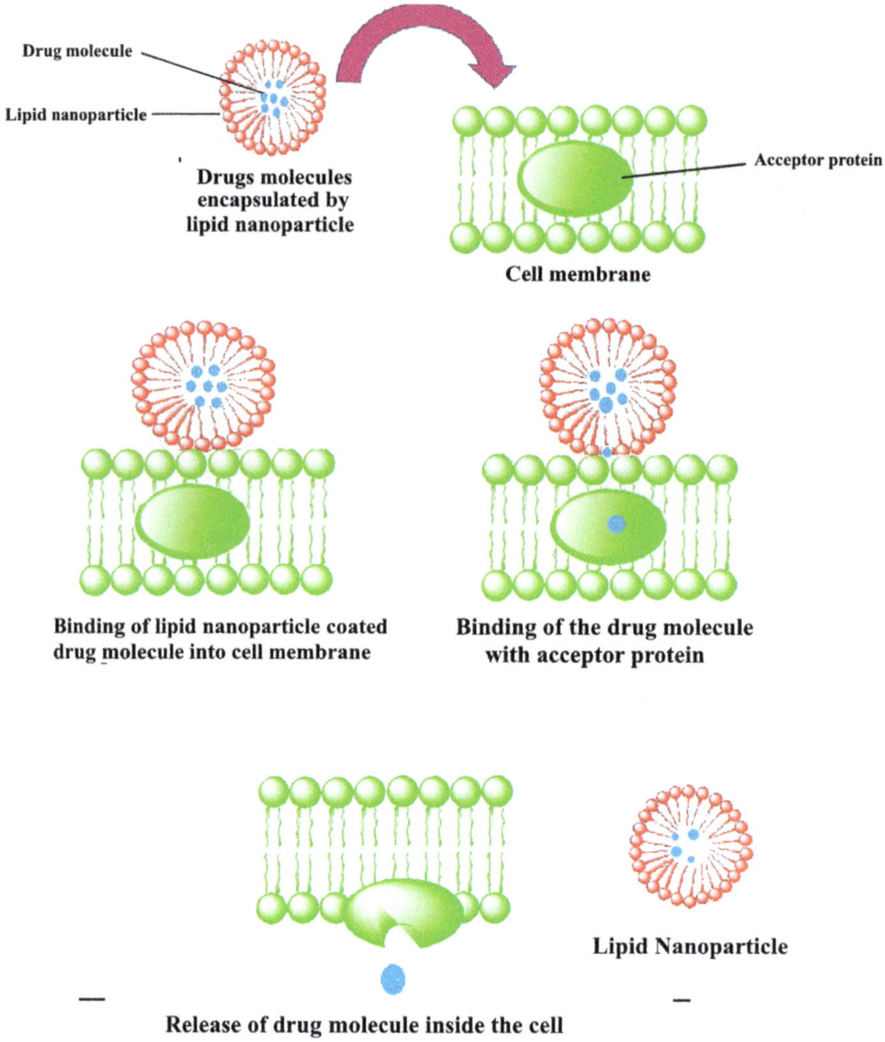

Figure 7.4. Schematic representation of delivery of lipid encapsulated drug molecule into the targeted cell.

tridentate, glyceryl tripalmitate, Kolliphor HS15 by a phase inversion-based technique [45]. These Q-NLCs have a probable aim at chemo-preventive use in breast cancer by decreasing the viability of breast cancer cells and inducing their apoptosis. They had depicted that aqueous solubility and stability of dietary flavonoid quercetin was strongly developed in occurrence with lipid nanocarriers and affectedly developed the anti-cancer activities by better Q content in those breast tumor cells [45]. Zhang *et al* had reported the formulation of a novel lipid-polymer hybrid NP (sub-100 nm) through a combination of nanoprecipitation and self-assembly [47]. They had used poly D,L-lactic-co-glycolic acid (PLGA) (which was ester-terminated) as a model hydrophobic polymer to form the polymeric core of the

NPs; PEG, which is covalently conjugated to 1,2-distearoyl-sn-glycero-3-phosphoethanolamine (DSPE), as a model hydrophilic polymer to form the stealth shell of the NPs and lecithin as a model lipid to form the lipid single-layered at the interface of the PLGA core and PEG shell. Since both PLGA and DSPE-PEG polymers have been approved by the FDA for medical use and lecithin is a natural lipid extracted from soybean, they had anticipated the lipid-polymer hybrid NPs would be biocompatible, biodegradable, and potentially safe as a drug carrier for clinical use. They designed PLGA-lipid-PEG hybrid NPs with tunable size and the surface charge has been used as robust anticancer docetaxel (Dtxl) drug delivery platform, with tunable and sustained drug release profile, excellent serum stability, high drug encapsulation yield, and potential for differential targeting of cells and tissues [47].

SLNs have elastic surface topology and useful properties that have gained them universal significance due to their several advantages, i.e. better stability pattern and inclusion of chemotherapeutic agents (figure 7.5) [38, 49, 56]. As compared with a traditional drug delivery system, SLNs has been extensively documented as pharmaceutical transporters for drug delivery, specifically for the targeted cells. SLNs have been used in various areas like targeted oral administration, drug delivery, protein–peptide delivery, ocular delivery, cosmetics, topical administration, and intravenous administration. In a novel drug delivery system, it has the main problem of delivering any drug in the brain because it is not easy to cross the blood–brain barrier, but the help of SLNs overcomes this problem. It has a potential approach because of its lipid behavior, and its size being in nanometers; it has also helped to achieve targeted drug delivery. It has reduced the medicine toxicity, enlarged movement period, biocompatibility, and few incidences of recognition by the reticuloendothelial system and subsequent clearance. Liposomes are considered to be the most successful drug-carrier system known to date. Polymeric nanocarriers, core–shell nanomedicine, metallic nanoparticles, liposomes, and SLNs can help to deliver drugs with heightened effectiveness and reduced toxicity and can overcome biological barriers, therefore improving anticancer activity in the treatment of breast cancer and triple-negative breast cancer, as compiled in table 7.1 [44, 50–58].

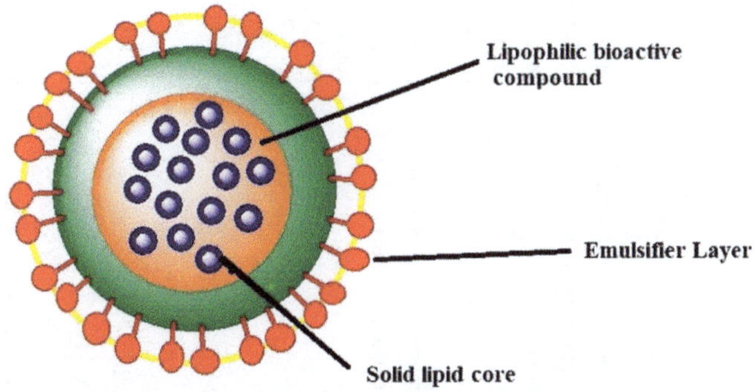

Figure 7.5. Schematic representation of lipophilic compound entrapped solid lipid NPs.

Table 7.1. Nanocarriers with potential applications in the treatment of breast cancer.

Type of Nanocarrier	Component of the delivery system	Drug	Therapeutic indication	Purpose	Finding
Polymeric NP and polymeric micelles	Polyethylene glycol (PEG)	Decitabine (DAC) doxorubicin Combination therapy	Triple-negative breast cancer (TNBC)	DNA hypermethylation inhibition	Best tumor-suppressive effects in inhibiting breast cancer growth [50]
core–shell nanomedicine 20 nm of particle diameter	poly(lactic-co-glycolic acid) PLGA nanocore encapsulating m-tetra (hydroxyphenyl)chlorin mTHPC	Dasatinib (a tyrosine kinase inhibitor)	Metastatic breast cancer cell	Synergistic cytotoxicity using Decitabine and a photo-sensitizer mTHPC	Disruption of Src kinase protein involved in the migration of metastatic cancer cells [51]
polymeric nanocarriers to treat breast cancer	methoxyl poly(ethylene glycol)-poly(d,l-lactide) copolymer (mPEG-PDLA)	Co-delivery of resveratrol (RES) and docetaxel (DTX) (prolonged release profiles)	Human breast adenocarcinoma cell line (MCF-7 cells	Synergetic therapy of BC IC_{50} of RES 23.0 μg ml^{-1}, IC_{50} of DTX 10.4 μg ml^{-1} but IC_{50} of 4.8 μg ml^{-1} Combination	The co-delivery of DTX and RES demonstrated potential synergism in the breast adenocarcinoma cell line MCF-7 cells [52]
Metallic NPs DOX-Hyd@AuNPs	Gold NPs via a poly (ethylene glycol) spacer	Doxorubicin	Breast cancer	Delivery drugs to breast cancer stem cells (BCSCs)	Showed greater potential to deliver DOX to breast cancer stem cells [53]
AuNRs@PAR-1 siRNA	AuNPs	siRNA	TNBC	Gene silencing of protease-activated receptor-1 (PAR-1) involved in tumor metastasis	Efficiently down-regulated PAR-1 expression [54]

(*Continued*)

Table 7.1. (*Continued*)

Type of Nanocarrier	Component of the delivery system	Drug	Therapeutic indication	Purpose	Finding
lipid-based nanocarriers	RGD–ECO/siβ3 NPs (ECO =1-aminoethyl)iminobis [N-oleicylsteinyl-1-aminoethyl) propionamide]	RGD peptide, β3 integrin	TNBC	To treat TNBC by delivering β3 integrin siRNA	Target BCSCs and cell surface of nucleolin which is overexpressed in TNBC cells [55]
ESC8-entrapped liposome	DODEAC, Cholesterol,	DOX, DEX, neuropilin-1	Breast cancer stem cell	To deliver an anticancer agent to BCSCs	Co-delivering DEX liposomes along with NRP-1(neuropilin-1) shRNA encoded plasmid was favorable to kill highly aggressive and drug-resistant BCSCs [44]
SLNs	SLNs using Compritol 888 ATO	Camptothecin	Breast cancer	To improve encapsulation efficiency and cytotoxicity	Improved targeting ability by SLNs in MCF-cell line [56]
lipid-based nanocarriers	NLCs	Quercetin	BC & TNBC	Improved Quercetin delivery by lipidic nanocarriers against BC	Facilitated cytotoxicity and apoptosis in MCF-7 and MDA-MB-231 cells [57].
LyP-1 containing lipid-based nanopharmaceuticals	LyP-1-containing self-micro emulsifying drug delivery system	LyP-1 peptide	TNBC	Reduction in p32 gene expressions	Improved *in vitro* cytotoxicity, reduction of tumor growth, and metastasis. Significant increase in cytotoxicity in p32-expressing 4T1 and MDA-MB-231 cells [58]

7.5 Bionanomaterials in imaging

The recent technological progress in nanomaterials and BNMs has become essential in producing high-resolution, high-contrast images preferred for correct, exact, and non-invasive diagnostics [59, 60]. BNMs show important imaging activities by delivering enormous imaging payloads and yielding greater sensitivity, design modularity, and enhancement of the multiplexing capacity [61]. In a few imaging modalities, BNMs, are not only ancillary contrast units but also a substitute for the unique and main source of image signals that make probable modality's survival. Contrast agents resulting from BNMs may find the close-fitting regulator over the delivery and significantly enlarged diagnostic sensitivity and specificity over traditional methodologies. These BNMs as imaging contrast agents can be separated into numerous major groups depending on the imaging modality, such as optical BNMs, magnetic BNMs, nuclear BNMs, and acoustic BNMs, which are likely to be clinically translated [61]. Capsids (usually from 20 to 400 nm in diameter) are the protein shells that enclose the viruses' genome. The appropriate size, the symmetry, and ease of structural manipulation make viral capsids unique nano-bio-templates linking biology and nanotechnology [11, 12]. Exceptional spectral properties of QDs allow ultrasensitive and long-term biolabeling. Li *et al* reported that QDs having inside viral shells of simian virus 40 (SV40) were used to inspect viral movement and localization inside mammalian cells, mimicking wild-type variant initial behavior and showing very different localization inside the cell [11]. When core–shell structure CdSe@CdZnS QDs are incubated with living cells, SVLP-QDs are revealed to enter the cells by caveolar endocytosis, travel along the microtubules, and gather in the endoplasmic reticulum. This technique copies the early contagion steps of SV40. This is the first example of viral imaging performances with encapsidated QDs in live cells [11]. The technique might serve as a novel alternative for many purposes, such as viral components and virus tracing, drug delivery probing, targeted NP delivery. So, SV40 VP1 might help adaptable building blocks for biocompatibilization and targeted delivery of various inorganic NPs.

7.6 Magnetic contrast-enhancing bionanomaterials

Magnetic resonance imaging (MRI) is an undisputed and powerful diagnostic tool in modern medical science. It is based on nuclear magnetic resonance (NMR) and subsequent relaxation of proton nuclear spins in an aqueous environment. The brain, central nervous system, and heart are a tool for tumors and cardiac functions. Without incision, it provides high-resolution images of soft tissues, and for this reason, it has been the primary choice for cellular and molecular imaging. Rare earth chelates compounds, especially Gd^{3+}-chelates, are most widely used and have a mainstay in clinics to enhance T1-weighted images by longitudinal relaxation of proton nuclear spins. Despite their success, they have several side effects. They have been shown to cause dangerous nephrogenic systemic fibrosis, leading to death in some cases. The metal chelates are known to cause lesions in the brain, kidney or liver of patients. The FDA has issued several warnings, and further studies are underway [62, 63]. A short blood half-life is combined with these, forcing the patients to uptake many doses for imaging [64]. These are mainly due to the retention of these chemical species by the body. Paramagnetic complexes dominate T1 relaxation-based contrasting agents, whereas T2 relaxation-based agents are mainly from the nanoparticulate origin. The nanosized superparamagnetic materials having a single magnetic domain are different classes of contrast agents due to their three distinct features discussed later in this section. Apart from the core's enhanced magnetic feature, they have canted spins on their surface. This thin layer, often called a dead layer, could be an oxidized form of the core's chemical composition or the same as that of the core. The word 'dead' has its origin related to its lowering effect on the particle's overall magnetization. Generally, it is antiferromagnetic, whereas the core can be ferro- or antiferromagnetic depending on the composition. Its thickness varies from the lattice parameter of the phase-in core or slightly less than it. The weakly responsive canting of spins reduces the net possible magnetization, which would have been there in its absence. Thus, it is obvious how it may affect clinical imaging. A typical coprecipitation route resulting in MNPs with such features and simultaneously having water dispersibility is shown in figure 7.6. As expected, the canted spin proportion decreases as the size of the core increases and becomes less important.

Though mostly canted spins' formation is unavoidable, a few synthesis procedures have been reported where coated particles are minimal or without dead layer [65, 66]. The enhanced surface area and quantum confinement effect on physicochemical properties enhance the contrasting ability of various inorganic NPs, leading to their numerous applications in magnetic resonance imaging contrast agents. One of the most widely employed materials amongst magnetic NPs (MNPs) for this purpose is nano-iron oxide (NIOs) which remains in the superparamagnetic state [67]. The NIOs are either degraded by natural mechanism, flushed out by the body system, or metabolized by different pathways to hemoglobin which is the prime reason behind their FDA approval for imaging. Apart from biocompatibility and biocompatibility issues, they significantly shorten the T2 relaxation times in

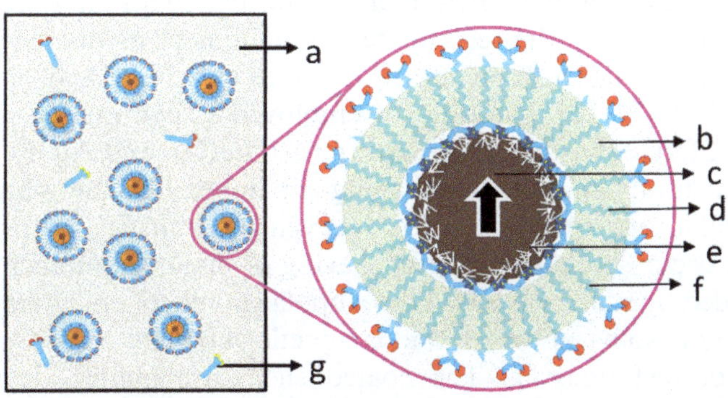

Figure 7.6. Water-based fluid containing MNPs and their constituents. (a) Water as a carrier medium, (b) Van der Waals force of attraction between hydrophobic tails, (c) ferromagnetic core, (d) hydrophobic part of coating material/stabilizer in the first layer, (e) antiferromagnetic dead layer, (f) hydrophobic part of coating material/dispersant in the second layer, (g) free coating material in dispersion.

body organs, viz., spleen, bone marrow, and liver, by providing strong contrasting effects in T2 weighted images. It occurs due to shorter transversal relaxation of proton nuclear spins in neighboring regions and decreased MR images' signal intensity. The other-dimensional characteristics of MNPs such as size, their distribution, crystallinity also matter for their application. The size and distribution of MNPs control their blood half-life and biodistribution during their application. NIOs < 50 nm have also been tested as blood-pool agents because of their easy distribution through intravascular and extracellular space. Further, the rheological properties of the final dispersion to be injected into the body may depend on many other factors [68, 69]. NIOs prepared from the coprecipitation route are generally chosen for clinical imaging. However, these NIOs suffer from poor dispersity and crystallinity. MNPs produced from the high-temperature decomposition of metal precursors in organic solvents overcome this problem by providing high resolution and imaging sensitivity. MNPs have given better results in imaging than coprecipitation methods. These MNPs have also been employed with T1 contrast agents but with limited success [70]. A majority of presently available imaging probes and contrast agents are either chemically or radioactively active. On the other hand, nonmagnetic NPs, especially QDs, exert their electronic and optical properties depending on their composition in these applications. The nanosized and molecular-sized contrasting agents have their contrasting mechanisms different from each other. There are three main requirements based on the components of NP-based MRI contrasting agents: (i) the core of NPs must have suitable above-mentioned properties; (ii) the coated shell should be compatible with water and biological systems; and (iii) the reactive moieties on the outer surface help in exploring the grafting of bioactive materials for targeting purpose. The hydrophilic outer surface is important for this application. The NPs are mainly prepared from the bottom-to-top approach in aqueous or organic solvents. The hydrophilic group forms coordinate bonds with metal ions of the NP surface and tail part having hydrophobic nature protrudes out in the space. Such scenarios require a second species to be present on the surface, which can be the same molecule as that of the first layer or different [71–73]. However, the functionalization with a hydrophilic group of ligands on the outer surface omits the second stage requirement as discussed above. The ligand exchange method is also one of the methods to achieve hydrophilicity on the outer surface of NPs [74, 75]. The typically employed T2 contrasting agents on NIOs are ferumoxides, ferucarbotran, ferumoxtran, Au–Fe_3O_4, and Au–FePt. The shortening of T2 relaxation enhances the imaging capability. The alloy-based materials, including bimetallic ferrite nanoparticles, are even good candidates for this task. The said shortening occurs because of the dephasing of magnetic moments due to field gradients provided by smaller NIOs. Thus, dipolar outer-sphere interaction between the nuclear proton spins of water and magnetic moment of NIOs becomes the platform for contrast imaging. The coated shells are mainly dextran-based or polyethylene glycolated, which are well known for stabilizing the NPs in aqueous solutions. The dextran surfaces of NPs with amine groups also enabled molecular imaging [76]. The NPs have certain advantages over conventional paramagnetic complex-based contrast agents, whether *in vivo* or *in vitro*. They are readily taken by both nonphagocytic cells and macrophage cells. They are good at targeted imaging because of the larger surface area, which can be conjugated with oligonucleotides and antibodies. The various other biomaterials facilitated with surface binding are peptides, viruses, proteins that enable internalization by an anionic cellular membrane.

7.7 Bionanomaterials as an anticancer agent

Conventional cancer therapeutics—especially treatment with radiation and chemotherapy—produces several familiar side effects, poses a threat to solid tissues, and seldom has outcomes within the disposal of cancer cells. BNMs offer trust to supply arrangements to the complex problems related to cancer treatment, in expansion to giving better capacity and efficiency in cancer cell destruction. Hydroxyapatite (HA) nanocrystals, N-(2-hydroxypropyl)meth-acrylamide (HPMA), magnetic NPs (iron oxide), metallic NPs (copper, zinc, and silver), nanoscale conjugated copolymer, γ-cyclodextrin, selenium, and liposomal NPs that have been observed and established over the last few years for bone tissue engineering and cancer treatment. Incorporating biosystems into nanotechnology has been taken up as a central and novel mission by many researchers in recent years. The surface modification of NPs with biological ligands, such as aptamers, arginine-glycine-aspartate (RGD) peptides, antibodies, folate, antibody-drug conjugate, transferrin, or antibody fragments, facilitates NP imaging, targeting, and internalization into specified cells, e.g. cancerous cells, and tumors [9, 77]. Folate is a renowned small molecule regularly used as a cancer cell-targeting ligand that binds to folate receptors with high affinity [77]. The chemical binding of folate onto the surface of NPs can expressively promote their targeted delivery into cancer cells that overexpress folate receptors. Cheng *et al* reported that Transferrin (Tf) is a major mammalian serum glycoprotein that can carry iron atoms into tissues [78]. Upon binding proteins, therapeutic drugs, or genetically by infusion of therapeutic proteins or peptides into the transferrin structure to the Tf receptor (TfR), the Tf/TfR complex is internalized by cells through receptor-mediated endocytosis [78]. TfR has been studied as a target for transporting anticancer drugs into cancer cells due to its overexpression by malignant tumor cells. TfR can be targeted by direct contact with Tf displayed on the nanomaterial surface [78, 79]. Radiation therapy is one of the oldest and best bets at the present time for cancer and tumor treatment. Among various types of cancer therapies, noninvasive phototherapy, mainly photodynamic therapy (PDT) and photothermal therapy (PTT) using BNMs looks promising [80, 81]. The term PDT refers to phototherapy followed by photochemotherapy in which the photosensitizers (PTSs) are employed to create highly reactive oxygen species (ROS) *in vivo* employing excitation by external electromagnetic radiation. ROS examples include but are not limited to singlet oxygen, hydroxyl radical, and peroxides, all of which irreversibly damage the targeted part in the biological system, viz., cancer and tumor cells. Oxidative stress can have specific effects on the cells, including oxidative destruction to proteins and DNA. An ideal photosensitizer should be excited in a particular narrow bandwidth of electromagnetic radiation at which there is no response from the tissue at the targeted location. The near IR-region (0.7–1.1 pm) serves this purpose in the human body as the photons corresponding to these radiations pass through negligible interaction with tissues and body fluids. The several limitations in the use of PTSs hamper their applications in PDT. The PDTs typically comprise water-soluble and partially or fully biocompatible metal-organic dyes. The major shortcoming is their rapid bio-degradation once they are injected into the body and/or degradation post-exposure to the laser. Many times, they also exhibit poor water solubility, which further hinders their application. Other limiting scenarios include their low efficiency in targeting tissues and poor excitation during clinical applications. The reasons for the latter include low absorption at cross-sections and low excitation coefficients at used wavelengths. As a solution to all of these problems, the systems based on NPs offer immense potential to improve the performance of PDTs [80] drastically.

Apart from PDT, PTT is the other widely used treatment method for cancer and tumors. PTT is a new approach to cancer therapy that transforms near-infrared (NIR) light to heat and possesses low side effects, noninvasiveness, and high spatiotemporal selectivity. Herein, the therapeutic agent absorbs energy in the form of photons and radiates a portion of the energy in the form of heat [80, 81]. The proximity of the therapeutic agent to the treatment site plays an important role here. The released heat causes the thermal ablation of unwanted cells. Thus, an increase in temperature causing tumor cells' death involves a disruption in cellular structure, necrosis, and/or apoptosis. Due to many available noble metal nanostructures (active in NIR) exhibiting plasmonic resonance, the development of PDTs has been phenomenal in recent years. In this respect, nano-gold in the form of spheres, rods, cages, and multifunctional nanoshells are a few to name which have been studied intensively. PTT and PDT using BNMs would be capable strategies to enhance the cancer therapeutic efficacy and reduce the injury to the neighboring healthy tissues.

Recently Hu *et al* have reported tumor-specific synergistic treatment using BNMs as a nanoplatform via immobilizing natural glucose oxidase on Cu-based layered double hydroxide (CuFe-LDH) nanosheets, which for the first time assimilates pH-responsive, acid-enhanced PTT, and heat-facilitated chemodynamic therapy concurrently [81]. Layered double hydroxides (LDHs) are a class of two-dimensional nanomaterial with useful properties, and the overall formula is expressed as $[M^{2+}{}_{1-x}M^{3+}{}_{x}(OH)_2]\ (A^{n-})_{x/n}\cdot mH_2O$ (M^{3+} and M^{2+} signify trivalent and divalent cations respectively, and A^{n-} acts as the transferrable interlaminar anion and can balance the charge of the host layer), and have been extensively explored as inorganic-biological merged BNMs owing to their decent biocompatibility [81]. Hu *et al* have described that LDHs having a high specific surface area, uniform shape, and changeable chemical composition, LDHs have been confirmed as brilliant drug transferers through specific cell imaging functions. Furthermore, LDHs can be restructured to yield adequate defects under acidic environments, which encourages photogenerated electron–hole pairs to comprehend efficient acid-enhanced NIR photothermal conversion [81].

Adjuvant to chemotherapy and radiation therapy, magnetic hyperthermia has emerged as one of the best possible cancers and tumor treatment alternatives.

Its therapeutic index makes it more promising, attracting numerous researchers towards it [82, 83]. MNPs have been employed with targeted drug delivery and killing of cancerous cells. As discussed in the previous section, the physical size of MNPs decides their magnetic nature. Depending on its numerical comparison with the core material's magnetic domain size, the MNP can be superparamagnetic, single domain with high coercivity, or multidomain like that of bulk magnetic material. Again because of the biological issues, NIOs are best suited for this purpose amongst all MNPs. Generally, at room temperature, the MNPs having a size equal to or less than single magnetic domain exhibit superparamagnetism where the moment of the whole particle is free for relaxation. At specified lower temperatures than room temperature, the same MNPs have ferromagnetic behavior with limited or no relaxivity of the particle's magnetic moment. In magnetism, this is referred to as a blocked state of MNPs. The relaxation mechanism of dispersed MNPs (in the superparamagnetic state) is governed by two mechanisms; Néels's relaxation and Brownian relaxation, and the particles are said to be unblocked in respect of their magnetic moments. The temperature at which the ratio of blocked and unblocked MNPs is 1:1 is regarded as blocking temperature [71]. Generally, in magnetic hyperthermia and drug delivery systems, the employed MNPs are in a superparamagnetic state with the opportunity of Brownian motion as a relaxation mechanism. The dispersion contains the MNPs, which are loaded with anticancer drugs by simple ligand exchange reactions or similar methods and later injected into blood vessels or directly in the body's region where treatment has to be carried out. The injected MNPs are traced to the desired region's vicinity with an external magnet producing a dc magnetic field. Once the loaded MNPs reach the infected tissues, they deliver the loaded drug whose kinetics and biochemistry play an important role. For hyperthermia, the part is exposed to a sinusoidal fluctuating ac magnetic field. The MNPs tend to align their moments in the applied field direction at any instant of time. To do so, when they are using the Brownian relaxation mechanism in fluidic surroundings present inside and outside cells, it will create friction. There are other mechanisms based on magnetic hysteresis and eddy current depending on several environmental factors. Subsequently, the infected region gets heated up by the field-controlled activity of MNPs. The frequency is adjusted, generating heat on harmful tumor/cancer cells and not healthy cells (figure 7.7). The MNPs provide a considerably high specific absorption rate, which makes the effort of researchers consistent in cancer treatments [82, 83].

7.8 Protein-based bionanomaterials and their utility

Beyond than their importance in Nature, proteins can be synthesized in the molecular biology lab and used within the lab as three-dimensional nano-scaffolds with tall basic and suitable modifications. Recently, the development of synthetic protein-based hybrid BNMs and protein-based nanocomposites have resulted in substantial improvements. The application of smart polypeptides and protein, i.e. mammalian elastin and collagen, keratins, insect-derived silk, and resilin entities as

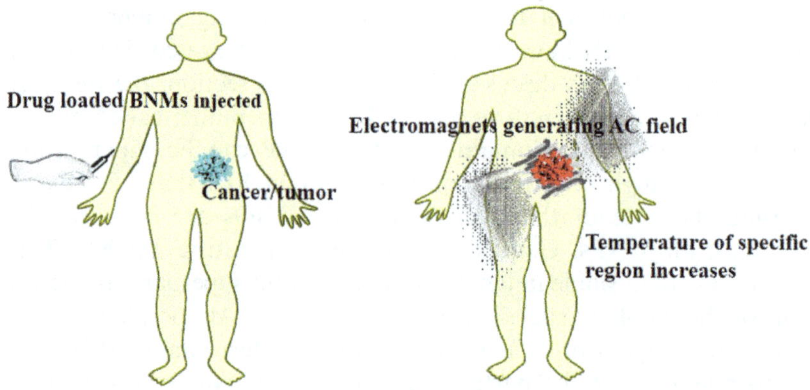

Figure 7.7. Schematic representation of magnetic hyperthermia treatment in the human body using BNMs.

supports in the fabrication of BNMs, provides a reasonable novel emerging material [84–86]. Bio templates of protein units and structural design with dissimilar sizes, such as bacteriophages, protein cages, protein membranes, protein fibers, and protein crystals, have been usually implemented for the manageable synthesis of protein-incorporated hybrid nanostructured materials. As a usual illustration of the bottom-up synthesis approach, proteins have been utilized as platforms for the nucleation of metal NPs and following the growth of metal NPs on the biomolecule's surface. As a typical example of a bottom-up synthesis approach, proteins have been used as platforms for the nucleation of metal ions and following the growth of metal NPs on the biological molecule's surface. Enzymes, peptides, and isolated proteins can be very practical for new BNM synthesis and device fabrications [84–86]. Biocompatible protein-based NMs are usually biodegradable, metabolizable, and are easy to functionalize for their addition to particular drugs and other targeting ligands.

Recently, Ahmed *et al* reported that the spherical and quasi-spherical silver NPs-β galactosidase hybrid (12.89 ± 0.16 nm) was operative as an antibacterial agent inhibiting the growth of *Escherichia coli, Pseudomonas aeruginosa* (gram-negative bacteria), and *Staphylococcus aureus* and *Staphylococcus epidermidis* (gram-positive bacteria), where gram-negative bacteria were more powerfully suppressed by these Ag NPs [87]. They had also reported that this silver NPs-β galactosidase hybrid also has industrial dye (acid dyes and direct or reactive) degeneration potential. Henceforth, Ag NPs-based BNMs can act as potential reducers of toxic dyes and help in wastewater bioremediation. According to their report, β-galactosidase from aspergillus oryzae was utilized to synthesize highly stable and well dispersed AgNPs where the enzyme itself acted as both the reducing and capping agent.

7.9 Nucleic acid associated bionanomaterials

Nanobioconjugates that comprise various well-designed NPs linked to biotic molecules have been used in several areas, for example, diagnostics, sensors, therapeutics, and bioengineering. Biological molecules, like DNA, have shown immense potential in the manufacture and building of nanolevel structures and devices. The hybrids of DNA or RNA and gold NPs can be employed for functional assemblies for various applications in medicine, diagnostics, or nano-electronics using biomarkers, specific imaging probes, or gene expression regulatory function. Mirkin *et al* have initially prepared a DNA gold NP hybrid (DNA–Au NPs) between 15 and 150 nm in diameter with a considerable therapeutic and diagnostic application [8, 88, 89]. Polyvalent oligonucleotides DNA–Au NPs conjugates have various optical properties due to their surface plasmon, and the large extinction coefficient made it one of the most useful elements in the medical field [8, 88, 89].

7.10 Utility of DNA—nanostructures

As a naturally occurring biomacromolecule, DNA for storage and transmission of all genetic information for life exhibits excellent biocompatibility and programmability. The DNA molecule has attractive features for use in nanoscience and nanotechnology: its tiny dimension, with a width of nearly 2 nm; its short helical pitch basic structural repeat of approximately 3.4–3.6 nm; and its toughness with a persistence length of nearly 50 nm [88–97]. This stiff DNA motif comprises two double helices associated with each other twice through crossover points. In the last few decades, numerous DNA nanostructures have been established, including one-, two- and three-dimensional nanomaterials and several DNA-based nanodevices; DNA arrays have been made. Biotechnologists, biologists, and biologically oriented physical scientists, and nanotechnologists work together and they have been established with specific structural and topological features that can be made from assembling DNA. Amongst numerous DNA assemblies, three-dimensional DNA nanostructures hold the potential to be the general nanocarriers for targeted and smart drug delivery. DNA nanostructure-based drug delivery systems, compared to traditional drug delivery systems, have several benefits, including programmable sequences, precise shape and size, high drug loading capability and passive delivery into live cells, exceptional biocompatibility, and biodegradability. Finally, the strict Watson–Crick base-pairing rules make it conceivable to assimilate functional nucleic acids (e.g. aptamers, nucleic acid probes, and DNAzymes) into DNA nanostructures [97]. All these characteristics favor the utilization of DNA nanostructures in cellular biophysics biomimetic systems, therapeutics, and diagnostics for human health-related applications. To date, a vast range of chemotherapeutic drug–DNA hybridized nanostructures has been advanced for the therapy involving anti-tumor activities. Usually, chemotherapeutic drug Doxorubicin, Daunorubicin, has been loaded to DNA nanostructures via intercalation and has been used in clinics for decades [94–96]. Recently Zhu and co-workers constructed aptamer-based DNA nanotrains as carriers for targeted chemotherapeutic drug transport in cancer therapy [94]. Aptamers are short, single-stranded oligonucleotides (DNA, RNA) molecules with precise binding properties with high affinity and specific recognition abilities against various non-nucleic acid targets across a variety of size scales from ions to cells, specific organs, and full protein [94–96]. Huang *et al* reported that the aptamers are directly assembled from DNA strands through base pairing, followed by chemotherapeutic drugs [96]. Recently, the aptamer-attached DNA nanotrains, a conjugate of different DNA double strands, were synthesized by Zhu *et al*, and then chemotherapeutic drug DOX was loaded to the nanotrains through the intercalation method [94]. The designs of drug–DNA hybridized systems, comprising the creation of nanostructures and the new ways to load drugs, impact drug delivery efficiency at a large scale [94–96]. New findings have concentrated on improving novel drug–DNA hybridized materials to gain more precision and efficiency in therapy for several diseases [94–97].

Peptide nucleic acids (PNAs B = nucleobase) are DNA/RNA synthetic analogs with 2-([2-Aminoethyl] amino) acetic acid backbone, whose effects in achiral and uncharged mimic and PNAs are better nucleic acid mimetics than many other oligonucleotides. They have several fascinating properties such as strengthened binding-affinity to complementary nucleic acids, increased biological stability, extraordinary thermal stability, and ionic strength, and unique hybridization relative to nucleic acids and improved cellular uptake has accelerated rapidly [98–100]. These unique physicochemical properties of PNA permit a novel approach of finding, which is a quicker and more consistent analytical procedure and novelties use in the pharmaceutical fields and molecular diagnostics. PNAs replace DNA as a probe for the biomolecular device in the cytogenetics, molecular genetic diagnostics, and various pharmaceutical potentials and the growth of biosensor/chip/array and many more analysis determinations. PNAs' physicochemical properties make them resistant to enzymatic cleavage and they do not degrade in biological environments. PNA partakes unique antisense and antigene properties, just owing to its inhibitory effect on translation and transcription, and it undergoes complementary binding to DNA or RNA with high affinity and specificity. Hence, many procedures utilizing PNA-based oligomers for the detection and treatment of several diseases such as AIDS, cancer, etc have been designed and developed to date. PNA is used for PCR reaction modulation/mutation in fluorescent *in situ* hybridization and microarray as a probe, also in many *in vitro* and *in vivo* assays [98–100].

7.11 Conclusion and prospects

Recently, nanoscience and nanotechnology have brought marvelous changes in different disciplines such as chemistry, biology, physics, material sciences, etc [101–104]. The use of nanotechnology in biology and medicine has led to wonderful growth in the past decades, and yet, as research activities in this scientific area are continuing with great speed, nano-biotechnology and nanomedicine are still proposing various exciting possibilities for the near future. Bionanotechnology is updating investigation and improvement in healthcare nanomedicines, nanotherapeutics, and nano-based drug delivery systems, environmental and agricultural domains. The synthesis of BNMs using biotic processes is very fast, environmentally friendly, and non-toxic [9, 10, 22, 23]. Already in the 1960s, artificial liposomes were suggested as carriers of proteins and drugs for the treatment of various diseases. Surface functionalized nanomaterials and BNMs have attracted great attention in the biomedical field for evolving the new generation of targeted drug-delivery systems, diagnoses, and treatments of various life-threatening diseases [22, 23]. An effective biological interface permits inorganic nanomaterials to efficiently mimic their biotic counterparts (e.g. synthetic receptors, biomimetic catalysts, combinatorial ligands, imprinted polymers, etc). In the near future, nanomaterials can be engineered using biotic material (e.g. microorganisms, organelles, cell receptors, enzymes, tissue) and biologically inferred material (for example, aptamers, recombinant antibodies, engineered proteins, and so forth) for diagnosis and therapeutic use, especially for making chemical and biological sensors and potential theragnostic agents. For an effective target recognition, inorganic nanomaterials can be functionalized with tumor-targeting moieties such as monoclonal antibodies (or their fragments), aptamers, proteins or peptide-based molecules, nucleic acids, and a variety of small molecules, i.e. folate. Such targeting ligands are expected to provide great affinity and precision toward target cells/tissues and ultimately contribute, with an important role, in increasing cellular uptake of BNMs through the internalization processes. Lipid-based nanoemulsified drug delivery systems have promising potential in enhancing the oral bioavailability of poorly soluble drugs [36–49]. The capacity of SLNs to consolidate drugs into nanocarriers offers a modern model in drug delivery conveyance that might be utilized for drug targeting [38, 49, 56]. SLNs hold incredible assurance for reaching the goals of controlled and efficient site-specific drug delivery. SLNs were developed as a promising method for the fruitful conveyance of hydrophobic drugs due to their versatile features and distinctive advantages. Lipid-based BNMs would be considered suitable vehicles to deliver an integrated, personalized approach to cancer diagnosis and therapy in future cancer disease management [36–49].

BNMs can play a key role in nanomedicine, as they can efficiently transport and provide imaging probes, therapeutic agents, or biological materials to targeted sites such as a specific organ, tissue, or even underlying cell. The *in situ* fabrication of useful BNMs is an existing challenge that has already shown great future potential. These BNMs are entirely biocompatible for biomedical applications. The biologically formed BNMs are used to treat contagious infections, cancer detection and diagnosis, cardiovascular and other illnesses. Presently, the key focus is to advancement of a multifunctional therapeutic BNMs platform with the highest targeting efficacy. The effectiveness of poorly soluble anticancer drugs can be improved with bio-conjugation. The engineered BNMs can be used to identify cancer-specific cells at the cellular level to deliver the drugs to the affected sites. These targeted delivery systems in nanoscience and nanotechnology may contribute extremely to *in vitro* and *in vivo* applications of BNMs in the field of nanomedicine. These targeted drug delivery techniques for various BNMs-based nanomedicines without toxicity will be able to diagnose several types of cancers. The BNMs for drug delivery may be potential natural nano-carriers and may have greater importance for theranostic systems. The biomimetic growth of nanomaterials in aqueous solutions is very useful when applied to therapeutics and medical imaging *in vivo* since these nanomaterials will be well dispersed in bodies that are currently very challenging. In recent times BNMs can be favorably utilized for fabricating novel diagnostic and electronic devices, including sensors, electronic noses, lab-on-a-chip, DNA chips, and micro total analysis systems (μ-TAS). Recently, lipid drug delivery systems have been given predictable consideration due to their inherent properties such as biocompatibility, self-assembly capabilities, and ability to cross the blood–brain barrier, particle size variability, and finally, cost-effectiveness, making lipid-based delivery systems much more attractive.

PTT employing radiation adsorbent in the NIR region is becoming an effective method for localized cancer treatment. The application of NIR adsorbent before PTT makes the fluence rate and irradiation time determination easier for the operator. Recently, the combination of thermal dosimetry using NIR adsorbent has been explored on ICG lactosome. However, testing the same with different types of cancer is yet to be explored [105]. The enormous contribution in the past two decades in magnetic hyperthermia has brought it to a platform that was not visible when establishing the technique in cancer treatment. The control of quality parameters and an increase in production of all BNMs also encompasses the field of magnetic hyperthermia. With the help of several seminal works, the time has come to decide a standard protocol in cancer treatment that characterizes the nanomaterials before any application. The scalable synthesis protocols need to be decided for BNMs for their industrial-scale productions. The critical step involving the functionalization of BNMs needs to be controlled properly. The reproducible yield at every step followed by purification of BNMs needs to be assured for closeness with trial results. The aqueous synthesis of BNMs would prove an eco-friendly approach rather than their exclusive synthesis in organic medium(s). The main challenge in both the former and latter methods remains about the precise control of synthesis parameters to produce BNMs with acceptable characteristics at the nano-level. The improving reproducibilities and higher scalable possibilities are the next steps in this direction. The long-term stability will decide the shelf-life and transport from the manufacturing spot to the site of delivery of BNMs. Here the importance of nanometrology will ultimately vindicate the properties of BNMs in organs over longer periods of months or years. The clinical results with mice, rabbits, and humans are not very encouraging, emphasizing their localized and delocalized studies on their biotransformation in microenvironments. The scarcity of non-ambiguous proofs of BNMs gives this field a well-specified direction for future research. The constitution and deployment of regulatory barriers in the form of authorities are the need of the hour for such advanced materials in biological applications. This will also reduce the cost and assure a deeper reach in the global markets for BNMs.

References

[1] Nagamune T 2017 Biomolecular engineering for nanobio/bionanotechnology *Nano Converg.* **4** 9

[2] Ho L W C, Liu Y, Han R, Bai Q and Choi C H J 2019 Nano–cell interactions of non-cationic bionanomaterials *Acc. Chem. Res.* **52** 1519–30

[3] Sapsford K E *et al* 2013 Functionalizing nanoparticles with biological molecules: developing chemistries that facilitate nanotechnology *Chem. Rev.* **113** 1904–2074

[4] Agasti S S, Rana S, Park M-H, Kim C K, You C-C and Rotello V M 2010 Nanoparticles for detection and diagnosis *Adv. Drug Delivery Rev.* **62** 316–28
[5] Nam J, Won N, Bang J, Jin H, Park J, Jung S, Jung S, Park Y and Kim S 2013 Surface engineering of inorganic nanoparticles for imaging and therapy *Adv. Drug Delivery Rev.* **65** 622–48
[6] Doane T L and Burda C 2012 The unique role of nanoparticles in nanomedicine: imaging, drug delivery, and therapy *Chem. Soc. Rev.* **41** 2885–911
[7] Nel A E, Madler L, Velegol D, Xia T, Hoek E M V, Somasundaran P, Klaessig F, Castranova V and Thompson M 2009 Understanding biophysicochemical interactions at the nano-bio interface *Nat. Mater.* **8** 543–57
[8] Wu X A, Choi C H J, Zhang C, Hao L and Mirkin C A 2014 Intracellular fate of spherical nucleic acid nanoparticle conjugates *JACS* **136** 7726–33
[9] Tran N T T, Wang T-H, Lin C-Y, Tsai Y-C, Lai C-H, Tai Y and Yung B Y M 2011 Direct synthesis of rev peptide-conjugated gold nanoparticles and their application in cancer therapeutics *Bioconjugate Chem.* **22** 1394–401
[10] Kim S *et al* 2019 Synthesis of DNA-templated copper nanoparticles with enhanced fluorescence stability for cellular imaging *Microchim. Acta* **186** 479
[11] Li F, Zhang Z-P, Peng J, Cui Z-Q, Pang D-W, Li K, Wei H-P, Zhou Y-F, Wen J-K and Zhang X-E 2009 Imaging viral behaviors in mammalian cells with self-assembled capsid–quantum-dot hybrid particles *Small* **5** 718–26
[12] Tagit O, de Ruiter M Â V, Brasch M, Ma Y and Cornelissen J J L M 2017 Quantum dot encapsulation in virus-like particles with tunable structural properties and low toxicity *RSC Adv.* **7** 38110–8
[13] Alqahtani M S, Alqahtani A, Al-Thabit A, Roni M and Syed R 2019 Novel lignin nanoparticles for oral drug delivery *J. Mater. Chem.* B **7** 4461–73
[14] Iravani S and Varma R S 2020 Greener synthesis of lignin nanoparticles and their applications *Green Chem.* **22** 612–36
[15] Hivare P, Panda C, Gupta S and Bhatia D 2021 Programmable DNA nanodevices for applications in neuroscience *ACS Chem. Neurosci.* **12** 363–77
[16] Kaur M, Arshad M and Ullah A 2018 In-situ nanoreinforced green bionanomaterials from natural keratin and montmorillonite (MMT)/cellulose nanocrystals (CNC) *ACS Sust. Chem. Eng.* **6** 1977–87
[17] Liu Y, Yu Q, Chang J and Wu C 2019 Nanobiomaterials: from 0D to 3D for tumor therapy and tissue regeneration *Nanoscale* **11** 13678–708
[18] Prasad Prajapati J, Das D, Katlakunta S, Maramu N, Ranjan V and Mallick S 2021 Synthesis and characterization of ultrasmall Cu_2O nanoparticles on silica nanoparticles surface *Inorg. Chim. Acta* **515** 120069
[19] Mallick S, Mukhi P, Kumari P, Mahato K R, Verma S K and Das D 2019 Synthesis, characterization and catalytic application of starch supported cuprous iodide nanoparticles *Catal. Lett.* **149** 3501–7
[20] Price W J and Whiteside P J 1977 General method for analysis of siliceous materials by atomic-absorption spectrophotometry and its application to macro- and micro-samples *Analyst* **102** 664–71
[21] Blackburn G, Scott T G, Bayer I S, Ghosh A, Biris A S and Biswas A 2013 Bionanomaterials for bone tumor engineering and tumor destruction *J. Mater. Chem.* B **1** 1519–34

[22] Maduraiveeran G 2020 Bionanomaterial-based electrochemical biosensing platforms for biomedical applications *Anal. Methods* **12** 1688–701

[23] Pavlovic M, Rouster P and Szilagyi I 2017 Synthesis and formulation of functional bionanomaterials with superoxide dismutase activity *Nanoscale* **9** 369–79

[24] Banerjee M, Mallick S, Paul A, Chattopadhyay A and Ghosh S S 2010 Heightened reactive oxygen species generation in the antimicrobial activity of a three component iodinated chitosan-silver nanoparticle composite *Langmuir* **26** 5901–8

[25] Mallick S, Sharma S, Banerjee M, Ghosh S S, Chattopadhyay A and Paul A 2012 Iodine-stabilized Cu nanoparticle chitosan composite for antibacterial applications *ACS Appl. Mater. Interf.* **4** 1313–23

[26] Mallick S, Sanpui P, Ghosh S S, Chattopadhyay A and Paul A 2015 Synthesis, characterization and enhanced bactericidal action of a chitosan supported core–shell copper–silver nanoparticle composite *RSC Adv.* **5** 12268–76

[27] Mallick S 2018 Synthesis and characterization of Cu and Ag-based mixed metal nanoparticle composite for antibacterial applications *Ind. J. Chem.–Section A* **57A** 1249–56

[28] Daglar B, Ozgur E, Corman M E, Uzun L and Demirel G B 2014 Polymeric nanocarriers for expected nanomedicine: current challenges and future prospects *RSC Adv.* **4** 48639–59

[29] Chen Y-x, Wei C-x, Lyu Y-q, Chen H-z, Jiang G and Gao X-l 2020 Biomimetic drug-delivery systems for the management of brain diseases *Biomater. Sci.* **8** 1073–88

[30] Verde E L, Landi G T, Carrião M S, Drummond A L, Gomes J A, Vieira E D, Sousa M H and Bakuzis A F 2012 Field dependent transition to the non-linear regime in magnetic hyperthermia experiments: comparison between maghemite, copper, zinc, nickel and cobalt ferrite nanoparticles of similar sizes *AIP Adv.* **2** 032120

[31] Hergt R, Dutz S and Zeisberger M 2010 Validity limits of the Néel relaxation model of magnetic nanoparticles for hyperthermia *Nanotechnology* **21** 015706

[32] Bealer E J, Kavetsky K, Dutko S, Lofland S and Hu X 2020 Protein and polysaccharide-based magnetic composite materials for medical applications *Int. J. Mol. Sci.* **21** 186

[33] Chen Y, Chen C, Rehman H U, Zheng X, Li H, Liu H and Hedenqvist M S 2020 Shape-memory polymeric artificial muscles: mechanisms, applications and challenges *Molecules* **25** 4246

[34] Liang Y-Y, Zhang L-M, Jiang W and Li W 2007 Embedding magnetic nanoparticles into polysaccharide-based hydrogels for magnetically assisted bioseparation *ChemPhysChem* **8** 2367–72

[35] Pan Y *et al* 2002 Bioadhesive polysaccharide in protein delivery system: chitosan nanoparticles improve the intestinal absorption of insulin *in vivo Int. J. Pharm.* **249** 139–47

[36] Torchilin V P 2005 Recent advances with liposomes as pharmaceutical carriers *Nat. Rev. Drug Discovery* **4** 145–60

[37] Torchilin V P 1985 Liposomes as targetable drug carriers *Crit. Rev. Ther. Drug Carrier Syst.* **2** 65–115

[38] Duan Y, Dhar A, Patel C, Khimani M, Neogi S, Sharma P, Siva Kumar N and Vekariya R L 2020 A brief review on solid lipid nanoparticles: part and parcel of contemporary drug delivery systems *RSC Adv.* **10** 26777–91

[39] Gregoriadis G, Leathwood P D and Ryman B E 1971 Enzyme entrapment in liposomes *FEBS Lett.* **14** 95–9

[40] Laing P, Bacon A, McCormack B, Gregoriadis G, Frisch B T and Schuber F 2006 The 'co-delivery' approach to approach to liposomal vaccines: application to the development of influenza-A and hepatitis-B vaccine candidates *J. Liposome Res.* **16** 229–35

[41] Symon Z, Peyser A, Tzemach D, Lyass O, Sucher E, Shezen E and Gabizon A 1999 Selective delivery of doxorubicin to patients with breast carcinoma metastases by stealth liposomes *Cancer* **86** 72–8

[42] Perez A T, Domenech G H, Frankel C and Vogel C L 2002 Pegylated liposomal doxorubicin (Doxil) for metastatic breast cancer: the Cancer Research Network, Inc., experience *Canc. Invest.* **20** 22–9

[43] O'Shaughnessy J A 2003 Pegylated liposomal doxorubicin in the treatment of breast cancer *Clin. Breast Canc.* **4** 318–28

[44] Ahmad A, Mondal S K, Mukhopadhyay D, Banerjee R and Alkharfy K M 2016 Development of liposomal formulation for delivering anticancer drug to breast cancer stem-cell-like cells and its pharmacokinetics in an animal model *Mol. Pharmaceutics* **13** 1081–8

[45] Sun M, Nie S, Pan X, Zhang R, Fan Z and Wang S 2014 Quercetin-nanostructured lipid carriers: Characteristics and anti-breast cancer activities *in vitro Colloids Surf.,* **B 113** 15–24

[46] Miller A D 2013 Lipid-based nanoparticles in cancer diagnosis and therapy *J. Drug Deliv.* **1** 1–9

[47] Zhang L, Chan J M, Gu F X, Rhee J-W, Wang A Z, Radovic-Moreno A F, Alexis F, Langer R and Farokhzad O C 2008 Self-assembled lipid-polymer hybrid nanoparticles: a robust drug delivery platform *ACS Nano* **2** 1696–702

[48] Barenholz Y 2012 Doxil®. The first FDA-approved nano-drug: Lessons learned *J. Contr. Rel.* **160** 117–34

[49] Chandra Bhatt P, Srivastava P, Pandey P, Khan W and Panda B P 2016 Nose to brain delivery of astaxanthin-loaded solid lipid nanoparticles: fabrication, radio labeling, optimization and biological studies *RSC Adv.* **6** 10001–10

[50] Li S-Y, Sun R, Wang H-X, Shen S, Liu Y, Du X-J, Zhu Y-H and Jun W 2015 Combination therapy with epigenetic-targeted and chemotherapeutic drugs delivered by nanoparticles to enhance the chemotherapy response and overcome resistance by breast cancer stem cells *J. Contr. Rel.* **205** 7–14

[51] Malarvizhi G L, Chandran P, Retnakumari A P, Ramachandran R, Gupta N, Nair S and Koyakutty M 2014 A rationally designed photo-chemo core–shell nanomedicine for inhibiting the migration of metastatic breast cancer cells followed by photodynamic killing *Nanomed. Nanotechnol. Biol. Med.* **1** 579–87

[52] Guo X, Zhao Z, Chen D, Qiao M, Wan F, Cun' D, Sun Y and Yang M 2019 Co-delivery of resveratrol and docetaxel via polymeric micelles to improve the treatment of drug-resistant tumors *Asian J. Pharm. Sci.* **14** 78–85

[53] Sun T-M *et al* 2014 Cancer stem cell therapy using doxorubicin conjugated to gold nanoparticles via hydrazone bonds *Biomaterials* **35** 836–45

[54] Zhang W, Meng J, Ji Y, Li X, Kong H, Wu X and Xu H 2011 Inhibiting metastasis of breast cancer cells *in vitro* using gold nanorod-siRNA delivery system *Nanoscale* **3** 3923–32

[55] Parvani J G, Gujrati M D, Mack M A, Schliemann W P and Lu Z-R 2015 Silencing β3 integrin by targeted ECO/siRNA nanoparticles inhibits EMT and metastasis of triple-negative breast cancer *Cancer Res.* **75** 2316–25

[56] Acevedo-Morantes C Y, Acevedo-Morantes M T, Suleiman-Rosado D and Ramírez-Vick J E 2013 Evaluation of the cytotoxic effect of camptothecin solid lipid nanoparticles on MCF7 cells *Drug Deliv.* **20** 338–48

[57] de Sousa Cunha F, dos Santos Pereira L N, de Costa e Silva T M P, de Sousa Luz R A and Nogueira Mendes A 2019 Development of nanoparticulate systems with action in breast and ovarian cancer: nanotheragnostics *J. Drug Targeting* **27** 732–41

[58] Timur S S *et al* 2019 Efficacy of a novel LyP-1-containing self-microemulsifying drug delivery system (SMEDDS) for active targeting to breast cancer *Eur. J. Pharm. Biopharm.* **136** 138–46

[59] Jonghoon K, Nohyun L and Taeghwan H 2017 Recent development of nanoparticles for molecular imaging *Phil. Trans. R. Soc.* A **375** 20170022

[60] Mehlenbacher R D, Kolbl R, Lay A and Dionne J A 2018 Nanomaterials for *in vivo* imaging of mechanical forces and electrical fields *Nat. Rev. Mater.* **3** 17080

[61] Smith B R and Gambhir S S 2017 Nanomaterials for *in vivo* imaging *Chem. Rev.* **117** 901–86

[62] Kanda T, Ishii K, Kawaguchi H, Kitajima K and Takenaka D 2014 High signal intensity in the dentate nucleus and globus pallidus on unenhanced T1-weighted MR images: relationship with increasing cumulative dose of a gadolinium-based contrast material *Radiology* **270** 834–41

[63] Ramalho J *et al* 2016 Gadolinium-based contrast agent accumulation and toxicity: an update *Am. J. Neuroradiol.* **37** 1192–8

[64] Aime S and Caravan P 2009 Biodistribution of gadolinium-based contrast agents, including gadolinium deposition *J. Magn. Reson. Imaging* **30** 1259–67

[65] Unni M *et al* 2017 Thermal decomposition synthesis of iron oxide nanoparticles with diminished magnetic dead layer by controlled addition of oxygen *ACS Nano* **11** 2284–303

[66] Roca A G *et al* 2009 Magnetite nanoparticles with no surface spin canting *J. Appl. Phys.* **105** 114309

[67] Na H B, Song I C and Hyeon T 2009 Inorganic nanoparticles for MRI contrast agents *Adv. Mater.* **21** 2133–48

[68] Chand M, Shankar A, Noorjahan, Jain K and Pant R P 2014 Improved properties of bidispersed magnetorheological fluids *RSC Adv.* **4** 53960–6

[69] Chand M, Kumar S, Shankar A, Sonia, Jain K, Singh S and Pant R 2013 The effect of size distribution on viscoelastic properties of ferrofluid *Magnetohydrodynamics* **49** 489–94

[70] Jeon M, Halbert M V, Stephen Z R and Zhang M 2020 Iron oxide nanoparticles as T1 contrast agents for magnetic resonance imaging: fundamentals, challenges, applications, and prospectives *Adv. Mater.* 1906539.

[71] Shankar A, Chand M, Basheed G A, Thakur S and Pant R P 2015 Low-temperature investigations on double surfactant water-based ferrofluid *J. Magn. Magn. Mater.* **374** 696–702

[72] Bao N, Shen L, Wang Y, Padhan P and Gupta A 2007 A facile thermolysis route to monodisperse ferrite nanocrystals *J. Am. Chem. Soc.* **129** 12374–5

[73] Frey N A, Peng S, Cheng K and Sun S 2009 Magnetic nanoparticles: synthesis, functionalization, and applications in bioimaging and magnetic energy storage *Chem. Soc. Rev.* **38** 2532–42

[74] Meerod S, Tumcharern G, Wichai U and Rutnakornpituk M 2008 Magnetite nanoparticles stabilized with polymeric bilayer of poly (ethylene glycol) methyl ether–poly (ε-caprolactone) copolymers *Polymer* **49** 3950–6

[75] Peng S and Sun S 2007 Synthesis and characterization of monodisperse hollow Fe_3O_4 nanoparticles *Angew. Chem. Int. Ed.* **46** 4155–8

[76] Otsuka H, Nagasaki Y and Kataoka K 2003 PEGylated nanoparticles for biological and pharmaceutical applications *Adv. Drug Deliv. Rev.* **55** 403–19
[77] Fernández M, Javaid F and Chudasama V 2018 Advances in targeting the folate receptor in the treatment/imaging of cancers *Chem. Sci.* **9** 790–810
[78] Cheng Y, Zak O, Aisen P, Harrison S C and Walz T 2004 Structure of the human transferrin receptor-transferrin complex *Cell* **116** 565–76
[79] Qian Z M, Li H, Sun H and Ho K 2002 Targeted drug delivery via the transferrin receptor-mediated endocytosis pathway *Pharmacol. Rev.* **54** 561–87
[80] Wang S *et al* 2015 Plasmonic copper sulfide nanocrystals exhibiting near-infrared photothermal and photodynamic therapeutic effects *ACS Nano* **9** 1788–800
[81] Hu T, Yan L, Wang Z, Shen W, Liang R, Yan D and Wei M 2021 A pH-responsive ultrathin Cu-based nanoplatform for specific photothermal and chemodynamic synergistic therapy *Chem. Sci.* **12** 2594–603
[82] Giustini A J, Petryk A A, Cassim S M, Tate J A, Baker I and Hoopes P J 2010 Magnetic nanoparticle hyperthermia in cancer treatment *Nano Life* **1**
[83] Lanier O L, Korotych O I, Monsalve A G, Wable D, Savliwala S, Grooms N W F, Nacea C, Tuitt O R and Dobson J 2019 Evaluation of magnetic nanoparticles for magnetic fluid hyperthermia *Int. J. Hyperth.* **36** 686–700
[84] Walsh T R and Knecht M R 2017 Biointerface structural effects on the properties and applications of bioinspired peptide-based nanomaterials *Chem. Rev.* **117** 12641–704
[85] Desai M S and Lee S-W 2015 Protein-based functional nanomaterial design for bioengineering applications *WIREs Nanomed. Nanobiotechnol.* **7** 69–97
[86] De la Rica R and Matsui H 2010 Applications of peptide and protein-based materials in bionanotechnology *Chem. Soc. Rev.* **39** 3499–509
[87] Ahmed F, Qayyum S and Husain Q 2018 Benign nano-assemblages of silver induced by β galactosidase with augmented antimicrobial and industrial dye degeneration potential *Mater. Sci. Eng.* C **91** 570–8
[88] Hurst S J, Hill H D and Mirkin C A 2008 Three-dimensional hybridization' with polyvalent DNA–gold nanoparticle conjugates *J. Am. Chem. Soc.* **130** 12192–200
[89] Dhar S, Daniel W L, Giljohann D A, Mirkin C A and Lippard S J 2009 Polyvalent oligonucleotide gold nanoparticle conjugates as delivery vehicles for platinum (IV) warheads *J. Am. Chem. Soc.* **131** 14652–3
[90] Douglas S M, Dietz H, Liedl T, Högberg B, Graf F and Shih W M 2009 Self-assembly of DNA into nanoscale three-dimensional shapes *Nature* **459** 414–8
[91] Rothemund P W K, Ekani-Nkodo A, Papadakis N, Kumar A, Fygenson D K and Winfree E 2004 Design and characterization of programmable DNA nanotubes *JACS* **126** 16344–52
[92] Seeman N C 2003 DNA in a material world *Nature* **421** 427–31
[93] Whitesides G M and Grzybowski B 2002 Self-assembly at all scales *Science* **295** 2418–21
[94] Zhu G, Zheng J, Song E, Donovan M, Zhang K, Liu C and Tan W 2013 Self-assembled, aptamer-tethered DNA nanotrains for targeted transport of molecular drugs in cancer theranostics *Proc. Natl Acad. Sci.* **110** 7998–8003
[95] Ryu Y, Hong C A, Song Y, Beak J, Seo B A, Lee J-j and Kim H-S 2020 Modular protein–DNA hybrid nanostructures as a drug delivery platform *Nanoscale* **12** 4975–81
[96] Huang X, Blum N T, Lin J, Shi J, Zhang C and Huang P 2021 Chemotherapeutic drug–DNA hybrid nanostructures for anti-tumor therapy *Mater. Horizons.* **8** 78–101

[97] Watson J D and Crick F H C 1953 Molecular structure of nucleic acids: a structure for deoxyribose nucleic acid *Nature* **171** 737–8

[98] Uhlmann E, Peyman A, Breipohl G and Will D W 1998 PNA: synthetic polyamide nucleic acids with unusual binding properties *Angew. Chem. Int. Ed.* **37** 2796–823

[99] Singh R P, Oh B-K and Choi J-W 2010 Application of peptide nucleic acid towards development of nanobiosensor arrays *Bioelectrochemistry* **79** 153–61

[100] Singh K R B, Sridevi P and Singh R P 2020 Potential applications of peptide nucleic acid in biomedical domain *Eng. Rep.* **2** e12238

[101] Sanna V and Sechi M 2020 Therapeutic potential of targeted nanoparticles and perspective on nanotherapies *ACS Med. Chem. Lett.* **11** 1069–73

[102] Singh K R B, Nayak V, Sarkar T and Singh R P 2020 Cerium oxide nanoparticles: properties, biosynthesis and biomedical application *RSC Adv.* **10** 27194–214

[103] Nayak V, Singh K R B, Singh A K and Singh R P 2021 Potentialities of selenium nanoparticles in biomedical science *New J. Chem.* **45** 2849–78

[104] Shanavas A, Jain N K, Kaur N, Thummuri D, Prasanna M, Prasad R, Naidu V G M, Bahadur D and Srivastava R 2019 Polymeric core–shell combinatorial nanomedicine for synergistic anticancer therapy *ACS Omega* **4** 19614–22

[105] Rubia-Rodríguez I *et al* 2021 Whither magnetic hyperthermia? A tentative roadmap *Materials* **14** 1–36

IOP Publishing

Bionanomaterials
Fundamentals and biomedical applications
Ravindra Pratap Singh and Kshitij RB Singh

Chapter 8

Bionanomaterials for tissue implant and regeneration

Jhansi Lakshmi Parimi, Venkata Sundeep Seesala, Ragavi Rajasekaran, Mamoni Banerjee, Santanu dhara, Padmavati Manchikanti, Jagadish Kumar Suluvoy and Praveen Kumar Chiruguri

The relentless bio-mimetic performance of nanomaterials within the advances of tissue engineering created the introduction of tissue implants, and regenerative medicine with the aim to build up biological substitutes that refurbish, sustain, or boost damaged tissue and organ functionality. Noteworthy research efforts have brought exhilarating unconventional materials to resolve varied issues related to traditional implants and tissue engineering materials for natural tissues. This highlights suitable candidates with superior biocompatibility and mechanical properties to enhance tissue growth for bone, cartilage, vascular, neural, skin and bladder implants. This review is an across-the-board assemblage of the progress made in this exhilarating, potential space of bioengineering efforts created to make scaffolds, tissues, and organs to regenerate human tissues to a degree of risks and reimbursement.

8.1 Introduction

Technological developments in the area of tissue engineering have brought a ray of hope for the regenerative approaches, which have the capability to support, correct and regenerate damaged tissues and organs. The pressing needs for the availability of substitutes for immediate implantation to replace or rejuvenate the functions of compromised, damaged or destroyed tissue/organs due to accidents urged for the development of complementary implants or prostheses to augment the native functional supports [1, 2]. For a tissue implant to mimic the functions of native tissue, it should meet the criteria of structural, functional and chemical features [3]. Hence, it is a combination of the efforts from tissue engineering, material science,

doi:10.1088/978-0-7503-3767-0ch8

and medical technologies (pharmaceuticals and biotechnology). Current clinical outcomes of tissue implants would have been mere dreams without the introduction of nanomaterials used for the construction and performance of the tissue constructs, i.e. scaffolds. This step forward brought the advantageous efforts to regenerative medicine from the targeted delivery of biomolecules and drugs to regeneration of the skin, cartilage, bone, cardiac muscles, etc [1, 2]. Moreover, it reduced the suffering posed due to the high cost of the autografts.

The instructive visualization of nano-enabled regenerative approaches for tissue implants was possible with the advancements in the dimensional (2D, 3D, and 4D) scaffold construction strategies like electrospinning and additive manufacturing [4]. Hence, the new generation nanobiomaterials were able to carry biomolecules, cells, growth factors along while maintaining the structural and functional mimicking of natural tissues

The advanced vision of the biomaterials at nanoscale made the simulation of micro- and macro-environments of the tissues possible. Together with the utilization of traditional and advanced fabrication techniques, molecular structures of the tissues could be fabricated together with the cells and growth factors required for the regeneration to take place. Further, precise control over the topography would be possible with electrospinning and other advanced bioprinting techniques where various nanobiostructures, in the form of fibre matrices, wires, spheres, grooves, multi-branching structures and composites can be developed to be used as tissue implants [4, 5]. Continuous efforts to develop complementary functional tissue implants are challenging and need efforts for the development of more resilient materials and characterization techniques

Owing to the presence of biologically active components, nanobiomaterials once fabricated possess the capability for directed targeting and simulating tissue regeneration *in vivo* [6]. Anisotropy, surface features, and traceability pay an important role for cell proliferation to happen. Once the process is initiated, the growth of the cells and tissue will happen *in situ* as shown in figure 8.1(a); identification of the molecular interaction in order to impart the self-healing potential and moderate targeting for the stem cell therapies are the prime goals of the nano enablement of the biomaterials. The schematic shown in figure 8.1(b) shows the depiction of the process. Continuing efforts in this direction could lead to the development of multifunctional, bioactive materials which can bring the potential advantage of self-healing and resorbable capability.

The objective of this chapter is to provide a review of the potential effects of the amalgamation of nanobiomaterial tissue-engineered implants. It describes the various biomaterials that have been researched for the construction of scaffolds, carriers, substrates, etc for different tissue engineering techniques. Special attention has been placed on identifying and presenting potential nano-enabled tissue implants for bone, nerve, muscle, skin tissue from the perspective of biomaterials. The importance of being biocompatible and consequences of incompatibility have been highlighted with long-term toxicity reference.

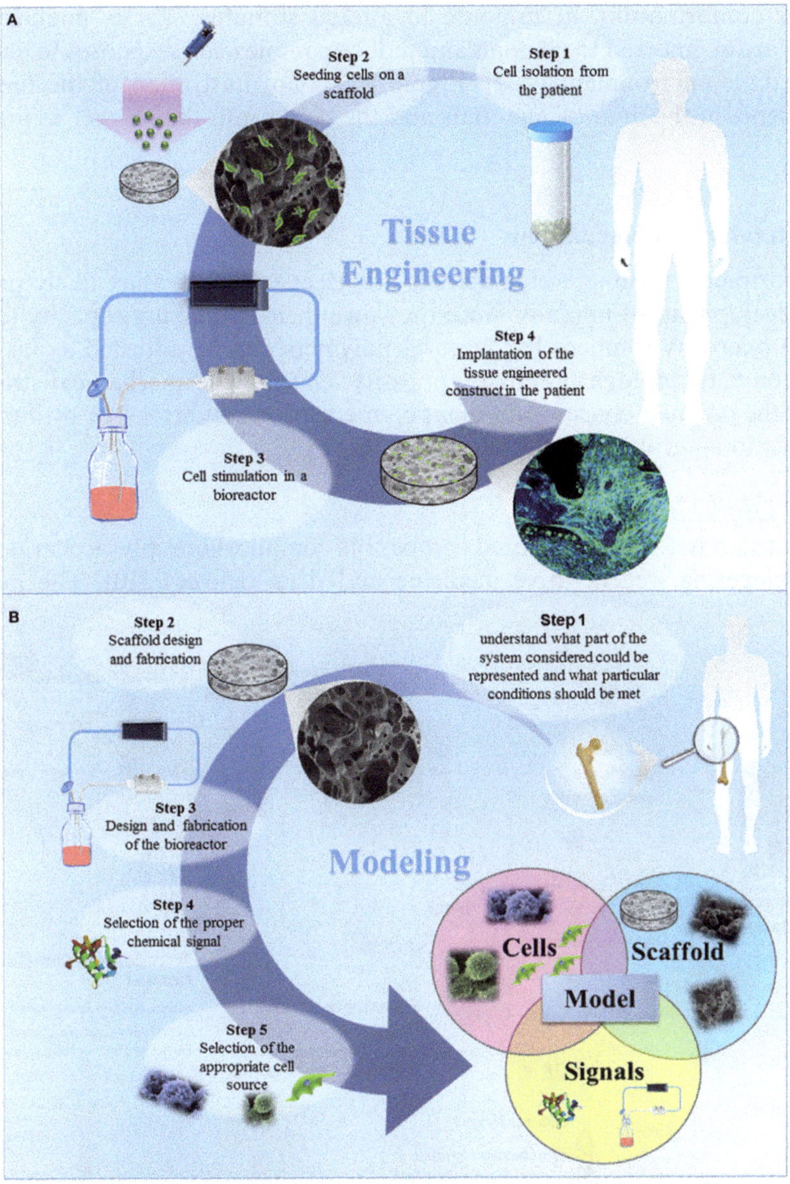

Figure 8.1. (a) The classical tissue engineering (TE) paradigm, a three-step platform involving, cells, scaffold and reactor, and (b) the TE approach for the development of *in vitro* models. A five-step modelling process, shows in the intricacies involved in the design and development of mimicking of model tissue. Adapted and reproduced with permission from [9].

8.2 Materials and structures

Use of biomaterials as prosthesis started in the 1960s, and around the 1980s a variety of dental and orthopedic applications, and bioactive drugs had entered the pharmacy. New generations of synthetic polymers being produced will change their molecular conformation, in response to altered stimulus. These 'intelligent' biomaterials are engineered to respond and induce complex cell responses to changes in the immediate environment [4, 7]. Figure 8.2 is an illustration of the timeline of developments in the area of materials and the debut into the market as interactive implants.

8.2.1 Natural origin biomaterials

Huge assortments of innate biomaterials are accessible possessing likely properties for the development of implants since they owe their mimicking capacity to that of the tissue microenvironment [8]. Natural polymers can be adjusted as far as their degradation rate, biological activity, porosity, charge, and mechanical strength by changing the polymer concentration or polymerization conditions, or by introducing useful functional groups for tissue compatibility [9].

8.2.1.1 Chitin/chitosan

Chitin/chitosan is a widely explored compatible complex homoplysaccharide used in tissue engineering, regenerative medicine and drug delivery [10]. The molecular

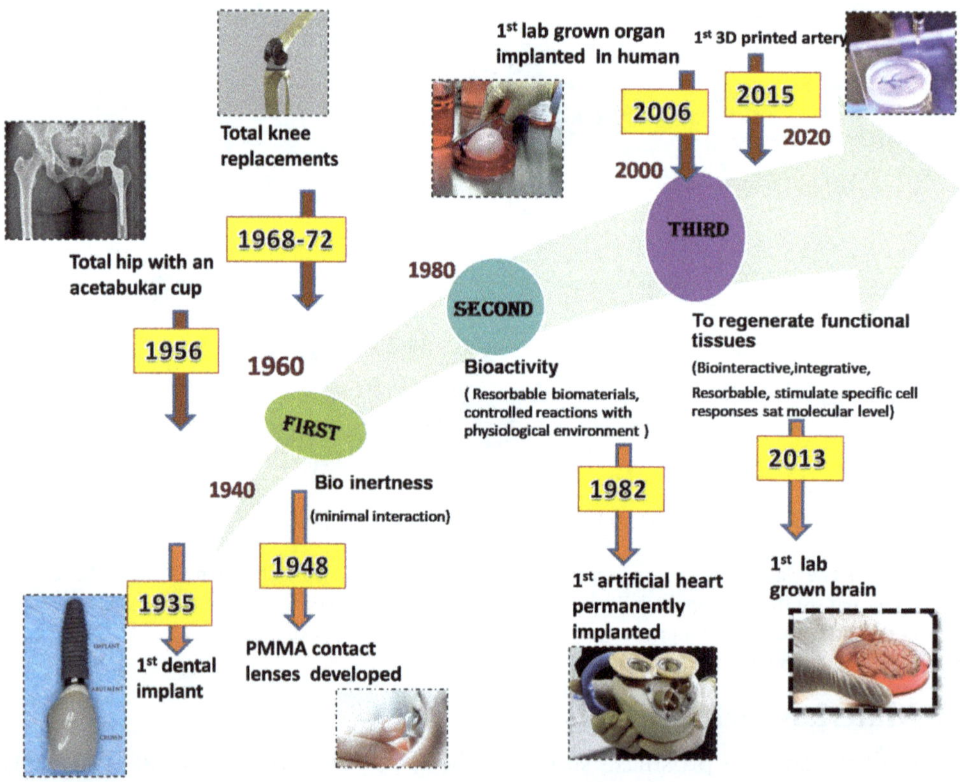

Figure 8.2. Evolutionary contribution of biomaterials to tissue implants and regeneration. Adapted figure and reproduced with modifications from [7], copyright (2012), with permission from Elsevier.

structure containing β(1/4) groups linked to *N*-acetyl-D-glucosamine, which has a structural similarity to that of glycosaminoglycans of the extra cellular matrix, provides the compatible involvement in the tissue regeneration to chitosan [11]. The crystallinity of the polymer depends on the degree of deacetylation of the polymer. The gel-forming nature of chitosan in acidic media and the visible swelling action by absorbing a substantial amount of water have made chitosan hydrogels a large 3D network of structures used in tissue regeneration that are very well explored as wound dressings, muscle implants, etc [12].

8.2.1.2 Collagen

Collagen is the most commonly used biomaterial and is an abundant structural protein produced from fibroblasts in the human body. It is involved in all three phases of the wound healing cascade; hence, its use in tissue engineering and regenerative medicine is irreplaceable [13–16]. Important logical evidence indicates that the chemotactic effects of collagen depend on the preservation of its local structure. Fibroblasts, for example, have integrin receptors that sense flawless regions of local collagen and fibronectin particles [17].

8.2.1.3 Alginate (AG)

Alginate is an anionic biocompatible, biodegradable, nonlinear natural polysaccharide biopolymer derived from marine algae (Phaeophyceae). The major structural components manuronic acid and glucuronic acid groups impart haemostatic potential, which is a beneficial feature of alginate-based dressings over non-alginate dressings because they create coagulation effects due to the existence of divalent cations in the gel (presence of calcium or zinc) [18]. Alginate is used in the fabrication of cellular scaffolds, wound dressings as well as controlled drug delivery systems, including hydrogels, microparticles [19]. In addition to hemostatic ability, alginate dressings possess a unique property, gelling capacity intiated by ion exchange process, i.e. material-tissue cross talk (Ca^{++} ions from alginate and Na^{+} $^{+}$ ions of tissue fluid react and form a gel) [20–22]. Because of this property, alginates are of first-hand use in the management of exudates, especially in exudative wounds management, stable, interactive hydrogels for tissue implants, etc.

8.2.1.4 Hyaluronic acid (HA)

Hyaluronic acid is the anionic, non-sulphated polysaccharide widely used in tissue engineering and regenerative medicine, because it is a native structural element of the extra cellular matrix [23, 24]. The prime reconstruction capability of hyaluronic acid is used in skin repair and regeneration, bone repair, cartilage repair along with the composite synthetic polymers.

8.2.1.5 Keratin

Keratin is also a native structural component abundantly found in the fur, nails, horns, feathers of wool, and epithelia of vertebrates [25]. It is very desirable for wound healing due to its intrinsic bioactivity, biocompatibility and physical properties [26]. Predominantly keratin is used for wound management and skin repair.

8.2.1.6 Silk

Silk fibroin and silk sericin are derivatives of *Bombyx mori*, biocompatible proteins that help in essential healing events [27]. Regenerative effects of silk proteins have recently been used to establish usable bioactive scaffolds and viable bio-artificial skin grafts and have demonstrated considerable promise in the treatment of hard-to-heal wounds [28]. With the introduction of modern medicine, silk sutures were commercialized, taking into account the mechanical properties of silk threads, as the knots created by silk threads were tight and simple to manage [29]. *Song et al* documented the use of silk sericin in wound dressings that had positive impact on cell development and tissue regeneration of human skin [30].

8.2.1.7 Fucoidan

Fucoidan is a sulphate polysaccharide with an anticoagulant property that has recently attracted a lot of attention and is behaving like heparin [31]. In addition to anticoagulant properties, it also has active potential for the management of inflammation, thrombosis, infection and cell proliferation [32]. Due to all these practical properties, it has recently found its role in the treatment of burn wounds and is in use with other copolymers for the preparation of dressings.

8.2.1.8 Homoglycans

Biochemically, homoglycans are polysaccharides (starch, cellulose, dextran) made up of a single form of sugar monomer that is replicated in the chain [33]. As biocompatible materials, they are used as modulators for cellular reactions involved in wound healing [34]. Cellulose is, among other things, the most available unplugged polysaccharide polymer derived from renewable sources and used, along with another polymer, to enhance the physical-chemical properties of the alteration in the preparation of wound dressing scaffolds, drug delivery carriers, etc. Bacterial cellulose (BC) is a biopolymer made up of pure cellulose, from bacteria showing the greater potential for mending at wider range of dimensions (macro to nano) [35]. The resistance provided by the BC implants for skin [36], cornea [37], cartilage [38], bone [39] along with the composites suitable for the native tissue composition and architecture are not only limited to effective anti-bacterial resistance but also chemical and physical compatibility with resilience to the micro environment.

8.2.1.9 Gelatin

Gelatin is present naturally in ligaments, tendons, and tissues [40]. Gelatin possesses anti-thrombogenic and anti-inflammatory properties suitable as a wound dressing due to its simple film-forming, air-permeability, biocompatibility, non-toxicity and haemostatic properties. DouDerm® dressings-3D network of sodium carboxymethyl cellulose (CMC), pectin and gelatin are by Convatec America [40]. Gelatin, HA and NCC porous, spongy hydrogels [41] Crosslinked foam, starch-gelatin-borax-erythromycin, currently improve mechanical strength and performance [42].

There are other biopolymers secreted from bacteria gellan gum, polyhydroxyalkanoates (PHAs) possessing high molecular weight, slow degrading materials used for tissue engineering and regenerative medicine extensively [43–45].

Gellan gum also acts like alginates by interacting with the mono- and divalent cations of the environmental fluid [46], whereas PHAs acts by interacting with the molecular environment by inducing the release of cytokines [47–49].

There are numerous numbers of non-polymeric naturally occurring substances like, graphene [50], calcium phosphates [51–53], silicates (marine sponge secretions) [54–57] and fibrin [55, 58–61] which are among the high performing new generation natural materials used in the regenerative medicine alone or in combination with synthetic polymers. These have shown improved mechanical, compatible properties to tissue implants ranging from bone to cardian and smooth muscle tissues and vascular grafting materials.

8.2.2 Synthetic origin biomaterials

Synthetic biomaterials are steadier and precisely mechanical compared with natural biomaterials, and therefore profitable for the creation of implants [62–64]. The main preferences of synthetic materials are: adaptable parameter control, molecular weight, degradation time, ability to adjust substance properties that subsequently can be changed to create derivatives with improved adhesion and cross-connecting capacity and the enormous scope of large-scale production capacity. Based on the degradation capacity, they are of two types: (i) degradable polymers, and (ii) non-degradable polymers.

8.2.2.1 Non-degradable synthetic polymers

Non-degradable synthetic polymers are biologically inert and are used to reduce the host response to the biomaterial to a minimum [63, 65]. These materials provide the source for different types of medical devices [65–67] such as sutures, orthopaedic implants [70, 71], fracture fixation devices, catheters and dialysis tubings, implantable carriers [69] for the long-term delivery of drugs [68, 69, 72], e.g. contraceptive hormones, etc.

A wide variety of polymeric biomaterials in this category, which are used for making the structures used for the tissue engineering and regeneration of damaged tissues and organs, include the following; polysiloxanes, PMMA (poly(methyl methacrylate)), PHEMA (poly(2-hydroxyethyl methacrylate)) [73, 74], polyurethanes (PUs) [75, 76], poly(tetrafluoroethylene) (PTFE), poly(N-isopropylacrylamide) (PNiPAAm), PEG (polyethylene glycol) and PEO (polyethylene oxide). A detailed list [77–88] of polymers along with their intended application area has been detailed in table 8.1.

8.2.2.2 Degradable synthetic polymers

Degradable synthetic polymers are predominantly used for the short duration implants for tissue regeneration and delivery of active bio molecules and drugs to the target site [89–91]. These are generally used for adhesion, suturing, delivery and fixation purposes [92–95]. Chemically they belong to polyesters of alpha-hydroxy acids (PLA (polylactic acid), PGA (polyglycolic acid), PLGA, PDLLA (poly DL-lactic acid)), aliphatic polyesters having lactone ring (poly(ε-caprolactone) (PCL)),

Table 8.1. Progressive synthetic polymers for the tissue implants.

Materials	Area of application	References
Poly(glycolic acid) PGA	Bone, cartilage, liver, tendon, urothelium and intestinal tissue engineering	[93–95]
Poly(L-lactic acid) PLLA	Bone, cartilage, ligament, neural tissue engineering	[92–94
Poly(D,L-lactic-co-glycolic acid) PLGA	Bone, cartilage, urothelium and neural tissue engineering	[97–99]
Poly(caprolactone) PCL	Bone and vessel tissue engineering	[96–99]
Poly(dioxanone)	Bone tissue engineering and orthopaedic applications	[100]
Polyurethanes	Soft tissue engineering and biomedical applications	[73–75]
polyphosphazenes	Cartilage, bone, liver and neural tissue engineering	[101–103]
Polysiloxanes (silicones)	Catheters, shunts, drains and tubular implants, such as artificial urethra.	[63–66]
Poly(methyl methacrylate) PMMA	Orthopaedic implantsocular lenses, hard contact lenses	[67, 78]
Poly(2-hydroxyethyl methacrylate) PHEMA	Soft contact lenses, intraocular lenses, controlled drug delivery, for the repair of female breasts and nasal cartilages, replica corneas, wound dressings.	[68–72]
Poly (N-isopropylacrylamide) (PNiPAAm)	Drug and cell delivery, articular cartilage	[76–78]
Poly(tetrafluoroethylene) (PTFE)	Vascular grafting material	[82]
Polyvinyl alcohol (PVA)	Menisci implant	[104]

polyphosphazenes and polyvinyl alcohol (PVA) [96–100]. All of them have specific mechanical strength depending upon the molecular weight, which is a predominant factor for the time-dependent delivery and tissue-specific degradation capacity optimization. They are used for the delivery of genes, drugs, growth factors, supportive templates as scaffolds for cell growth and proliferation and tissue regeneration of damaged tissues and organs [101–106].

8.2.3 Biopolymers based nanostructures for tissue implants and regeneration

Advances in the development of nanoparticles (NPs) and involvement in influence over nanoscale structures have had a crucial effect on the designing of scaffolds for tissue replacement and delivery of medicines and bio molecules to provide customizable features. The distribution capacity for directed/stimuli response, and specific authority over action have rendered it conceivable for their usage to boost design

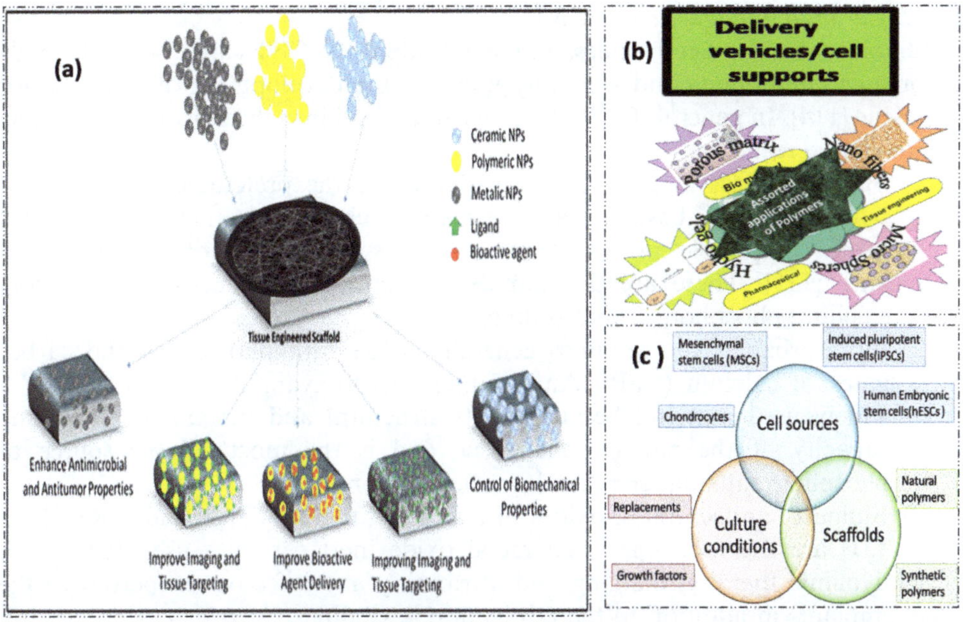

Figure 8.3. Biopolymers based nanostructures for tissue implants and regeneration; (a) examples of different types of NPs, (b) assorted applications of polymers, and (c) tissue engineering triad. (a) Adapted from [289], copyright (2015), with permission from Frontiers.

depending on the application [107]. An illustration depicting various nanostructures has been given in figure 8.3(a).

8.2.3.1 Metallic nanoparticles

The significant role performed by metallic NPs made of gold or silver in tissue engineering and regenerative medicine is irreplaceable. They are used for the functionalizations, tracing, tracking and destructing of target cells, tissues and delivery systems [108, 109].

8.2.3.1.1 Gold nanoparticles (AuNPs)

AuNPs are colloids of gold particles of nanometer scale. The surface of the gold particles offers great possibilities for functionalization, owing to the high reactive complementary group's capability for the conjugation of several ligands, ranging from biomolecules to various drug molecules for selective targeting and delivery. For tissue implants, these are loaded along with the implant via additive manufacturing techniques used for the tracing and tracking of the position, reactivity, etc of the implant, post-implantation [110, 111].

8.2.3.1.2 Silver nanoparticles (AgNPs)

AgNPs are the colloid of silver nanometer particles and are one of the most commonly used metallic NPs, primarily for their antimicrobial properties, in the biomedical field [112, 113].

8.2.3.2 Ceramic nanoparticles (CNPs)

In addition to metals, metal oxides, and metal sulphides, CNPs are essentially made of inorganic compounds and generally used for the development of implants for bone tissue [114]. In general, CNPs may be categorized into three groups depending upon the tissue reactivity.

(1) Bioactive glass nanoceramics (n-BGCs) are the preferable, materials for bone and dental tissue regeneration approaches due to their non-immunogenic, compatible, proliferative capabilities along with antibacterial resistance [115]. These are the complex structural forms made with silicon, calcium, phosphorous and sodium ions.

(2) Bioresorbable nanoceramics generally made with phosphates and carbonates of calcium (CaP). Among these, hydroxyapatite (HAp) [116] is a widely used material because of its structural and functional mimicking capacity of the native bone tissue and is the most soluble source of phosphate salts under neutral or alkaline conditions.

(3) Bioinert nanoceramics, oxides of zinc and titanium (TiO_2 and ZnO) [117–121] are the most preferred metal oxide inert ceramics used for photodynamic therapy, imaging and attributing anti-infective properties to the implants in addition to the fabrication flexibilities.

8.2.3.3 Magnetic nanoparticles (MNPs)

Oxides of iron, Fe_3O_4 and Fe_2O_3 are widely used magnetic NPs in tissue engineering and regenerative medicine for cell imaging purposes [122]. Many times, these are used for the destruction of diseased or abnormal cells like cancerous cells [123]. By including them in the implant, there is great flexibility of location of the implant after implantation and verification of the performance and movement through imaging, especially useful for nerve conduits for the verification of cell guidance to have improved clinical outcomes with less toxic effects.

8.2.3.4 Polymeric nanoparticles (PNPs)

PNPs are the most imperative nanobiomaterials for tissue engineering and regenerative medicine (TERM). The suppleness of tailoring the physical (morphology, solubility, degradation rate, strength), (chemistry and reactivity) and biological features (low cytotoxicity, strong biocompatibility, higher EPR effect) make them a preferred choice for drug delivery and tissue engineering platforms [124, 125]. Several studies have reported the use of these systems for the development of stimuli-responsive nanoengineered systems reports Most of the latest PNP systems are engineered to be responsive to various physicochemical stimuli systems to track, trace, and target the desired target cells or tissue of interest, allowing high precision and reliability distribution or targeting systems for TERM applications [126]. One among them is the development of smart indicator dressings.

8.2.3.4.1 Polymeric nanomaterials for the delivery of active substances

Delivery of active compounds at the target tissue site is the major challenge of TERM and the success of the encapsulating material always plays an important role in the performance, hence, polymeric nanomaterials designed to deliver the intended active component or indicator may be either in the form of swellable matrices, nanofiber scaffolds, or microparticles/spheres [127–130]. Porous matrixes are shown in figures 8.3(b) and (c). Recent studies are focusing on the use of plasma proteins as delivery carriers to target specific tissue and cell targets [131, 132]. Use of polymer conjugates with functionalized surfaces with the desired target ligands to meet the target tissue demand is the developing trend which shows the superior flexibility of these materials for tissue engineering applications.

8.2.4 Biomaterials for cell supports

As temporary ECM, polymers as scaffolds play a critical function, but seldom act as supports to damaged tissue micro and macro for the promotion of cell proliferation and tissue regeneration, as shown in figures 8.3(a)–(c). The evolving nanobiomaterials are capable of performing multiple roles, as support systems, delivery vehicles, growth promoters, rejuvenating materials for the native environment. Collagen, which is the ECM's key protein component, is known to be the ideal material of choice. Collagen-based scaffolds are in use for cartilage restoration, long bone breaks, and improvement of regeneration of many tissues [133]. In addition to collagen, chitosan-based materials are of interest for orthopaedic tissue implants and in muscle tissue engineering [134–136]. The polycationic existence and predictive degradation rate are helpful for the distribution to the target tissues [137–141]. Another potentially used cell transport method explored to stimulate the development of different tissues is alginate.

8.2.5 Bionanocomposites

It is possible to define nanocomposites as a template with special arrangement possessions, loaded with composite filling materials of a low dimension (size less than 100 nm) [142]. These substances, with the generally familiar name 'fillers', are used to modify or apply features, for the tracking, mimicking and targeting of the micro and macro tissue environment, such as signal-carrying capacity, tissue-specific compatibility, etc to the templates.

8.2.5.1 Metalic nanofillers

Metalic nanomaterials, like gold (Au), silver(Ag) and iron oxide(Fe_2O_3), are used to impart tracking, targeting and damaging tissue or cells of interest. An injectable scaffold developed by *Smith et al,* using AuNPs of below 100 nm showed enhanced tissue remodelling while encouraging the cell proliferation by making the ROS levels low [143, 144]. Iron oxide NPs for tracking and AgNPs for their commendable antibacterial activity are extensively in use for multi-functional performance of tissue constructs.

8.2.5.2 Ceramic nanofillers

Ceramic nanofillers used to impart additional chitosan with HAP nanopowders are a typical example of ceramic nanofiller polymer reinforcement [145, 146]. Cellulose, is another important biomaterial used along with nanoHAP to develop synthetic bone tissue scaffolds [147], zinc-HAP [148], PCL-TiO_2 [149], diopside-TiO_2 [150].

8.2.5.3 Carbon-based nanofillers

Among the carbon-based nanofillers, carbon nanotubes (CNTs) have been used extensively. Along with polymers for nerve, cardiac and muscle tissue implants [151–156]. CNTs are used to impart impulse transmission capacity and flexible mechanical strength without reacting to the native environment.

8.2.5.4 Cellulose-based nanofillers

Cellulose-based nanofillers are gaining increased interest owing to their abundance, natural mimicking of extra cellular matrix components. Use of these reduces the chances of foreign body response of the implants [157, 158]. These are available in three different forms, nanocrystals and nanofibrils and cellulose derived from bacteria, bacterial cellulose [36, 159, 160]. These fillers impart commendable mechanical strength, hence are widely used for skin, bone and vascular implants without indulging tissue compatibility issues.

8.2.5.5 Sol–gel nanocomposites

Sol–gel nanocomposites are the most used biomaterial because of their flexibility for customization as per the release pattern required for the drugs, templates for the cell and molecular interactions, support systems for the damaged tissues or organs [161–163].

A brief list of composites, biodegradable polymers used in making implants has been given in table 8.1. One among them is bioactive glass, with its great surface reactivity potential widely used to mimic the bone tissue environment. This when it is combined with other polymers of natural/synthetic origin shows improved performance, not only limited to its mechanical and surface reactivity but also improved biodegradability, compatibility and tissue interaction. Most widely explored polymers in combination are PLA [164] and poly(lactic-co-glycolic acid) [165] or polycaprolactone (PCL).

8.3 Strategies available for making tissue implants

Morphology and structure of the scaffold is the prime influential parameter for the complementary mimicry at the cellular level [166]. By keeping the local environment biochemical and signalling molecule involved, tissue implants are being made to mimic the target tissue regeneration.

Complementary tissue constructs fabrication, hence should meet the functional requirements of the target tissue to meet the demands at both to provide a native compatible environment. Strategies for developing scaffolds are mainly grouped into two categories:

(1) conventional methods;
(2) rapid prototyping (RP) methods, which are otherwise well known as additive manufacturing methods.

The scaffolds produced by each method will produce different characteristics. Depending upon the requirements these methods are used in combination or alone to prepare the scaffolds [167, 168]. Additive manufacturing methods, as shown in figure 8.4, provide a stable structurally mimicking architecture for tissue implants. Recent developments in this direction with the inclusion of simultaneous imaging and 3D fabrication made the debut of customizabe implants.

8.3.1 Conventional/traditional methods

Traditional methods used for the fabrication of scaffolds used for tissue engineering and regeneration include sol–gel technologies (solvent casting and practical leaching, gas foaming, thermal-induced phase separation), freeze-drying and electrospinning.

8.3.1.1 Sol–gel technologies

Solution–gelation type processing technologies, like solvent casting and practical leaching, gas foaming, and thermal-induced phase separation, are the most frequently used traditional methods for the fabrication of scaffolds used in tissue

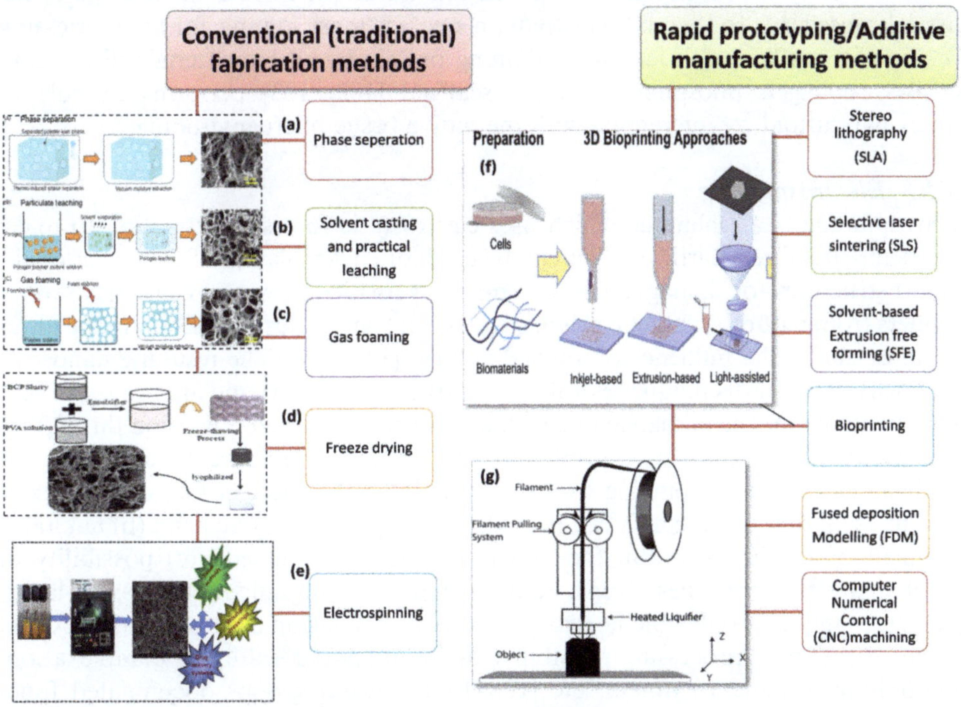

Figure 8.4. Conventional and rapid prototyping fabrication technologies for tissue engineered scaffolds. (a) Phase separation, (b) solvent casting and practical leaching, (c) gas foaming, (d) freeze drying, (e) electrospinning, (f) schematic diagrams showing the bio printing approaches; (A) inkjet-based bio printing systems, (B) extrusion-based bio printing systems, (C) DLP-based bio printing and (D) TPP-based bio printing platforms, and (g) fused deposition modeling. (a), (b), (c), and (e) reproduced from [290], copyright (2019), with permission from Elsevier. (f) Reproduced from [291], copyright (2018), with permission from Elsevier. (g) Reproduced from [292], copyright (2015), with permission from Elsevier.

engineering processes. These methods produce mesoporous structures, as shown in figure 8.4(a) [169–171].

The sol–gel based approach is used in all the sectors of healthcare because of the anticipated enhancement of natural tissue regeneration [172, 173]. The materials synthesised by this approach are used to immobilize bio molecules, anti-infective agents via entrapment or encapsulation into the matrix. This can be used for the prevention of prosthetic joint infections [174], for the synthesis of bone cement [175], artificial tissue and ligaments [176], and dental implants.

Among the new generation biomaterials prepared by this process are mesoporous bioactive glasses (MBGs), which have exceptional osteoconductivity, osteo-stimulation and degradation rate. The recent attempt of research in this direction has mainly focused on the fabrication of 3D foam scaffolds [177–179].

8.3.1.2 Freeze-drying

Fabrication of scaffolds using lyophilisation is a process in which the polymer solution blend is cooled to freezing point and the solutes will be separated in the ice phase, i.e. freezing and drying is the most widely used technique [180, 181]. The schematic process is clearly shown in figure 8.4(d). In this technique there is no damage to the material caused due to thermal sensitivity, hence it is most suitable for the fabrication of composite scaffolds fabrication containing protein-based biomaterials. For example, BG—collagen phosphatidyl serine scaffold [182, 183] performs its role as mimicking scaffold by interacting with the native tissue microenvironment.

8.3.1.3 Electrospinning

Electrospinning is a technique which uses electrostatic forces of attraction to make nanometer-size fibres, particles. This can be used for encapsulation of active materials, support structures for damaged tissues, templates for the growth of cells, etc. Several polymers from natural, synthetic origin singly or in composites are used to make ultra-fine fibres, under the influence of applied voltage [184–187]. The resulting nanoscale structures out of this technique resembles the structure of ECM and are proven to be a good facilitator for the exchange of gases, cell permeability and migration through its commendable presence or pores in its network, as shown in figure 8.4(c).

Advantages of electrospinning over other methods of nanofiber fabrication techniques are: (a) simple setup which can be scaled up as per the requirement; (b) tailorable alignment of the fibres within the matrix (random or aligned); (c) possibility of immobilizing bio molecules, drugs, active organic or inorganic materials; (d) layer-by-layer designing; (e) flexible horizontal, vertical dimension control through X and Y controls; (f) post-processing possibility of the prepared scaffolds, complexation, cross-linking, plasma treatment, etc [188–190]. Several groups documented functional tissue scaffolds ranging from skin, bone, nerve, muscle vascular grafts, etc [191–195], with incorporation into biological molecular tissues.

8.3.1.4 Rapid prototyping/additive manufacturing methods

Rapid prototyping methods are the newer technologies that allow for more control of scaffold geometry construction. The most important developments in the manufacture of scaffolds are solid free-form manufacturing (SFF) technologies, three-dimensional printing (3D), fused deposition modelling, 3D plotting or direct-write bioprinting [196]. 3D printing uses inkjet printing liquid binder fluid on a powder bed, as shown in figures 8.4(g) and (h).

For the printing of 3D scaffolds, which are suitable for tissue engineering and regeneration, advanced additive manufacturing techniques involving biological components during printing have come into focus and changed the fate of tissue implants. The printing of biomolecules automatically on a substrate to fabricate a heterogeneous performing architecture is called 'bioprinting'. The polymer material along with the loaded cells is called bio-ink. These bio-inks are generally sol–gel preparations, hydrogels, etc. A detailed illustration of the process has been shown in figure 8.4(f).

There are five different types of bioprinting methods in use for the fabrication of 3D tissue implants based on the model used for printing of cells onto a substrate: (1) ink-jet-based bioprinting [197] used for the printing of a live mammalian cell by using thermal and piezoelectric sensors models; (2) pressure-assisted bioprinting [198], by using this technique, layered 3D structures can be made by using thermal, or chemical cross-linking methods; (3) laser-assisted bio printing [199], a pulsed laser beam is used to deposit the material precisely on the surface of the substrate; (4) solenoid valve-based printing [200], used for printing of cells for skin repair; (5) acoustic-jet printing [201], which allows pico-litre quantity of bio-ink suitable for genetic materials, growth factors, cellular factors loading.

8.3.2 Outcome of complementary scaffold fabrication techniques (figure 8.3(a))

(1) Anisotropic and gradient scaffolds, which are high performance, smart materials for acclimatisation with their surrounding environment are a highly commendable achievement of the advanced fabrication techniques like additive manufacturing and additive electrospraying techniques. The scaffolds or structures made out of additive manufacturing technologies are flexible at the length scale and provide augmentative gradient features to the implants, hence they will be in a position to perform the role of substitute tissues [6, 197–208]. Several studies reported the use of alignment flexibility, hence structural mimicking, which allow making the tissue conduits for cornea, skin, tendon, nerve, muscle, etc.

(2) Surface feature manipulation, which is the most important property, influences the reactivity with the tissue micro- and macroenvironment. Surface roughness, compatibility, attraction can be manipulated pre- and post-fabrication. These features influence cell migration, toxicity and differentiation [209–212]. Any discretion of the surface features influences the cell–material interactions, since nano-biointerface reactions are predominant for the acceptance of implants; otherwise, it creates long term reactions like foreign body response (FBR).

(3) Development of injectable scaffolds is the technological breakthrough in the regenerative medicine which allowed the control of morphological features

in situ [213–215]. A few examples of this kind are stents, catheters, and ceramic implants, etc.

(4) Structures having the capability to track and image are the regeneration advancements towards the tracking capability for the identification of potential toxicity, if any, after implantation [216–218].

8.4 Potential tissue-engineered implants: a biomaterial perspective

The key objective of tissue implant engineering is to organize materials that can be applied to defective tissue sites and to allow the patient's cells to be remodelled. The active material architecture is a 3D scaffold which is a template for the cell interactions to happen. The porous architecture for cellular and vascular filtration and multiscale organisation makes a major contribution to the performance of the implants [219–222]. There is no one-size-fits-all configuration that is suitable for all applications of tissue engineering.

8.4.1 Bone tissue

For the designing and fabrication of bone implants a thorough understanding and knowledge of the compatible anatomy and physiology of the bone tissue and the complementary materials available for the compatible mimicking are required. By using a combination of traditional and additive manufacturing techniques, bone implants are being made to meet the tissue demands. Bone tissue implants need to have sufficient mechanical strength to withstand the load and should be free from degradation due to wear and tear while facilitating the regeneration of the tissue. Bioceramics, both crystalline amorphous forms of bioglass, polymers from natural and synthetic origin, like collagen, are used to make implants for bone tissue; since they mimic native extracellular components and architecture, they promote osteogenesis [223, 224]. In addition to these biologically active materials, currently carbon-based materials such as graphene and CNTs are in exploration, owing to the greater mechanical strength, signal transmission capacity, and are showing remarkable performance [223, 225, 226]. These materials not only provide required mechanical strength, but also help in the growth and proliferation of cellular components by directing the molecular fractions within the microenvironment and support the ingrowth of the blood vessels too owing to the presence of pores. Many reports have shown the superior performance of these kinds of implants, among them are [227–229]. Synthetic polymers which release acidic degradation components are prone to cause long-term implant degradation; hence resorbable materials are more preferred.

8.4.2 Neural tissue

Neural tissue regeneration is one of the important contributions of biomaterials, and gave a new face to high-performance nanobiomaterials. Nervous systems generally involve brain, spinal cord and retina. Any injury which might be due to sudden blockage within the nerve, or damage due to accidents or degeneration due to defects, etc needs corrections or replacements depending upon the extent of damage [230, 231].

For this kind of situation, nano-enabled approaches, utilization of biomaterials for the delivery of molecules and support systems enabling for the correction of a cascade of events are available and under development.

8.4.2.1 Spinal cord

Biomaterial based stumps can be placed within the direction of the nerves. Schwann cells, NSPCs and NSPcs are incorporated into these implants. Nanostructured implant nerve conduits, which are aligned in the directed growth of the axon are showing good results, are in use. Acute spinal injuries are currently being treated by using injectable cells in the form of suspension dispersions in the polymer matrix into the surrounding damage site to overcome the drawback of the remyelination of the spare axons. Nanoscale architecture is crucial to neuronal function, and collagen and chitosan are explored to meet the temporary demands of spinal injuries. Among the synthetic polymers, hydrogel nerve guiding tubular implants made of poly(2-hydroxyethyl methacrylate-*co*-methyl methacrylate) (P[HEMA/MMA]) [232]. P(HEMA/MMA) [233] shows potential compatibility.

8.4.2.2 Brain

Regeneration and repair of the brain has remained a key challenge for decades. Advancements in material science with the advent of nanotechnology brought nerve autographs, which are substitutes used to repair wounded peripheral nerves owing to their low risk of immunological rejection [234]. PLA-NSCs (neural stem cells) aligned nanofibers are being used to treat peripheral nervous system (PNS) injury.

CNTs, having the potential capability of conducting potential are a gifted feature for the signal transmission within or between the neurons. Graphene-based 3D conductive scaffolds are in demand for neuroregeneration because of their electrical and electrochemical performance [235, 236]. Nano-enabled materials and architectures provide several functionalities, including the monitoring and activation of electrical activity, the identification of neurotransmitters, neuromodulators and other neurologically important biomolecules, and the capacity to monitor medication distribution and regeneration.

8.4.2.3 Eye

8.4.2.3.1 Retina

Regenerative retinal degeneration treatment relies on pharmacotherapy. Advances in anti-vascular endothelial growth factor (anti-VEGF) therapies have been made. Ozurdex, is a PLGA-based implant for the management of macular oedema [237, 238]. More recent advances in retinal pigment epithelium (RPE) based delivery [239] include the use of solid synthetic injectable membranes.

8.4.2.3.2 Cornea

The cornea is the most sensitive and important part of the eye, and any injury or damage to the cornea leads to partial or total loss of vision. For this, there are no solutions available, other than replacements for the cornea or corneal implants [240–242].

Implant construction for the cornea is challenging since it demands the strength, and transparency (optical) of the corneal tissue. Poly(N-isoproplyacrylamide), a temperature-responsive hydrophobic polymer dependent epithelial cell layer, has been designed and transplanted directly to the eye without sutures exhibiting a compact, stratified structure [243–245]. For more than a decade, research and developments in corneal tissue engineering of collagen and non-collagen based engineered matrices, which are available in the form of cell sheets, sponges, films, sealants, have been showing improved morphological and biochemical functional similarity by forming a continuous layer more or less similar to native basal epithelium [246–250]. Studies using the materials which will get degraded, not shrunk during the period of stay are under development, by using different molecular weight ratios of PLGA in combination with other optically active or photoactive and transparent polymers [251–253].

8.4.3 Muscle tissue

Muscle tissue (skeletal, smooth and cardiac) anomalies causing substantial loss of muscle, need further surgical reconstruction. Engineered tissues are of hope for the recreation of the microarchitecture of the extracellular matrix. 2D and 3D electrospinning architectures using biodegradable polymers from natural and synthetic origin, like protein-based, polysaccharide-based, synthetic lactide and lactones, and PVA, are the most widely used successful muscular implants currently in use [254–259]. Seeding of myoblasts on parallel nanofiber surfaces to create structural bilayer mimicking is the most fascinating and remarkable contribution in this field

8.4.3.1 Cardiac tissue

Tissue reconstruction of the cardiac muscle is a challenging approach and involves the most demanding feature needed, i.e. contractility [260, 261]. In this direction biodegradable/non-biodegradable polymer from natural origins having better biodegradability, renewability, and low toxicity are used. Cardiac patches based on collagen with added electroconductive properties have been tested for their therapeutic ability [262, 263]. Graphene, a carbon-based material, having greater mechanical strength together with electrical and conducting capacity is best suited for cardiac implants. Gelatin-PCL-graphene implants, having desirable electrical conductivity and biological properties, are the only composite scaffold dependent implants that have been tested for cardiac tissue engineering [264–268]. The electrical properties of inserted grafts pose major obstacles for the reconstruction of infracted heart tissue. which includes the design of nano-engineered aligned collagen fibres. There are also AgNP- and AuNP-based cardiac patches for MI repair. In addition to these, cell sheet technology is also an emerging platform used for this purpose.

8.4.3.2 Cartilage

Cartilage is a semi-solid dedicated connective tissue. It is designed to bear weight, give support, torsion, bending, and resists tension [269]. Research and developments about synthetic materials, repair procedures, and technologies like 3D printing have brought major changes to artificial cartilage implant medical procedures [270]. Hallux rigidus is a joint condition found at the base of the big toe. It induces discomfort and tension in the joint, and over time, it becomes more and more painful to bend the foot. Cartiva is an 8–10 mm PVA disk implant that would be inserted with a small (1–1.5 mm) protrusion to act as a spacer in the first MTP joint. Implants designed to substitute or manage the muscle loss are supposed to provide 3D network, which is similar to the native structural environment for the guidance, movement and growth of the cells [271–273]. Chondrocytes are FDA-approved cells for cartilage treatment; MSCs are used where chondrocytes are not available [274]. There exist different types of implants, including fibrous structured implants, porous sponges, woven or nonwoven meshes, etc.

8.4.3.3 Meniscus

The meniscus is a thin crescent-shaped band of think, fibrous cartilage which acts as a shock absorber between the surfaces of the knees [275]. Major limitations of conventional implants are lack of adaptability in restoring the native morphology, biochemical composition, ultra structure and cellular phenotypes as per the individual patient needs [276]. Cell-free matrix (dECM) model is a successful implant which possesses the ultra structural, biochemical composition and bioactive cues of native non-immunogenic foreign cells [277, 278]. There exist many efforts in the use of polymer-based constructs for the delivery of dECM in the form of hydrogel to the injured site.

8.4.4 Skin

Skin substitutes are the heterogeneous group of substances which give support to temporary or permanent closure [279]. Currently in use from the long term to recent past, they belong to different catergories: limited time impermeable materials, one-layer long-lasting skin substitutes and combinatorial substitutes [280]. Human amniotic membrane, since 1910 has provided epidermal barrier function. Currently, this single-layer biologic material is being replaced by animal origin grafts [281] because of their long-lasting capacity, but with limited use at present.

Dermal and epidermal skin substitutes containing most importantly fibroblasts, epidermal keratinocyte, respectively, called 'cultured epidermal autografts', are mostly used in full-thickness burns [282]. Several natural, synthetic biocompatible and biodegradable polymers are in use for making scaffolds which are available in the form of hydrogels, 2D and 3D structures, nanofibrous scaffolds, 3D printed structures, foams, porous scaffolds [283]. There are many reports of biomaterials and engineered skin substitutes in the patent literature, which describe a diverse array of products including collagen impregnated scaffolds dressings with immobilized growth factor gradients and *in vitro* cultured skin substitutes. A brief list of commercially available skin implants is given in table 8.2.

Table 8.2. Commercially available biomaterial tissue implants.

Application	Product	Composition	Company
Skin	Apligraft	Neonatal fibroblasts—bovine type I collagen matrix.	Organogenesis
	Trans	Nylon mesh seeded with neonatal human foreskin fibroblasts	Advanced Tissue sciences
	Cyte	Human fibroblasts—extracellular matrix—polyglactin mesh	Advanced Tissue Sciences
	Dermagraft	scaffold	Integra Lifesciences
	Integra™	bovine collagen and chondroitin-6-sulfate GAG—silicone	Corporation
	Epicel	polymer	Genzyme
	Allopatch	Sheets of autologous keratinocytes attached to a petrolatum	CONMED
		gauze support	
		Human dermal allograft	
Cartilage/meniscus	Carticel (ACI)	Autologous cartilaginious matrix with chondrocytes	Genzyme
	Neocart	autologous bioengineered neocartilage	Histogenics
	VeriCart	ready-to-use collagen scaffold	Cartiva Inc.
	Cartiva	Synthetic poly vinyl alcohol (PVA) implant	Orteq Sports
	Actifit®	synthetic hybrid of polycaprolactone (80%) and polyurethane	Medicine Ltd
	Menaflex	(20%)	Aetna(ReGen Biologics)
	The Collagen meniscus	Collagen	Stryker Corporation
	implant (CMI)	type-I collagen fibers derived from bovine Achilles tendons	
Bone	Osteocel	Allograft cellular bone graft	Osiris therapeutics
	Pura-matrix	Peptide Hydrogel	Corning Life sciences
Blood vessels	Lifeline	Patients own cells	Cytograft Tissue engineering
	Omniflow	Cross-linked ovine collagen cross linked with a polyester mesh endoskeleton	Bionova

Cardiac	Anginera	living three-dimensional engineered human tissue	Theregen
	CardioWrap	amorphous bioresorbable copolymer 70:30	MAST biosurgery
	CryoValve	Poly(L-lactide-co-D,L-lactide)	Cryolife
		Aortic Allografts	
Retina	ECT Implant	PLGA—dexamethasone	Neurotech
	Ozurdex	Dexamethasome intravitreal implant	Allergan

8.5 Challenges in clinical translation

Soon after product's development it must be tested for safety and efficacy before it can be advanced to the clinic. The aim of the pre-clinical testing of the implant is to set down the scientific basis for the use of the device in a particular clinical investigation. This includes animal models, methods for measuring implantation and survival, and immunological profile testing. To be considered biocompatible, robust implants and all tissue-engineered implants need to follow the requirements set out to prevent or mitigate interaction with body fluids, especially blood, should not elicit any reaction with the proteins and other natural structural components, (like matrix), should not cause inflammation, and should not have other non-native material introduction issues.

Biocompatibility is the first and foremost element to be considered as an obstacle for clinical translation. The tissue implants to be eligible for translation to clinical phase should meet certain requirements, biological equivalence guidelines. They include concerns regarding the safety (with host and environment), toxicity, functionality tests. To be biocompatible, tissue-engineered implants should not display reactivity to the immune system, FBR, which will be activated shortly after implantation at any blood biomaterial interface. FBR is the end-stage product of a sequence of immunological and vascular responses of the body to foreign objects which eventually result in the deterioration of the implanted unit [284]. This results in a privileged microenvironment that persists for the lifespan of every inserted device. To mitigate this effect, surface treatment and use of resorbable materials is in use and better results are shown. This means that the implant can be non-immunogenic to the extent practicable.

Another problem is the production of materials that mitigate the immune response and promote encroachment [285]. The patient's immunogenicity towards tissue engineered implants is a major contributor to the non-compliance of the products. Hence properly modelled systems for the characterization of the various proposed reactions *in vitro* and *in vivo* to mitigate this major obstacle need fine-tuning and further upgrading.

Manufacturing and scalability is another problem. Considering the importance of tissue engineering and regenerative medicine contributions and performance for the health and welfare of society, the FDA established a robust policy agenda for regenerative medicine in 2017. Studies to reduce the inflammatory response to inserted products would be critical to the therapeutic effectiveness of any corneal reconstruction.

8.6 Long-term toxicity and side effects

Inflammation of the implant–host tissue interface is the principal source of long-term toxicity of biodegradable implants [286]. In addition to these related implant causes, FBR also leads to geometry, surface chemistry and wettability. FBR can contribute to osteolysis and sarcoma due to the degradation products of the implant material.

Long-term toxicity of products typically occurs due to deterioration during post-implant residence. The breakdown can be due to mechanical (creep, wear, stress breakage, fracture), electrochemical (corrosion), chemical and biochemical issues. An example is low tolerance of Teflon (polytetrafluroethylene) to wear and tear and its inappropriate use for joint implants and artificial valves [287]. The architecture of the implant is also vital to its success.

Implants should rely on potential triggering factors for implant malfunction or device failure. Corneal transplantation deficiencies are associated with extreme immune rejection rates [288]. Other issues include inadequate pre-clinical animal research models, wrong materials during processing, mechanical failure during implantation, poor patient–prosthesis interactions.

A list of biodegradable materials used in implants and associated FBR-producing capacity, etc has been mentioned in table 8.3.

8.7 Commercial tissue implants

The emergence of biomaterials to be part of reconstructive operations that are compatible and less inefficient is a praiseworthy scientific advance in the area of reconstructive medicine and tissue engineering. Important advances in detailed surgical techniques have been rendered for more aesthetic and consistent outcomes. These interactive bioimplants are meant for tissue substitution and regeneration and have the capability to mimic physiological functions. Commercially available bioimplants are based on target application and need, and are made from different sources of materials. A few among them are skin substitutes, cardiac implants,

Table 8.3. Biodegradable synthetic polymers producing FBR (foreign body response).

Biodegradable material	Type of implant	Properties that influence FBR	Side effect
Poly(α-esters): PGA PLLA, PDLLA, PLLAHA, PLLA-TCP PLGA PDO PGA-TMC	Pins, Screws, Plates, Rods, Tacks, Suture anchors, Spine cages, and scaffolds	Hydrophobic Implant fragmentation & particle generation	Fluid accumulation Sinus formation Swelling Osteolysis Synovitis Cyst formation (human studies)
Collagen Collagen-HA Collagen-TCP	Injectable gels and Foams for BTE	Biological	none
Calcium Phosphate TCP, HA	Bone cements Scaffolds	Slow degradation Particle generation	None

implants for shoulders, knees and extremities, etc. A list of commercially available FDA approved biomaterial tissue implants is given in table 8.3.

8.8 Conclusion and prospects

In a wider context, the futuristic vision of nanotechnology, which offered a ray of hope for cellular and molecular structures, was feasible with the development of third-generation biomaterials and provides a theoretical basis for the creation of multi-functional scaffolds. In conclusion, from the thorough analysis of the BNMs used for interactive tissue implant scaffolding in this chapter our attention is drawn to the following causes, which have led to the progress of the materials and have continued to contribute and we are hoping for potential advances in laying more building blocks.

I. A detailed catalogue of nanoscale or nanostructured biomaterials developed for their intelligent, multifunctional ability at the cellular level and regeneration can be tailored to be patient-specific while considering the underlying medical conditions, if any.
II. Intelligent scaffolds (micro/nanoscale regulation) are designed to regulate cell behaviour and operate differently for the benefit of efficiency of implants. More detailed control of the parameters for avoiding or improving the longevity of the tissue implants is needed.
III. Understanding the requirement of need for the development of stimuli-responsive synthetic polymers, bioactive nanocoatings, and testing models required to evaluate and identify the pitfalls.
IV. Need for the development of novel technologies which enables the systems for the delivery of sequential delivery vehicles.
V. Need for the understanding and further studies of interactions and effects of materials at the nano–bio interface.
VI. Flexible toxicity testing models for the pre-clinical evaluation of engineered structures

Finally, the potential aim of regenerative medicine is the prospect of using bioactive triggers as a therapeutic therapy to stimulate genes, restoring the integrity of tissues as they mature. This idea may have appeared impossible just a few years ago, 'a substance that would not be resisted by living tissues, robust, adaptable, non-toxic to patients' environmental, chemical and biological well-being' [1–3, 7, 9].

Acknowledgements

The authors wish to thank the Department of Science and Technology (DST) for the WOS-B research fellowship (Dr Jhansi Lakshmi Parimi) and Ministry of Human Resource and Development (MHRD), Government. of India for providing the research fellowship (Venkata Sundeep. Seesala). The authors would also like to thank Indian Institute of Technology Kharagpur, India, and Department of Biotechnology, Vignan's Foundation for Science, Technology & Research, Vadlamudi for the generous support of the studies which contributed to this review.

References

[1] Ratner B D, Hoffman A S, Schoen F J and Lemons J E 2013 Introduction – biomaterials science *Biomaterials Science: Introduction to Materials* 3rd edn (Amsterdam: Elsevier)

[2] Yang Y, Chawla A, Zhang J, Esa A, Jang H L and Khademhosseini A 2019 Applications of nanotechnology for regenerative medicine; healing tissues at the nanoscale *Principles of Regenerative Medicine* (New York: Academic) pp 485–504

[3] Fathi-Achachelouei M, Knopf-Marques H, Ribeiro da Silva C E, Barthès J, Bat E, Tezcaner A and Vrana N E 2019 Use of nanoparticles in tissue engineering and regenerative medicine *Front. Bioeng. Biotechnol* **24** 113

[4] Velu R, Calais T, Jayakumar A and Raspall F 2020 A comprehensive review on bio-nanomaterials for medical implants and feasibility studies on fabrication of such implants by additive manufacturing technique *Materials* **13** 92

[5] Pryjmaková J, Kaimlová M, Hubáček T, Švorčík V and Siegel J 2020 Nanostructured materials for artificial tissue replacements *Int. J. Mol. Sci.* **21** 2521

[6] Kryscio D R and Peppas N A 2009 Mimicking biological delivery through feedback-controlled drug release systems based on molecular imprinting *AIChE J* **55** 1311–24

[7] Rabkin E and Schoen F J 2002 Cardiovascular tissue engineering *Cardiovasc. Pathol* **11** 305–17

[8] Mogoşanu G D and Grumezescu A M 2014 Natural and synthetic polymers for wounds and burns dressing *Int. J. Pharmaceut* **463** 127–36

[9] Caddeo S, Boffito M and Sartori S 2017 Tissue engineering approaches in the design of healthy and pathological *in vitro* tissue models *Frontiers Bioeng. Biotechnol* **5** 40

[10] Rodríguez-Vázquez M, Vega-Ruiz B, Ramos-Zúñiga R, Saldaña-Koppel D A and Quiñones-Olvera L F 2015 Chitosan and its potential use as a scaffold for tissue engineering in regenerative medicine *BioMed. Res. Int.* **2015** 821279

[11] Costa-Pinto A R, Vargel I, Tuzlakoglu K, Correlo VM, Sol P C, Faria S, Piskin E, Reis R L and Neves NM 2014 Influence of scaffold composition over *in vitro* osteogenic differentiation of hBMSCs and *in vivo* inflammatory response *J. Biomater. Appl* **28** 1430–42

[12] Beşkardeş I G, Demirtaş T T, Durukan M D and Gümüşderelioğlu M 2015 Microwave-assisted fabrication of chitosan–hydroxyapatite superporous hydrogel composites as bone scaffolds *J. Tissue Eng. Regen. Med* **9** 1233–46

[13] Dong C and Lv Y 2016 Application of collagen scaffold in tissue engineering: recent advances and new perspectives *Polymers* **8** 42

[14] Zhang Q, Lu H, Kawazoe N and Chen G 2014 Pore size effect of collagen scaffolds on cartilage regeneration *Actabiomaterialia* **10** 2005–13

[15] Jha B S, Ayres C E, Bowman J R, Telemeco T A, Sell S A, Bowlin G L and Simpson D G 2011 Electrospun collagen: a tissue engineering scaffold with unique functional properties in a wide variety of applications *J. Nanomater.* **2011** 348268

[16] Islam A, Chapin K, Younesi M and Akkus O 2015 Computer aided bio manufacturing of mechanically robust pure collagen meshes with controlled macro porosity *Biofabrication* **7** 035005

[17] Greiling D and Clark RA 1997 Fibronectin provides a conduit for fibroblast transmigration from collagenous stroma into fibrin clot provisional matrix *J. Cell Sci.* **110** 861–70

[18] Segal H C, Hunt B J and Gilding K 1998 The effects of alginate and non-alginate wound dressings on blood coagulation and platelet activation *J. Biomater. Appl* **12** 249–57

[19] Thu H E, Zulfakar M H and Ng S F 2012 Alginate based bilayer hydrocolloid films as potential slow-release modern wound dressing *Int. J. Pharmaceut* **434** 375–83
[20] Dabiri G, Damstetter E and Phillips T 2016 Choosing a wound dressing based on common wound characteristics *Adv. Wound Care* **5** 32–41
[21] Boateng J S, Matthews K H, Stevens H N and Eccleston G M 2008 Wound healing dressings and drug delivery systems: a review *J. Pharmaceutical Sci.* **97** 2892–923
[22] Aderibigbe B A and Buyana B 2018 Alginate in wound dressings *Pharmaceutics* **10** 42
[23] Dreifke M B, Jayasuriya A A and Jayasuriya AC 2015 Current wound healing procedures and potential care *Mater. Sci. Eng.: C.* **48** 651–62
[24] Maeda N, Miao J, Simmons T J, Dordick J S and Linhardt R J 2014 Composite polysaccharide fibers prepared by electrospinning and coating *Carbohydr. Polym.* **102** 950–5
[25] Wang J, Hao S, Luo T, Cheng Z, Li W, Gao F, Guo T, Gong Y and Wang B 2017 Feather keratin hydrogel for wound repair: preparation, healing effect and biocompatibility evaluation *Coll. Surf. B: Biointerf* **149** 341–50
[26] Basu P, Kumar U N and Manjubala I 2017 Wound healing materials—a perspective for skin tissue engineering *Curr. Sci.* **112** 2392–404
[27] Chouhan D and Mandal B B 2020 Silk biomaterials in wound healing and skin regeneration therapeutics: From bench to bedside *ActaBiomaterialia* **103** 24–51
[28] Altman G H, Diaz F, Jakuba C, Calabro T, Horan R L, Chen J, Lu H, Richmond J and Kaplan DL 2003 Silk-based biomaterials *Biomaterials* **24** 401–16
[29] Postlethwait R W, Willigan D A and Ulin A W 1975 Human tissue reaction to sutures *Ann. Surgery* **181** 144
[30] Song A, Rane A A and Christman K L 2012 Antibacterial and cell-adhesive polypeptide and poly (ethylene glycol) hydrogel as a potential scaffold for wound healing *Actabiomaterialia* **8** 41–50
[31] Luthuli S, Wu S, Cheng Y, Zheng X, Wu M and Tong H 2019 Therapeutic effects of fucoidan: a review on recent studies *Mar. Drugs* **17** 487
[32] Murakami K *et al* 2010 Hydrogel blends of chitin/chitosan, fucoidan and alginate as healing-impaired wound dressings *Biomaterials* **31** 83–90
[33] Lee K Y, Jeong L, Kang Y O, Lee S J and Park W H 2009 Electrospinning of polysaccharides for regenerative medicine *Adv. Drug Del. Rev.* **61** 1020–32
[34] Kennedy J F, Methacanon P, Lloyd L L, Paterson M and Knill CJ 1997 Carbohydrate polymers as wound management aids *Carbohydrate Polymers* **34** 422
[35] Klemm D, Schumann D, Udhardt U and Marsch S 2001 Bacterial synthesized cellulose—artificial blood vessels for microsurgery *Progress Pol. Sci.* **26** 1561–603
[36] Picheth G F, Pirich C L, Sierakowski M R, Woehl M A, Sakakibara C N, de Souza C F, Martin A A, da Silva R and de Freitas R A 2017 Bacterial cellulose in biomedical applications: A review *Int. J. Biol. Macromol* **104** 97–106
[37] de Sousa R B, Vieira E G, Meneguin A B, Sábio R M, Furtini J A, da Silva and Filho EC 2018 Recent advances in methods of synthesis and applications of bacterial cellulose/calcium phosphates composites in bone tissue engineering: biomaterials; Biocomposites; Tissue Engineering; Bacterial cellulose Calcium Phosphates *Int. J. Adv. Medical Biotechnol. – IJAMB* **1** 11–20
[38] Goncalves S, Padrao J, Rodrigues I P, Silva J P, Sencadas V, Lanceros-Mendez S, Girao H, Dourado F and Rodrigues L R 2015 Bacterial cellulose as a support for the growth of retinal pigment epithelium *Biomacromolecules* **16** 1341–51

[39] Wei B, Yang G and Hong F 2011 Preparation and evaluation of a kind of bacterial cellulose dry films with antibacterial properties *Carbohydr. Polym.* **84** 533–8

[40] Poursamar S A, Hatami J, Lehner A N, da Silva C L, Ferreira F C and Antunes A P 2015 Gelatin porous scaffolds fabricated using a modified gas foaming technique: Characterisation and cytotoxicity assessment *Mater. Sci. Eng.: C.* **48** 63–70

[41] Yin F, Lin L and Zhan S 2019 Preparation and properties of cellulose nanocrystals, gelatin, hyaluronic acid composite hydrogel as wound dressing *J. Biomater. Sci., Polymer Edn* **30** 190–201

[42] Tavakoli J 2017 Physico-mechanical, morphological and biomedical properties of a novel natural wound dressing material *J. Mech. Behav. Biomed. Mater.* **65** 373–82

[43] Stevens L R, Gilmore K J and Wallace G G 2016 Tissue engineering with gellan gum *Biomater. Sci.* **4** 1276–90

[44] Silva-Correia J, Miranda-Gonçalves V, Salgado A J, Sousa N, Oliveira J M, Reis R M and Reis R L 2012 Angiogenic potential of gellan-gum-based hydrogels for application in nucleus pulposus regeneration: *in vivo* study *Tissue Eng. Part* A **18** 1203–12

[45] Oliveira J T, Martins L, Picciochi R, Malafaya P B, Sousa R A, Neves N M, Mano J F and Reis R L 2010 Gellan gum: a new biomaterial for cartilage tissue engineering applications *J. Biomed. Mater. Res. Part A: Off. J. Soc. Biomater., Jap. Soc. Biomater. Aus. Soc. Biomater. Kor. Soc. Biomater.* **93** 852–63

[46] Vashisth P, Nikhil K, Roy P, Pruthi P A, Singh R P and Pruthi V 2016 A novel gellan–PVA nanofibrous scaffold for skin tissue regeneration: fabrication and characterization *Carbohyd. Polym.* **136** 851–9

[47] Akkineni A R, Ahlfeld T, Lode A and Gelinsky M 2016 A versatile method for combining different biopolymers in a core/shell fashion by 3D plotting to achieve mechanically robust constructs *Biofabrication* **8** 045001

[48] Możejko-Ciesielska J and Kiewisz R 2016 Bacterial polyhydroxyalkanoates: still fabulous? *Microbiol. Res.* **192** 271–82

[49] Hayati A N, Rezaie H R and Hosseinalipour S M 2011 Preparation of poly (3-hydroxybutyrate)/nano-hydroxyapatite composite scaffolds for bone tissue engineering *Mater. Lett.* **65** 736–9

[50] Samy S M, Silva N A and Correlo V M *et al* 2013 Development and characterization of PHB-HV based 3D scaffolds for a tissue engineering and cell-therapy combinatorial approach for spinal cord Injury regeneration *Macromol. Biosci.* **3** 1567–92

[51] Kumar A M, Suresh B, Ramakrishna S and Kim KS 2015 Biocompatible responsive polypyrrole/GO nanocomposite coatings for biomedical applications *RSC Adv.* **5** 99866–74

[52] Cox S C, Thornby J A, Gibbons G J, Williams M A and Mallick K K 2015 3D printing of porous hydroxyapatite scaffolds intended for use in bone tissue engineering applications *Mater. Sci. Eng.: C.* **47** 237–47

[53] Zhou C, Ye X, Fan Y, Ma L, Tan Y, Qing F and Zhang X 2014 Biomimetic fabrication of a three-level hierarchical calcium phosphate/collagen/hydroxyapatite scaffold for bone tissue engineering *Biofabrication* **6** 035013

[54] Franco P Q, João C F, Silva J C and Borges J P 2012 Electrospun hydroxyapatite fibers from a simple sol–gel system *Mater. Lett.* **67** 233–6

[55] Zeimaran E, Pourshahrestani S, Djordjevic I, Pingguan-Murphy B and Kadri N A 2015 Towler Mr Bioactive glass reinforced elastomer composites for skeletal regeneration: a review *Mater. Sci. Eng.: C.* **53** 175–88

[56] Jr Jones 2013 Review of bioactive glass: from Hench to hybrids *Actabiomaterialia* **9** 4457–86
[57] Deliormanlı A M 2015 Preparation, *in vitro* mineralization and osteoblast cell response of electrospun 13–93 bioactive glass nanofibers *Mater. Sci. Eng.: C.* **53** 262–71
[58] Jockenhoevel S, Zund G, Hoerstrup S P, Chalabi K, Sachweh J S, Demircan L, Messmer B J and Turina M 2001 Fibrin gel–advantages of a new scaffold in cardiovascular tissue engineering *Eur. J. Cardio-thoracic Surg* **19** 424–30
[59] Ahmed T A, Dare E V and Hincke M 2008 Fibrin: a versatile scaffold for tissue engineering applications *Tissue Eng. Part B: Rev.* **14** 199–215
[60] Ehrbar M, Metters A, Zammaretti P, Hubbell J A and Zisch A H 2005 Endothelial cell proliferation and progenitor maturation by fibrin-bound VEGF variants with differential susceptibilities to local cellular activity *J. Contr. Rel* **101** 93–109
[61] Jackson M R 2001 Fibrin sealants in surgical practice: an overview *Am. J. Surg* **182** S1–S7
[62] Jia Y, Zhang H, Yang S, Xi Z, Tang T, Yin R and Zhang W 2018 Electrospun PLGA membrane incorporated with andrographolide-loaded mesoporous silica nanoparticles for sustained antibacterial wound dressing *Nanomedicine* **13** 2881–99
[63] Hench L L and Polak J M 2002 Third-generation biomedical materials *Science* **295** 1014–7
[64] Ratner B D, Hoffman A S, Schoen F J and Lemons JE *Biomaterials Science: An Introduction to Materials in Medicine* (Amsterdam: Elsevier)
[65] https://www.covalon.com/purchase-products/periopertative-carescar-dressing
[66] https://www.medica-tradefair.com/vis/v1/en/exhibitors/medcom2019.2615021
[67] Ovington L G 2007 Advances in wound dressings *Clinics Dermatol.* **25** 33–8
[68] Langer R S and Peppas NA 1981 Present and future applications of biomaterials in controlled drug delivery systems *Biomaterials* **2** 201–14
[69] Lloyd A W, Faragher R G and Denyer S P 2001 Ocular biomaterials and implants *Biomaterials* **22** 769–85
[70] Hendriks J G, Van Horn J R, Van Der Mei H C and Busscher H J 2004 Backgrounds of antibiotic-loaded bone cement and prosthesis-related infection *Biomaterials* **25** 545–56
[71] Saha S and Pal S 1984 Mechanical properties of bone cement: a review *J. Biomed. Mater. Res.* **18** 435–62
[72] Wichterle O and Lim D 1960 Hydrophilic gels for biological use *Nature* **185** 117–8
[73] Lu S and Anseth K S 1999 Photopolymerization of multilaminated poly (HEMA) hydrogels for controlled release *J. Contr. Rel.* **57** 291–300
[74] Young C D, Wu J R and Tsou TL 1998 Fabrication and characteristics of polyHEMA artificial skin with improved tensile properties *J. Mem. Sci.* **146** 83–93
[75] Gunatillake P A, Martin D J, Meijs G F, McCarthy S J and Adhikari R 2003 Designing biostable polyurethane elastomers for biomedical implants *Aust. J. Chem.* **56** 545–57
[76] Gogolewski S 1989 Selected topics in biomedical polyurethanes. A review *Coll. Polym. Sci.* **267** 757–85
[77] Kotz P, Fisher J, McCluskey P, Hartwell S D and Dharma H 2009 Use of a new silver barrier dressing ALLEVYN? Ag in exuding chronic wounds. *Int. Wound J.* **6** 186–94
[78] Hoffman A S 2002 Hydrogels for biomedical applications *Adv. Drug Deliv. Rev* **54** 3–12
[79] Ibusuki S, Fujii Y, Iwamoto Y and Matsuda T 2003 Tissue-engineered cartilage using an injectable and in situ gelablethermoresponsivegelatin: fabrication and *in vitro* performance *Tiss. Eng.* **9** 371–84

[80] Ibusuki S, Iwamoto Y and Matsuda T 2003 System-engineered cartilage using poly (N-isopropylacrylamide)-grafted gelatin as in situ-formable scaffold: *in vivo* performance *Tiss. Eng.* **9** 1133–42
[81] Langer R, Brem H and Tapper D 1981 Biocompatibility of polymeric delivery systems for macromolecules *J. Biomed. Mater. Res.* **15** 267–77
[82] Bhatia P, Nangia S, Aggarwal S and Tewari C 2011 Implanon: subdermal single rod contraceptive implant *J. Obst. Gynecol. Ind.* **61** 422
[83] Wagner M S, Arias R D and Nucatola D L 2007 The combined etonogestrel/ethinylestradiol contraceptive vaginal ring *Exp. Opin. Pharmacother* **8** 1769–77
[84] Xue L and Greisler H P 2003 Biomaterials in the development and future of vascular grafts *J. Vasc. Surg* **37** 472–80
[85] Pasut G and Veronese F M 2007 Polymer–drug conjugation, recent achievements and general strategies *Prog. Polym. Sci.* **32** 933–61
[86] Jeong B, Bae Y H, Lee D S and Kim S W 1997 Biodegradable block copolymers as injectable drug-delivery systems *Nature* **388** 860–2
[87] Elbert D L and Hubbell J A 1996 Surface treatments of polymers for biocompatibility *Ann. Rev. Mater. Sci.* **26** 365–94
[88] Gref R, Minamitake Y, Peracchia M T, Trubetskoy V, Torchilin V and Langer R 1994 Biodegradable long-circulating polymeric nanospheres *Science* **263** 1600–3
[89] Harris J M and Chess R B 2003 Effect of pegylation on pharmaceuticals *Nat. Rev. Drug Discov.* **2** 214–21
[90] Xue L and Greisler H P 2003 Biomaterials in the development and future of vascular grafts *J. Vasc. Surg.* **37** 472–80
[91] Behravesh E, Yasko A W, Engel P S and Mikos A G 1999 Synthetic biodegradable polymers for orthopaedic applications *Clin. Orthopaed. Rel. Res. (1976–2007)* **367** S118–S29
[92] Nguyen K T and West J L 2002 Photopolymerizable hydrogels for tissue engineering applications *Biomaterials* **23** 4307–14
[93] Seal B L, Otero T C and Panitch A 2001 Polymeric biomaterials for tissue and organ regeneration *Mater. Sci. Eng.: R: Rep* **34** 147–230
[94] Perumal G, Pappuru S, Chakraborty D, Nandkumar A M, Chand D K and Doble M 2017 Synthesis and characterization of curcumin loaded PLA—Hyperbranched polyglycerol electrospun blend for wound dressing applications *Mater. Sci. Eng.: C.* **76** 1196–204
[95] Siafaka P I, Barmbalexis P and Bikiaris DN 2016 Novel electrospunnanofibrous matrices prepared from poly (lactic acid)/poly (butylene adipate) blends for controlled release formulations of an anti-rheumatoid agent *Eur. J. Pharmaceut. Sci.* **88** 12–25
[96] Mir M, Ali M N, Barakullah A, Gulzar A, Arshad M, Fatima S and Asad M. 2018 Synthetic polymeric biomaterials for wound healing: a review *Progress Biomater.* **7** 1–21
[97] Langer R and Vacanti J P 1993 Tissue engineering *Science* **260** 920–6
[98] Wang Y, Wang C, Xie Y, Yang Y, Zheng Y, Meng H, He W and Qiao K 2019 Highly transparent, highly flexible composite membrane with multiple antimicrobial effects used for promoting wound healing *Carbohyd. Polym.* **222** 114985
[99] Ajmal G, Bonde G V, Thokala S, Mittal P, Khan G, Singh J, Pandey V K and Mishra B 2019 Ciprofloxacin HCl and quercetin functionalized electrospun nanofiber membrane: fabrication and its evaluation in full thickness wound healing. Artificial Cells *Nanomed. Biotechnol.* **47** 228–40

[100] Ghaee A, Karimi M, Lotfi-Sarvestani M, Sadatnia B and Hoseinpour V 2019 Preparation of hydrophilic polycaprolactone/modified ZIF-8 nanofibers as a wound dressing using hydrophilic surface modifying macromolecules *Mater. Sci. Eng.: C.* **103** 109767

[101] Rodríguez F J, Gómez N, Perego G and Navarro X 1999 Highly permeable polylactide-caprolactone nerve guides enhance peripheral nerve regeneration through long gaps *Biomaterials* **20** 1489–500

[102] Martins J A, Lach A A, Morris H L, Carr A J and Mouthuy P-A 2020 Polydioxanone implants: A systematic review on safety and performance in patients *J. Biomater. Appl.* **34** 902–916

[103] Andrianov A K and Payne L G 1998 Protein release from polyphosphazene matrices *Adv. Drug Del. Rev.* **31** 185–96

[104] Langone F, Lora S, Veronese F M, Caliceti P, Parnigotto P P, Valenti F and Palma G 1995 Peripheral nerve repair using a poly (organo) phosphazene tubular prosthesis *Biomaterials* **16** 347–53

[105] Laurencin C T, El-Amin S F, Ibim S E, Willoughby D A, Attawia M, Allcock H R and Ambrosio A A 1996 A highly porous 3-dimensional polyphosphazene polymer matrix for skeletal tissue regeneration *J. Biomed. Mater. Res.: Off. J. Soc. Biomater. Jap. Soc. Biomater.* **30** 133–8

[106] Tang Y, Lan X, Liang C, Zhong Z, Xie R, Zhou Y, Miao X, Wang H and Wang W 2019 Honey loaded alginate/PVA nanofibrous membrane as potential bioactive wound dressing *Carbohyd. Polym.* **219** 113–20

[107] Yang Y, Chawla A, Zhang J, Esa A, Jang H L and Khademhosseini A 2019 Applications of nanotechnology for regenerative medicine; healing tissues at the nanoscale *Principles of Regenerative Medicine* (New York: Academic) pp 485–504

[108] Dobson J 2006 Gene therapy progress and prospects: magnetic nanoparticle-based gene delivery *Gene Ther.* **13** 283–7

[109] Mody V V, Siwale R, Singh A and Mody H R 2010 Introduction to metallic nanoparticles *J. Pharm. Bioall. Sci* **2** 282

[110] Kang B, Mackey M A and El-Sayed M A 2010 Nuclear targeting of gold nanoparticles in cancer cells induces DNA damage, causing cytokinesis arrest and apoptosis *J. Am. Chem. Soc.* **132** 1517–9

[111] Rai M, Yadav A and Gade A 2009 Silver nanoparticles as a new generation of antimicrobials *Biotechnol. Adv.* **27** 76–83

[112] Prabhu S and Poulose E K 2012 Silver nanoparticles: mechanism of antimicrobial action, synthesis, medical applications, and toxicity effects *Int. Nano Lett.* **2** 32

[113] Singh D, Singh S, Sahu J, Srivastava S and Singh Mr 2016 Ceramic nanoparticles: Recompense, cellular uptake and toxicity concerns *Artif. Cells, Nanomed. Biotechnol.* **44** 401–9

[114] Jones Jr 2015 Reprint of: review of bioactive glass: from Hench to hybrids *Actabiomaterialia* **23** S53–S82

[115] Yao C, Zhu J, Xie A, Shen Y, Li H, Zheng B and Wei Y 2017 Graphene oxide and creatine phosphate disodium dual template-directed synthesis of GO/hydroxyapatite and its application in drug delivery *Mater. Sci. Eng.: C.* **73** 709–15

[116] Yin Z F, Wu L, Yang H G and Su Y H 2013 Recent progress in biomedical applications of titanium dioxide *Phy. Chem. Chem. Phys* **15** 4844–58

[117] Yu Q, Sun J, Zhu X, Qiu L, Xu M, Liu S, Ouyang J and Liu J 2017 Mesoporous titanium dioxide nanocarrier with magnetic-targeting and high loading efficiency for dual-modal imaging and photodynamic therapy *J. Mater. Chem. B.* **5** 6081–96

[118] Shrestha B K, Shrestha S, Tiwari A P, Kim J I, Ko S W, Kim H J, Park C H and Kim C S 2017 Bio-inspired hybrid scaffold of zinc oxide-functionalized multi-wall carbon nanotubes reinforced polyurethane nanofibers for bone tissue engineering *Mater. Des* **133** 69–81
[119] Bhowmick A, Banerjee S L, Pramanik N, Jana P, Mitra T, Gnanamani A, Das M and Kundu P P 2018 Organically modified clay supported chitosan/hydroxyapatite-zinc oxide nanocomposites with enhanced mechanical and biological properties for the application in bone tissue engineering *Int. J. Biol. Macromol.* **106** 11–9
[120] Gupta A K and Gupta M 2005 Synthesis and surface engineering of iron oxide nanoparticles for biomedical applications *Biomaterials* **26** 3995–4021
[121] Li X, Wei J, Aifantis K E, Fan Y, Feng Q, Cui F Z and Watari F 2016 Current investigations into magnetic nanoparticles for biomedical applications *J. Biomed. Mater. Res. Part* A **104** 1285–96
[122] Tang Z, He C, Tian H, Ding J, Hsiao B S, Chu B and Chen X 2016 Polymeric nanostructured materials for biomedical applications *Prog. Polymer Sci.* **60** 86–128
[123] Lale S V, Aravind RG A, Kumar A and Koul D S V 2014 AS1411 aptamer and folic acid functionalized pH-responsive ATRP fabricated pPEGMA–PCL–pPEGMA polymeric nanoparticles for targeted drug delivery in cancer therapy *Biomacromolecules* **15** 1737–52
[124] Cheng R, Meng F, Deng C, Klok H A and Zhong Z 2013 Dual and multi-stimuli responsive polymeric nanoparticles for programmed site-specific drug delivery *Biomaterials* **34** 3647–57
[125] Veiseh O, Tang B C, Whitehead K A, Anderson D G and Langer R 2015 Managing diabetes with nanomedicine: challenges and opportunities *Nat. Rev. Drug Discov.* **14** 45–57
[126] Affolter-Zbaraszczuk C, Ozcelik H, Meyer F, Gallet O, Lavalle P, Ball V, Ghimbeu C M, Schaaf P and Knopf-Marques H 2017 Hybrid extracellular matrix microspheres for development of complex multicellular architectures *RSC Adv.* **7** 5528–32
[127] Santo V E, Duarte A R, Gomes M E, Mano J F and Reis RL 2010 Hybrid 3D structure of poly (d, l-lactic acid) loaded with chitosan/chondroitin sulfate nanoparticles to be used as carriers for bio macromolecules in tissue engineering *J. Supercrit. Fluids* **54** 320–7
[128] Perez R A, Won J E, Knowles J C and Kim H W 2013 Naturally and synthetic smart composite biomaterials for tissue regeneration *Adv. Drug Del. Rev.* **65** 471–96
[129] Gaharwar A K, Peppas N A and Khademhosseini A 2014 Nanocomposite hydrogels for biomedical applications *Biotechnol. Bioeng.* **111** 441–53
[130] Tezcaner A, Baran E T and Keskin D 2016 Nanoparticles based on plasma proteins for drug delivery applications *Curr. Pharmaceut. Des.* **22** 3445–54
[131] Malafaya P B, Silva G A and Reis R L 2007 Natural–origin polymers as carriers and scaffolds for biomolecules and cell delivery in tissue engineering applications *Adv. Drug Del. Rev.* **59** 207–33
[132] Suh J K and Matthew H W 2000 Application of chitosan-based polysaccharide biomaterials in cartilage tissue engineering: a review *Biomaterials* **21** 2589–98
[133] Di Martino A, Sittinger M and Risbud M V 2005 Chitosan: a versatile biopolymer for orthopaedic tissue-engineering *Biomaterials* **26** 5983–90
[134] Lee J Y, Nam S H, Im S Y, Park Y J, Lee Y M, Seol Y J, Chung C P and Lee S J 2002 Enhanced bone formation by controlled growth factor delivery from chitosan-based biomaterials *J. Contr. Rel.* **78** 187–97
[135] Paige K T, Cima L G., Yaremchuk M J, Vacanti J P and Vacanti C A 1995 Injectable cartilage *Plastic Reconstr. Surg.* **96** 1390–1398

[136] Perteghella S *et al* 2017 Fabrication of innovative silk/alginate micro carriers for mesenchymal stem cell delivery and tissue regeneration *Int. J. Mol. Sci.* **18** 1829
[137] Drury J L and Mooney D J 2003 Hydrogels for tissue engineering: scaffold design variables and applications *Biomaterials* **24** 4337–51
[138] Mosahebi A, Simon M, Wiberg M and Terenghi G 2001 A novel use of alginate hydrogel as Schwann cell matrix *Tiss. Eng.* **7** 525–34
[139] Glicklis R, Shapiro L, Agbaria R, Merchuk J C and Cohen S 2000 Hepatocyte behavior within three-dimensional porous alginate scaffolds *Biotechnol. Bioeng.* **67** 344–53
[140] Smith S E, Snider C L, Gilley D R, Grant D N, Sherman S L, Ulery B D, Grant D A and Grant S A 2017 Homogenized porcine extracellular matrix derived injectable tissue construct with gold nanoparticles for musculoskeletal tissue engineering applications *J. Biomater. Nanobiotechnol.* **8** 125
[141] Kumar S, Raj S, Jain S and Chatterjee K 2016 Multifunctional biodegradable polymer nanocomposite incorporating graphene-silver hybrid for biomedical applications *Mater. Des.* **108** 319–32
[142] Bhowmick S and Koul V 2016 Assessment of PVA/silver nanocomposite hydrogel patch as antimicrobial dressing scaffold: synthesis, characterization and biological evaluation *Mater. Sci. Eng.: C* **59** 109–19
[143] Tomoaia G, Soritau O, Tomoaia-Cotisel M, Pop L B, Pop A, Mocanu A, Horovitz O and Bobos L D 2013 Scaffolds made of nanostructured phosphates, collagen and chitosan for cell culture *Powder Technol.* **238** 99–107
[144] Kim H L, Jung G Y, Yoon J H, Han J S, Park Y J, Kim D G, Zhang M and Kim D J 2015 Preparation and characterization of nano-sized hydroxyapatite/alginate/chitosan composite scaffolds for bone tissue engineering *Mater. Sci. Eng.: C.* **54** 20–5
[145] Gouma P, Xue R, Goldbeck C P, Perrotta P and Balázsi C 2012 Nano-hydroxyapatite—Cellulose acetate composites for growing of bone cells *Mater. Sci. Eng.: C.* **32** 607–12
[146] Lee E J, Kwak D H and Kim D J 2015 Mechanical properties of cellulose acetate/hydroxyapatite nanoparticle composite fiber by electro-spinning process *J. Cer. Proc. Res.* **16** 330–4
[147] Huang Y, Zhang X, Qiao H, Hao M, Zhang H, Xu Z, Zhang X, Pang X and Lin H 2016 Corrosion resistance and cytocompatibility studies of zinc-doped fluorohydroxyapatite nanocomposite coatings on titanium implant *Ceramics Int.* **42** 1903–15
[148] Kiran A, Kumar T S, Sanghavi R, Doble M and Ramakrishna S 2018 Antibacterial and bioactive surface modifications of titanium implants by PCL/TiO_2 nanocomposite coatings *Nanomaterials* **8** 860
[149] Khandan A, Abdellahi M, Ozada N and Ghayour H 2016 Study of the bioactivity, wettability and hardness behaviour of the bovine hydroxyapatite-diopside bio-nanocomposite coating *J. Taiwan Inst. Chem. Eng.* **60** 538–46
[150] Jell G, Verdejo R, Safinia L, Shaffer M S, Stevens M M and Bismarck A 2008 Carbon nanotube-enhanced polyurethane scaffolds fabricated by thermally induced phase separation *J. Mater. Chem.* **18** 1865–72
[151] Pan L, Pei X, He R, Wan Q and Wang J 2012 Multiwall carbon nanotubes/polycaprolactone composites for bone tissue engineering application *Coll. Surf. B: Biointerf.* **93** 226–34
[152] Tan W, Twomey J, Guo D, Madhavan K and Li M 2010 Evaluation of nanostructural, mechanical, and biological properties of collagen–nanotube composites *IEEE Trans. NanoBiosci.* **9** 111–20

[153] Chen L, Hu J, Shen X and Tong H 2013 Synthesis and characterization of chitosan–multiwalled carbon nanotubes/hydroxyapatite nanocomposites for bone tissue engineering *J. Mater. Sci.: Mater. Med.* **24** 1843–51

[154] Akasaka T, Yokoyama A, Matsuoka M, Hashimoto T, Abe S, Uo M and Watari F 2009 Adhesion of human osteoblast-like cells (Saos-2) to carbon nanotube sheets *Bio-medical Mater. Eng.* **19** 147–53

[155] Im O, Li J, Wang M, Zhang L G and Keidar M 2012 Biomimetic three-dimensional nanocrystalline hydroxyapatite and magnetically synthesized single-walled carbon nanotube chitosan nanocomposite for bone regeneration *Int. J. Nanomed.* **7** 2087

[156] Moon R J, Schueneman G T and Simonsen J 2016 Overview of cellulose nanomaterials, their capabilities and applications *JOM* **68** 2383–94

[157] Roman M 2015 Toxicity of cellulose nanocrystals: a review *Industr. Biotechnol.* **11** 25–33

[158] Lin N and Dufresne A 2014 Nanocellulose in biomedicine: Current status and future prospect *Eur. Polym. J* **59** 302–25

[159] Schumann D A, Wippermann J, Klemm D O, Kramer F, Koth D, Kosmehl H, Wahlers T and Salehi-Gelani S 2009 Artificial vascular implants from bacterial cellulose: preliminary results of small arterial substitutes *Cellulose* **16** 877–85

[160] Hench L L, Splinter R J, Allen W C and Greenlee T K 1971 Bonding mechanisms at the interface of ceramic prosthetic materials *J. Biomed. Mater. Res.* **5** 117–41

[161] Peter M, Binulal N S, Soumya S, Nair S V, Furuike T, Tamura H and Jayakumar R 2010 Nanocomposite scaffolds of bioactive glass ceramic nanoparticles disseminated chitosan matrix for tissue engineering applications *Carbohyd. Polym.* **79** 284–9

[162] Xu C, Su P, Chen X, Meng Y, Yu W, Xiang A P and Wang Y 2011 Biocompatibility and osteogenesis of biomimetic Bioglass-Collagen-Phosphatidylserine composite scaffolds for bone tissue engineering *Biomaterials* **32** 1051–8

[163] Mota J, Yu N, Caridade S G, Luz G M, Gomes M E, Reis R L, Jansen J A, Walboomers X F and Mano J F 2012 Chitosan/bioactive glass nanoparticle composite membranes for periodontal regeneration *Actabiomaterialia* **8** 4173–80

[164] Kim H W, Kim H E and Knowles J C 2006 Production and potential of bioactive glass nanofibers as a next-generation biomaterial *Adv. Funct. Mater.* **16** 1529–35

[165] Tsang V L and Bhatia S N 2005 Fabrication of three-dimensional tissues *Tissue Engineering II* (Berlin: Springer) pp 189–205

[166] Roseti L, Parisi V, Petretta M, Cavallo C, Desando G, Bartolotti I and Grigolo B 2017 Scaffolds for bone tissue engineering: state of the art and new perspectives *Mater. Sci. Eng.: C.* **78** 1246–62

[167] Abdelaal O A and Darwish S M 2013 Review of rapid prototyping techniques for tissue engineering scaffolds fabrication *Characterization and Development of Biosystems and Biomaterials* (Berlin: Springer) pp 33–54

[168] Owens G J, Singh R K, Foroutan F, Alqaysi M, Han C M, Mahapatra C, Kim H W and Knowles J C 2016 Sol–gel based materials for biomedical applications *Prog. Mater. Sci.* **77** 1–79

[169] Rosenholm J M, Sahlgren C and Lindén M 2010 Towards multifunctional, targeted drug delivery systems using mesoporous silica nanoparticles–opportunities & challenges *Nanoscale* **2** 1870–83

[170] Yang P, Gai S and Lin J 2012 Functionalized mesoporous silica materials for controlled drug delivery *Chem. Soc. Rev.* **41** 3679–98

[171] Sumida K, Liang K, Reboul J, Ibarra I A, Furukawa S and Falcaro P 2017 Sol–gel processing of metal–organic frameworks *Chem. Mater.* **29** 2626–45

[172] Chen F M and Liu X 2016 Advancing biomaterials of human origin for tissue engineering *Progress Polym. Sci.* **53** 86–168

[173] Meseguer-Olmo L, Ros-Nicolás M J, Vicente-Ortega V, Alcaraz-Baños M, Clavel-Sainz M, Arcos D, Ragel C V, Vallet-Regí M and Meseguer-Ortiz C 2006 A bioactive sol-gel glass implant for *in vivo* gentamicin release *Exp. Model Rabbit. J. Orthopaed. Res.* **24** 454–60

[174] Aguilera-Correa J J, Garcia-Casas A, Mediero A, Romera D, Mulero F, Cuevas-López I, Jiménez-Morales A and Esteban J 2020 A new antibiotic-loaded sol–gel can prevent bacterial prosthetic joint infection: from *in vitro* studies to an *in vivo* model *Front. Microbiol* **10** 2935

[175] Lin M C, Chen C C, Wu I T and Ding S J 2020 Enhanced antibacterial activity of calcium silicate-based hybrid cements for bone repair *Mater. Sci. Eng.: C.* **110** 110727

[176] Li H, Li J, Jiang J, Lv F, Chang J, Chen S and Wu C 2017 An osteogenesis/angiogenesis-stimulation artificial ligament for anterior cruciate ligament reconstruction *Actabiomaterialia* **54** 399–410

[177] Baino F, Fiume E, Miola M and Verné E 2018 Bioactive sol-gel glasses: processing, properties, and applications *Int. J. Appl. Cer. Technol* **15** 841–60

[178] Baino F, Fiume E, Miola M, Leone F, Onida B and Verné E 2019 Fe-doped bioactive glass-derived scaffolds produced by sol–gel foaming *Mater. Lett.* **235** 207–11

[179] Sharifianjazi F, Parvin N and Tahriri M 2017 Synthesis and characteristics of sol–gel bioactive SiO_2–P_2O_5–CaO–Ag_2O glasses *J. Non-Crys. Sol* **476** 108–13

[180] Roseti L, Parisi V, Petretta M, Cavallo C, Desando G, Bartolotti I and Grigolo B 2017 Scaffolds for bone tissue engineering: state of the art and new perspectives *Mater. Sci. Eng.: C.* **78** 1246–62

[181] Aranaz I, Gutiérrez M C, Ferrer M L and Del Monte F 2014 Preparation of chitosan nanocompositeswith a macroporous structure by unidirectional freezing and subsequent freeze-drying *Mar. Drugs* **12** 5619–42

[182] Nasiri B and Mashayekhan S 2017 Fabrication of porous scaffolds with decellularized cartilage matrix for tissue engineering application *Biologicals* **48** 39–46

[183] Lu T, Li Y and Chen T 2013 Techniques for fabrication and construction of three-dimensional scaffolds for tissue engineering *Int. J. Nanomed.* **8** 337

[184] Liao S, Li B, Ma Z, Wei H, Chan C and Ramakrishna S 2006 Biomimetic electrospun nanofibers for tissue regeneration *Biomed. Mater.* **1** R45

[185] Zou B, Liu Y, Luo X, Chen F, Guo X and Li X 2012 Electrospun fibrous scaffolds with continuous gradations in mineral contents and biological cues for manipulating cellular behaviors *Actabiomaterialia* **8** 1576–85

[186] Venugopal J R, Low S, Choon AT, Kumar A B and Ramakrishna S 2008 Nanobioengineered electrospun composite nanofibers and osteoblasts for bone regeneration *Artif. Org* **32** 388–97

[187] Zhang K, Wang X, Jing D, Yang Y and Zhu M 2009 Bionic electrospun ultrafine fibrous poly (L-lactic acid) scaffolds with a multi-scale structure *Biomed. Mater.* **4** 035004

[188] Chronakis I S 2005 Novel nanocomposites and nanoceramics based on polymer nanofibers using electrospinning process—a review *J. Mater. Proc. Technol* **167** 283–93

[189] Kai D, Prabhakaran M P, Jin G and Ramakrishna S 2011 Polypyrrole-contained electrospun conductive nanofibrous membranes for cardiac tissue engineering *J. Biomed. Mater. Res. Part* A **99** 376–85
[190] Asran A S, Henning S and Michler G H 2010 Polyvinyl alcohol–collagen–hydroxyapatite biocompositenanofibrous scaffold: Mimicking the key features of natural bone at the nanoscale level *Polymer* **51** 868–76
[191] Puperi D S, Kishan A, Punske Z E, Wu Y, Cosgriff-Hernandez E, West J L and Grande-Allen K J 2016 Electrospun polyurethane and hydrogel composite scaffolds as biomechanical mimics for aortic valve tissue engineering *ACS Biomater. Sci. Eng* **2** 1546–58
[192] Xue Y, Ravishankar P, Zeballos M A, Sant V, Balachandran K and Sant S 2020 Valve leaflet-inspired elastomeric scaffolds with tunable and anisotropic mechanical properties *Polym. Adv. Technol* **31** 94–106
[193] Zhu B, Li W, Lewis R V, Segre C U and Wang R 2015 E-spun composite fibers of collagen and dragline silk protein: fiber mechanics, biocompatibility, and application in stem cell differentiation *Biomacromolecules* **16** 202–13
[194] Sarhan W A, Azzazy H M and El-Sherbiny I M 2016 Honey/chitosan nanofiber wound dressing enriched with Allium sativum and Cleome droserifolia: enhanced antimicrobial and wound healing activity *ACS Appl. Mater. Interf* **8** 6379–90
[195] HPS A K, Saurabh C K, Adnan A S, Fazita M N, Syakir M I, Davoudpour Y, Rafatullah M, Abdullah C K, Haafiz M K and Dungani R 2016 A review on chitosan-cellulose blends and nanocellulose reinforced chitosan biocomposites: Properties and their applications *Carbohyd. Polym.* **150** 216–26
[196] Zhou G, Liu S, Ma Y, Xu W, Meng W, Lin X, Wang W, Wang S and Zhang J 2017 Innovative biodegradable poly (L-lactide)/collagen/hydroxyapatite composite fibrous scaffolds promote osteoblastic proliferation and differentiation *Int. J. Nanomed.* **12** 7577
[197] Chia H N and Wu BM 2015 Recent advances in 3D printing of biomaterials *J. Biol. Eng.* **9** 1–4
[198] Chang C C, Boland E D, Williams S K and Hoying J B 2011 Direct-write bioprinting three-dimensional biohybrid systems for future regenerative therapies *J. Biomed. Mater. Res. Part B: Appl. Biomater.* **98** 160–70
[199] Seitz H, Deisinger U, Leukers B, Detsch R and Ziegler G 2009 Different calcium phosphate granules for 3-D printing of bone tissue engineering scaffolds *Adv. Eng. Mater.* **11** B41–6
[200] Guillemot F and et al 2010 High-throughput laser printing of cells and biomaterials for tissue engineering *Actabiomaterialia* **6** 2494–500
[201] Bakhshinejad A and D'souza R M A brief comparison between available bio-printing methods *2015 IEEE Great Lakes Biomedical Conference (GLBC)* 2015 May 14 (Piscataway, NJ: IEEE) pp 1–3
[202] Calvert P and Boland T 2012 Biopolymers and Cells *Inkjet Technol. Dig. Fabric* 275
[203] Akar B, Jiang B, Somo S I, Appel A A, Larson J C, Tichauer K M and Brey E M 2015 Biomaterials with persistent growth factor gradients *in vivo* accelerate vascularized tissue formation *Biomaterials* **72** 61–73
[204] Callahan L A, Ganios A M, Childers E P, Weiner S D and Becker M L 2013 Primary human chondrocyte extracellular matrix formation and phenotype maintenance using RGD-derivatized PEGDM hydrogels possessing a continuous Young's modulus gradient *Actabiomaterialia* **9** 6095–104

[205] Chen L, Song W, Markel D C, Shi T, Muzik O, Matthew H and Ren W 2016 Flow perfusion culture of MC3T3-E1 osteogenic cells on gradient calcium polyphosphate scaffolds with different pore sizes *J. Biomater. Appl.* **30** 908–18

[206] De Mulder E L, Buma P and Hannink G 2009 Anisotropic porous biodegradable scaffolds for musculoskeletal tissue engineering *Materials* **2** 1674–96

[207] Shirazi S F, Gharehkhani S, Mehrali M, Yarmand H, Metselaar H S, Kadri N A and Osman N A 2015 A review on powder-based additive manufacturing for tissue engineering: selective laser sintering and inkjet 3D printing *Sci. Technol. Adv. Mater.* **16** 033502

[208] Wu J, Du Y, Watkins S C, Funderburgh J L and Wagner W R 2012 The engineering of organized human corneal tissue through the spatial guidance of corneal stromal stem cells *Biomaterials* **33** 1343–52

[209] Ariyasinghe N R, Lyra-Leite D M and McCain M L 2018 Engineering cardiac microphysiological systems to model pathological extracellular matrix remodeling *Am. J. Physiol. – Heart Circul. Physiol.* **315** H771–89

[210] Chen C S, Mrksich M, Huang S, Whitesides G M and Ingber D E 1997 Geometric control of cell life and death *Science* **276** 1425–8

[211] Kilian K A, Bugarija B, Lahn B T and Mrksich M 2010 Geometric cues for directing the differentiation of mesenchymal stem cells *Proc. Nat. Acad. Sci.* **107** 4872–7

[212] Deligianni D D, Katsala N D, Koutsoukos P G and Missirlis Y F 2000 Effect of surface roughness of hydroxyapatite on human bone marrow cell adhesion, proliferation, differentiation and detachment strength *Biomaterials* **22** 87–96

[213] Huang H H, Ho C T, Lee T H, Lee T L, Liao K K and Chen F L 2004 Effect of surface roughness of ground titanium on initial cell adhesion *Biomol. Eng.* **21** 93–7

[214] Rezwan K, Chen Q Z, Blaker J J and Boccaccini A R 2006 Biodegradable and bioactive porous polymer/inorganic composite scaffolds for bone tissue engineering *Biomaterials* **27** 3413–31

[215] Xu H H, Weir M D, Burguera E F and Fraser A M 2006 Injectable and macroporous calcium phosphate cement scaffold *Biomaterials* **27** 4279–87

[216] Krebs M D, Sutter K A, Lin A S, Guldberg R E and Alsberg E 2009 Injectable poly (lactic-co-glycolic) acid scaffolds with in situ pore formation for tissue engineering *Actabiomaterialia* **5** 2847–59

[217] Griffin D R, Weaver W M, Scumpia P O, Di Carlo D and Segura T 2015 Accelerated wound healing by injectable microporous gel scaffolds assembled from annealed building blocks *Nat. Mater.* **14** 737–44

[218] Lusic H and Grinstaff M W 2013 X-ray-computed tomography contrast agents *Chem. Rev.* **113** 1641–66

[219] Tang J, Sheng Y, Hu H and Shen Y 2013 Macromolecular MRI contrast agents: structures, properties and applications *Prog. Polym. Sci.* **38** 462–502

[220] Wahsner J, Gale E M, Rodríguez-Rodríguez A and Caravan P 2018 Chemistry of MRI contrast agents: current challenges and new frontiers *Chem. Rev.* **119** 957–1057

[221] Bez M and et al 2017 In situ bone tissue engineering via ultrasound-mediated gene delivery to endogenous progenitor cells in mini-pigs *Sci. Transl. Med.* **9**

[222] Du Y, Guo J L, Wang J, Mikos A G and Zhang S 2019 Hierarchically designed bone scaffolds: from internal cues to external stimuli *Biomaterials* **218** 119334

[223] Jin S S and et al 2019 A biomimetic hierarchical nanointerface orchestrates macrophage polarization and mesenchymal stem cell recruitment to promote endogenous bone regeneration *ACS Nano* **13** 6581–95

[224] Stuckensen K and et al 2018 Tissue mimicry in morphology and composition promotes hierarchical matrix remodeling of invading stem cells in osteochondral and meniscus scaffolds *Adv. Mater.* **30** 1706754
[225] Damaraju S M, Shen Y, Elele E, Khusid B, Eshghinejad A, Li J, Jaffe M and Arinzeh T L 2017 Three-dimensional piezoelectric fibrous scaffolds selectively promote mesenchymal stem cell differentiation *Biomaterials* **149** 51–62
[226] Takizawa T and et al 2018 Titanium fiber plates for bone tissue repair *Adv. Mater.* **30** 1703608
[227] Pobloth A M and et al 2018 Mechanobiologically optimized 3D titanium-mesh scaffolds enhance bone regeneration in critical segmental defects in sheep *Sci. Transl. Med* **10** aam8828
[228] Zhang B, Filion T M, Kutikov A B and Song J 2017 Facile stem cell delivery to bone grafts enabled by smart shape recovery and stiffening of degradable synthetic periosteal membranes *Adv. Funct. Mater.* **27** 1604784
[229] Wei D X, Dao J W and Chen G Q 2018 A micro-ark for cells: highly open porous polyhydroxyalkanoate microspheres as injectable scaffolds for tissue regeneration *Adv. Mater.* **30** 1802273
[230] Lin Z and et al 2018 Precisely controlled delivery of magnesium ions thru sponge-like monodisperse PLGA/nano-MgO-alginate core-shell microsphere device to enable in-situ bone regeneration *Biomaterials* **174** 1–6
[231] Leterrier C, Potier J, Caillol G, Debarnot C, Boroni F R and Dargent B 2015 Nanoscale architecture of the axon initial segment reveals an organized and robust scaffold *Cell Rep.* **13** 2781–93
[232] Katayama Y, Montenegro R, Freier T, Midha R, Belkas J S and Shoichet M S 2006 Coil-reinforced hydrogel tubes promote nerve regeneration equivalent to that of nerve autografts *Biomaterials* **27** 505–18
[233] Oudega M, Gautier S E, Chapon P, Fragoso M, Bates M L, Parel J M and Bunge M B 2001 Axonal regeneration into Schwann cell grafts within resorbable poly (α-hydroxyacid) guidance channels in the adult rat spinal cord *Biomaterials* **22** 1125–36
[234] Novikov L N, Novikova L N, Mosahebi A, Wiberg M, Terenghi G and Kellerth J O 2002 A novel biodegradable implant for neuronal rescue and regeneration after spinal cord injury *Biomaterials* **23** 3369–76
[235] Tschernutter M, Schlichtenbrede F C, Howe S, Balaggan K S, Munro P M, Bainbridge J W, Thrasher A J, Smith A J and Ali R R 2005 Long-term preservation of retinal function in the RCS rat model of retinitis pigmentosa following lentivirus-mediated gene therapy *Gene Ther.* **12** 694–701
[236] Das T P 1996 Transplantation of neural retina in patients with retinitis pigmentosa *Invest. Ophthalmol. Vis. Sci* **37** S96
[237] Keirstead H S, Nistor G, Bernal G, Totoiu M, Cloutier F, Sharp K and Steward O 2005 Human embryonic stem cell-derived oligodendrocyte progenitor cell transplants remyelinate and restore locomotion after spinal cord injury *J. Neurosci* **25** 4694–705
[238] Pacella E, Vestri A R, Muscella R, Carbotti M R, Castellucci M, Coi L, Turchetti P and Pacella F 2013 Preliminary results of an intravitreal dexamethasone implant (Ozurdex®) in patients with persistent diabetic macular edema *Clin. Ophthalmol. (Auckland, New Zealand)* **7** 1423

[239] Liu Y, Wang R, Zarembinski T I, Doty N, Jiang C, Regatieri C, Zhang X and Young M J 2013 The application of hyaluronic acid hydrogels to retinal progenitor cell transplantation *Tiss. Eng. Part* A **19** 135–42

[240] Mitrousis N, Tam R Y, Baker A E, van der Kooy D and Shoichet M S 2016 Hyaluronic acid-based hydrogels enable rod photoreceptor survival and maturation *in vitro* through activation of the mTOR pathway *Adv. Funct. Mater.* **26** 1975–85

[241] Shah A, Brugnano J, Sun S, Vase A and Orwin E 2008 The development of a tissue-engineered cornea: biomaterials and culture methods *Ped. Res.* **63** 535–44

[242] Yang J, Yamato M, Nishida K, Hayashida Y, Shimizu T, Kikuchi A, Tano Y and Okano T 2006 Corneal epithelial stem cell delivery using cell sheet engineering: not lost in transplantation *J. Drug Targ.* **14** 471–82

[243] Higa K, Shimmura S, Kato N, Kawakita T, Miyashita H, Itabashi Y, Fukuda K, Shimazaki J and Tsubota K 2007 Proliferation and differentiation of transplantable rabbit epithelial sheets engineered with or without an amniotic membrane carrier *Invest. Ophthalmol. Vis. Sci.* **48** 597–604

[244] Orwin E J and Hubel A 2000 In vitro culture characteristics of corneal epithelial, endothelial, and keratocyte cells in a native collagen matrix *Tiss. Eng.* **6** 307–19

[245] Bryant M R, Szerenyi K, Schmotzer H and McDonnell P J 1994 Corneal tensile strength in fully healed radial keratotomy wounds *Invest. Ophthalmol. Vis. Sci.* **35** 3022–31

[246] Chen J, Li Q, Xu J, Huang Y, Ding Y, Deng H, Zhao S and Chen R 2005 Study on biocompatibility of complexes of collagen–chitosan–sodium hyaluronate and cornea *Artif. Org.* **29** 104–13

[247] Zhong S P, Teo W E, Zhu X, Beuerman R, Ramakrishna S and Yung L Y 2007 Development of a novel collagen–GAG nanofibrous scaffold via electrospinning *Mater. Sci. Eng.:* C **27** 262–6

[248] Zorlutuna P, Tezcaner A Y, Kıyat I, Aydınlı A and Hasırcı V 2006 Cornea engineering on polyester carriers *Biomed. Mater. Res.* A **79** 104–13

[249] Liu Y, Gan L, Carlsson D J, Fagerholm P, Lagali N, Watsky M A, Munger R, Hodge W G, Priest D and Griffith M 2006 A simple, cross-linked collagen tissue substitute for corneal implantation *Invest. Ophthalmol. Vis. Sci.* **47** 1869–75

[250] Derderian C A, Olivier W A, Baux G, Levine J and Gurtner G C 2003 Microvascular free-tissue transfer for traumatic defects of the upper extremity: a 25-year experience *J. Reconstr. Microsurg* **19** 455–62

[251] Khademhosseini A 2008 *Micro and Nanoengineering of the Cell Microenvironment: Technologies and Applications* (Boston, MA: Artech House)

[252] Zhang L and Webster T J 2009 Nanotechnology and nanomaterials: promises for improved tissue regeneration *Nano Today* **4** 66–80

[253] Beier J P, Klumpp D, Rudisile M, Dersch R, Wendorff J H, Bleiziffer O, Arkudas A, Polykandriotis E, Horch R E and Kneser U 2009 Collagen matrices from sponge to nano: new perspectives for tissue engineering of skeletal muscle *BMC Biotechnol.* **9** 34

[254] Robbie K, Beydaghyan G, Brown T, Dean C, Adams J and Buzea C 2004 Ultrahigh vacuum glancing angle deposition system for thin films with controlled three-dimensional nanoscale structure *Rev. Scient. Instr.* **75** 1089–97

[255] Zhao C, Andersen H, Ozyilmaz B, Ramaprabhu S, Pastorin G and Ho H K 2015 Spontaneous and specific myogenic differentiation of human mesenchymal stem cells on polyethylene glycol-linked multi-walled carbon nanotube films for skeletal muscle engineering *Nanoscale* **7** 18239–49

[256] Hosoyama K, Ahumada M, McTiernan C D, Davis D R, Variola F, Ruel M, Liang W, Suuronen E J and Alarcon E I 2018 Nanoengineeredelectroconductive collagen-based cardiac patch for infarcted myocardium repair *ACS Appl. Mater. Interf.* **10** 44668–77

[257] Elsayed Y, Lekakou C, Labeed F and Tomlins P 2016 Fabrication and characterisation of biomimetic, electrospungelatin fibre scaffolds for tunica media-equivalent, tissue engineered vascular grafts *Mater. Sci. Eng.:* C **61** 473–83

[258] Izadifar M, Babyn P, Kelly M E, Chapman D and Chen X 2017 Bioprinting pattern-dependent electrical/mechanical behavior of cardiac alginate implants: characterization and ex vivo phase-contrast micro tomography assessment *Tissue Eng. Part C: Methods* **23** 548–64

[259] Aussel A and et al 2017 Chitosan-based hydrogels for developing a small-diameter vascular graft: *in vitro* and *in vivo* evaluation *Biomed. Mater.* **12** 065003

[260] Baei P, Jalili-Firoozinezhad S, Rajabi-Zeleti S, Tafazzoli-Shadpour M, Baharvand H and Aghdami N 2016 Electrically conductive gold nanoparticle-chitosan thermosensitive hydrogels for cardiac tissue engineering *Mater. Sci. Eng.: C.* **63** 131–41

[261] Liu Y, Wang S and Zhang R 2017 Composite poly (lactic acid)/chitosan nanofibrous scaffolds for cardiac tissue engineering *Int. J. Biol. Macromol* **103** 1130–7

[262] Wang T, Ji X, Jin L, Feng Z, Wu J, Zheng J, Wang H, Xu Z W, Guo L and He N 2013 Fabrication and characterization of heparin-grafted poly-L-lactic acid–chitosan core–shell nanofibers scaffold for vascular gasket *ACS Appl. Mater. Interf.* **5** 3757–63

[263] Chen X, Feng B, Zhu D Q, Chen Y W, Ji W, Ji T J and Li F 2019 Characteristics and toxicity assessment of electrospungelatin/PCL nanofibrous scaffold loaded with graphene *in vitro* and *in vivo Int. J. Nanomed.* **14** 3669

[264] Pieper J S, Van Der Kraan P M, Hafmans T, Kamp J, Buma P, Van Susante J L, Van Den Berg W B, Veerkamp J H and Van Kuppevelt T H 2002 Crosslinked type II collagen matrices: preparation, characterization, and potential for cartilage engineering *Biomaterials* **23** 3183–92

[265] Litwiniuk M, Krejner A, Speyrer M S, Gauto A R and Grzela T 2016 Hyaluronic acid in inflammation and tissue regeneration *Wounds* **28** 78–88

[266] Gao Y *et al* 2014 The ECM-cell interaction of cartilage extracellular matrix on chondrocytes *BioMed. Res. Int.* **2014** 648459

[267] Martel-Pelletier J, Wildi L M and Pelletier JP 2012 Future therapeutics for osteoarthritis *Bone* **51** 297–311

[268] Kon E, Roffi A, Filardo G, Tesei G and Marcacci M 2014 Scaffold-based cartilage treatments: with or without cells? A systematic review of preclinical and clinical evidence *Arthrosc.: J. Arthrosc. Rel. Surg.* **31** 767–75

[269] De Coninck T, Elsner J J, Linder-Ganz E, Cromheecke M, Shemesh M, Huysse W, Verdonk R, Verstraete K and Verdonk P 2014 In-vivo evaluation of the kinematic behavior of an artificial medial meniscus implant: A pilot study using open-MRI *Clin. Biomech.* **29** 898–905

[270] Verdonk R, Verdonk P, Huysse W, Forsyth R and Heinrichs E L 2011 Tissue ingrowth after implantation of a novel, biodegradable polyurethane scaffold for treatment of partial meniscal lesions *Am. J. Sp. Med.* **39** 774–82

[271] Lyons L P, Hidalgo Perea S, Weinberg J B, Wittstein J R and McNulty A L 2020 Meniscus-derived matrix bioscaffolds: effects of concentration and cross-linking on meniscus cellular responses and tissue repair *Int. J. Molecular Sci.* **21** 44

[272] Ruprecht J C, Waanders T D, Rowland C R, Nishimuta J F, Glass K A, Stencel J, DeFrate L E, Guilak F, Weinberg J B and McNulty A L 2019 Meniscus-derived matrix scaffolds promote the integrative repair of meniscal defects *Scient. Rep.* **9** 1–3
[273] Wright K A, Nadire K B, Busto P, Tubo R, McPherson J M and Wentworth B M 1998 Alternative delivery of keratinocytes using a polyurethane membrane and the implications for its use in the treatment of full-thickness burn injury *Burns* **24** 7–17
[274] Vig K, Chaudhari A, Tripathi S, Dixit S, Sahu R, Pillai S, Dennis V A and Singh S R 2017 Advances in skin regeneration using tissue engineering *Int. J. Mol. Sci.* **18** 789
[275] Shevchenko R V, James S L and James S E 2010 A review of tissue-engineered skin bioconstructs available for skin reconstruction *J. Roy. Soc. Interf.* **7** 229–58
[276] Gruss J S and Jirsch D W 1978 Human amniotic membrane: a versatile wound dressing *Can. Med. Assoc. J* **118** 1237
[277] Halim A S, Khoo T L and Yussof S J 2010 Biologic and synthetic skin substitutes: an overview *Indian J. Plastic Sur.: Offic. Publ. Assoc. Plastic Surg. Ind.* **43** S23
[278] Hesketh M, Sahin K B, West Z E and Murray R Z 2017 Macrophage phenotypes regulate scar formation and chronic wound healing *Int. J. Mol. Sci.* **18** 1545
[279] Wisconsin Alumni research Foundation 2011 *US7935364*
[280] Stratatech Corp. 2006 *US0258001*
[281] Morais J M, Papadimitrakopoulos F and Burgess D J 2010 Biomaterials/tissue interactions: possible solutions to overcome foreign body response *AAPS J* **12** 188–96
[282] Anderson J M, Rodriguez A and Chang D T 2008 Foreign body reaction to biomaterials *Semin. Immunol.* 20 86–100
[283] Charnley J, Kamangar A and Longfield M D 1969 The optimum size of prosthetic heads in relation to the wear of plastic sockets in total replacement of the hip *Med. Biol. Eng.* **7** 31–9
[284] Silver M D and Wilson G J 1977 The pathology of wear in the Beall model 104 heart valve prosthesis *Circulation* **56** 617–22
[285] Hanle D D, Harrison E C, Yoganathan A P, Allen D T and Corcoran W H 1989 In vitro flow dynamics of four prosthetic aortic valves: a comparative analysis *J. Biomechan.* **22** 597–607
[286] Hicks C R, Fitton J H, Chirila T V, Crawford G J and Constable I J 1997 Keratoprostheses: advancing toward a true artificial cornea *Surv. Ophthalmol.* **42** 175–89
[287] Assil K K and Quantock A J 1993 Wound healing in response to keratorefractive surgery *Surv. Ophthalmol.* **38** 289–302
[288] Smolin G and Goodman D 1988 Corneal graft reaction *Int. Ophthalmol. Clin.* **28** 30–6
[289] Zuidema J M, Provenza C, Caliendo T, Dutz S and Gilbert R J 2015 Magnetic NGF-releasing PLLA/iron oxide nanoparticles direct extending neurites and preferentially guide neurites along aligned electrospun microfibers *ACS Chem. Neurosci.* **18** 1781-8
[290] Qian Z, Radke D, Jia W, Tahtinen M, Wang G and Zhao F 2019 Bioengineering scaffolds for regenerative engineering *Encyclopedia of Biomedical Engineering* ed R Narayan (Amsterdam: Elsevier) pp 444–61
[291] Ma X, Liu J, Zhu W, Tang M, Lawrence N, Yu C, Gou M and Chen S 2018 3D bioprinting of functional tissue models for personalized drug screening and in vitro disease modeling *Adv. Drug Deliv. Rev.* **132** 235–51
[292] Carneiro O S, Silva A F and Gomes R 2015 Fused deposition modeling with polypropylene *Mater. Des.* **83** 768–76

IOP Publishing

Bionanomaterials
Fundamentals and biomedical applications
Ravindra Pratap Singh and Kshitij RB Singh

Chapter 9

Molecularly imprinted bionanomaterials and their biomedical applications

Semra Akgönüllü, Monireh Bakhshpour and Adil Denizli

Molecularly imprinted polymers (MIPs) have recently gained numerous applications in various domains, namely pharmaceutical, medical, environmental, food control, and homeland security. In particular, MIP-based bionanomaterials have created an attractive vision for biomedical applications by forming specific cavities for targets. Moreover, this is an inexpensive, quick, easy-to-use, highly sensitive, and selective sensing approach, especially for theranostics, diagnosis, and screening applications. Hence, this chapter aims at discussing the principle of molecular imprinting technique, the combination of MIP-based bionanomaterials, the recent advances and strategies in molecular imprinting methods, and their biomedical applications.

9.1 Introduction

Numerous approaches have been utilized to mimic the specific binding-related interactions between natural molecules and this interaction phenomenon over the years [1]. Billions of dollars are invested in natural antibody marketing almost every year to provide the request for diagnosis and treatment. However, natural antibodies are high-cost and they still show poor stability. The application of molecular imprinting techniques has been identified as a sustainable technique that could be applied for antibody mimicking and eliminating the disadvantages of using a natural antibody [2]. One of the studies in this area was developed by Mosbach and their research group [3]. They displayed that crosslinked polymers prepared using diazepam or theophylline as target molecules, displaying selectivity and specificity comparable to those of antibodies. The molecularly imprinted polymers were also called 'plastic antibodies' or 'synthetic antibodies' [3, 4].

Molecularly imprinted polymers (MIPs) are synthetic polymers pre-arranged for a target analyte [5]. MIPs can be capable of creating specific and selective cavities for various target analytes such as antibodies, enzymes, proteins, and hormones.

doi:10.1088/978-0-7503-3767-0ch9

Recently, MIPs have attracted increasing attention as selectivity recognition elements with application in sensing and/or separation of several molecules in various materials [6, 7]. MIPs have drawn attention owing to their infinite advantages such as high stability, selectivity, sensitivity, and affinity to the target analytes, low-cost, ease of integration. However, MIPs have some disadvantages such as the lack of conductive activity, large particle formation, heterogeneous distribution, and partial embedding of the binding sites. For example, magnetic MIPs have been synthesized to increase conductivity capability [8–10]. As a result, to improve their analytical performance and overcome some disadvantages, different bionanomaterials are combined with molecular imprinting techniques.

9.2 Molecularly imprinted polymers

9.2.1 Synthesis of MIPs

Molecular recognition has been the subject of most chemical research because of its importance in processes such as separation, catalysis, the main type of detection (which is essential for biological processes and currently the detection system). MIPs are generally utilized as a receptor for target molecules. Therefore, they are called analogs of the antibody–antigen system [11].

The molecular imprinting technique is based on the polymerization of the appropriate crosslinker around a target molecule with a specially selected functional monomer [12–15]. Several procedures are involved in the application of MIPs, especially during synthesis. However, all procedures follow the same fundamental steps: (i) a polymer matrix containing a target or template molecule that is covalently or non-covalently attached to the functional monomers is fabricated; (ii) the target molecule is extracted from the polymer matrix (desorption or regeneration step), specific binding sites to the target molecule are formed; and (iii) when the MIP interacts with the sample containing the target molecule, the only target molecule is specifically bound to the cavity in the complex medium. Figure 9.1 shows a typical protocol for the preparation of MIPs; generally, the

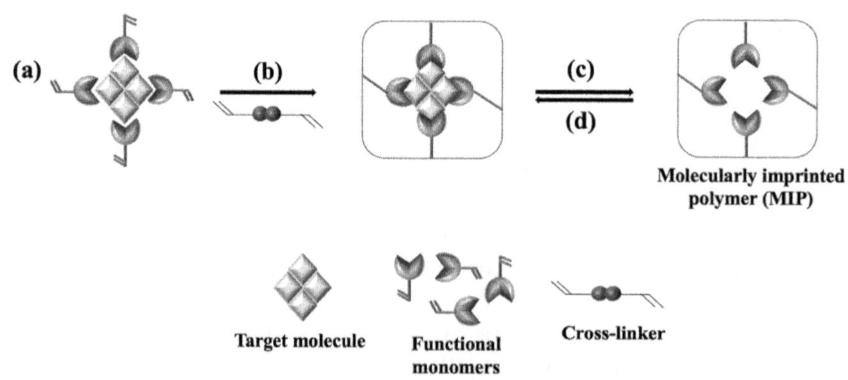

Figure 9.1. Schematic illustration of MIPs synthesis: (a) pre-complex; (b) polymerization; (c) removing of target; and (d) rebinding of target.

process contains the target molecule, various functional monomers and the crosslinker, also an initiator and a solvent.

The solvents have a significant role as a porogen in MIPs. The functional groups are obtained using functional monomer for specific recognition regions in the structure of polymers. Then, the polymerization is done using crosslinking monomers. In the end, the target molecule is efficiently removed to create specific recognition regions complementary to target molecules. Thus, MIPs that mimic the characteristics and functions of natural antibodies are capable of interacting with the target molecule [2].

In MIPs, specific recognition regions can be created for different targets molecules such as enzymes [16], amino acids [17], proteins [18], oligonucleotides [19], hormones [20], drugs [21], bacteria [22], viruses [23], pesticides [24], toxins [25], metal ions [26], antibiotics [27] and suchlike. MIPs have different advantages such as simple synthesis, preparation, and storage, highly stable structure, low cost, high reusability performance and user-friendliness. In particular, they are perfect materials for use in medical applications [28].

Although the imprinting of low molecular weight target molecules (oligopeptides, amino acids, nucleotides, antibiotics, hormones, sugars, peptides, mycotoxins, and drugs) is conceived as simple, the imprinting process toward polypeptides or macromolecular molecules (e.g., protein) is still complex. Typical challenges include preserving the natural protein conformation during imprinting, heterogeneous binding caused by multiple functional regions, slow mass transfer because of macromolecular structure, and permanent embedding of proteins. These challenges can be overcome using techniques such as surface imprinting, bulk imprinting and epitope imprinting approach. MIPs have been used in various areas such as purification, separation, biomarker detection, drug delivery, disease treatment, and so on [2].

9.2.2 Surface imprinting

With the surface imprinting technique, binding sites are created at the surface of the polymer matrix [29]. The specific recognition sites are more easily reachable with suitable binding kinetics in this method. Namely, target/polymer binding are not diffusion limited [30, 31]. Therefore, this technique is a phenomenon that is applicable particularly for imprinting of macromolecules. Fewer template molecules are utilized in the surface imprinting technique because in conventional imprinting techniques the target molecule is only used in the surface coating step. The main disadvantage of the surface imprinting technique in the biosensor design is that it shows lower sensitivity compared to bulk imprinting due to the reduced number of recognition sites [32]. This technique is broadly utilized for different types of target molecules such as microorganisms, proteins, cells, and virus. Figure 9.2(a) shows a summary of the preparation of specific cavities for the target molecules with surface imprinting technique.

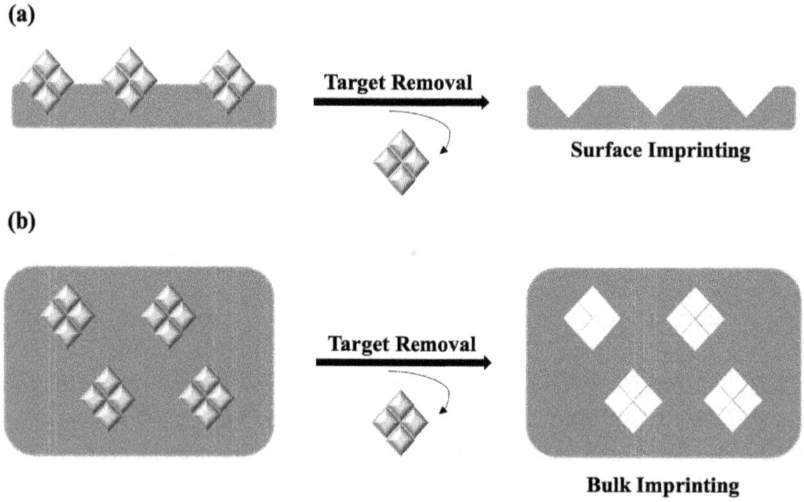

Figure 9.2. (a) Schematic representation of surface imprinting technology and (b) bulk imprinting technology.

9.2.3 Bulk imprinting

In the bulk imprinting technique, a target analyte is imprinted as a whole in the polymer. After the polymerization the target molecule needs to be completely removed from the polymer matrix. Small particles can be formed by crushing these polymers. In this way, target-specific three-dimensional recognition sites are obtained selectively within the polymer matrix. Bulk imprinting is usually chosen for imprinting of micro molecules, as binding and removing of the target molecule is easier and reversible. It is also an advantage for the reusability of the imprinted polymer matrix [32, 33]. The bulk imprinting technique is summarized in figure 9.2(b).

Keeping the three-dimensional conformational stability of a macro-molecule during the polymerization is a major difficulty. Macromolecules are embedded in matrices deep enough to cause restriction or inaccessibility. These recognition sites may be suitable for smaller polypeptides [34, 35]. Removal of the target molecule from the MIP can also be a problem. Alternative imprinting techniques have been developed to overcome these challenges [31].

9.2.4 Epitope imprinting

In immunology, epitopes are specific sites within the protein structures. Thanks to the epitope imprinting method, it is not necessary to imprint the whole of the protein [36]. In epitope imprinting, a part structure or a fragment of the protein macromolecule is utilized as a pseudo-template to synthesize imprint-based polymers [37]. So far, surface and bulk imprinting have been mentioned. For the first time, Minoura and Rachkov suggested an epitope imprinting technique for the recognition of peptides [38]. The short characteristic peptides are utilized as targets rather than entire proteins. Shea and group reported a milestone study in epitope imprinting method for protein recognition [39]. Since then, epitope imprinting has been broadly adopted

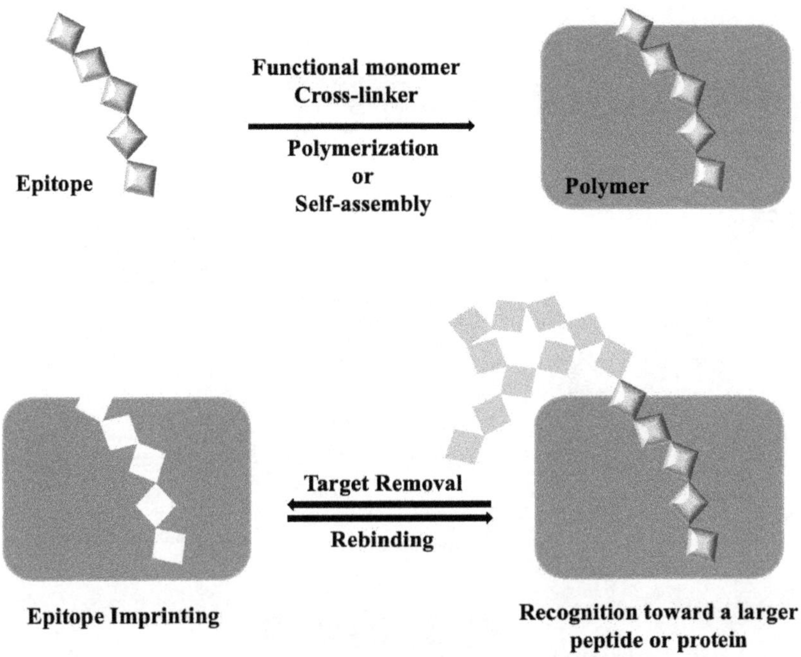

Figure 9.3. Schematic representation of epitope imprinting technology.

to overcome these limitations [40]. Figure 9.3 shows a summary of the epitope imprinting technique.

9.3 Bionanomaterials

Bionanomaterials are novel materials at the nanoscale level used for biomedical applications. These nano size-based structure materials with dimensions 1–1000 nm size are used frequently for clinical, biomedical, and biosensor applications. The bionanomaterials have superior properties over conventional biomaterials due to their nanometer size characteristics, maximizing interface adhesion [41]. These bionanomaterials have been utilized in many fields related to their applications, processing, modeling, and characterization. Also, the bionanomaterials have been known as nano-size polymers, nanocomposites, metals, nanostructured ceramics, and self-assembled materials. These materials enable increasing the surface area thanks to the nano-size properties. Bionanomaterials usually display prominent optical, mechanical, and electrical features compared to other macroscopic and/or microscopic structures. Nanotechnology-based biomaterials can be employed for bio-imaging, drug delivery, biosensors and other biomedical applications. This chapter aims to discuss the unique applications of bionanomaterials in biomedical systems, giving the reader a bird's-eye view of bionanomaterials' applications [42]. This chapter focuses on those models that research in biomedicine can provide for the design of MIP-based nanomaterials and their various biomedical applications (figure 9.4).

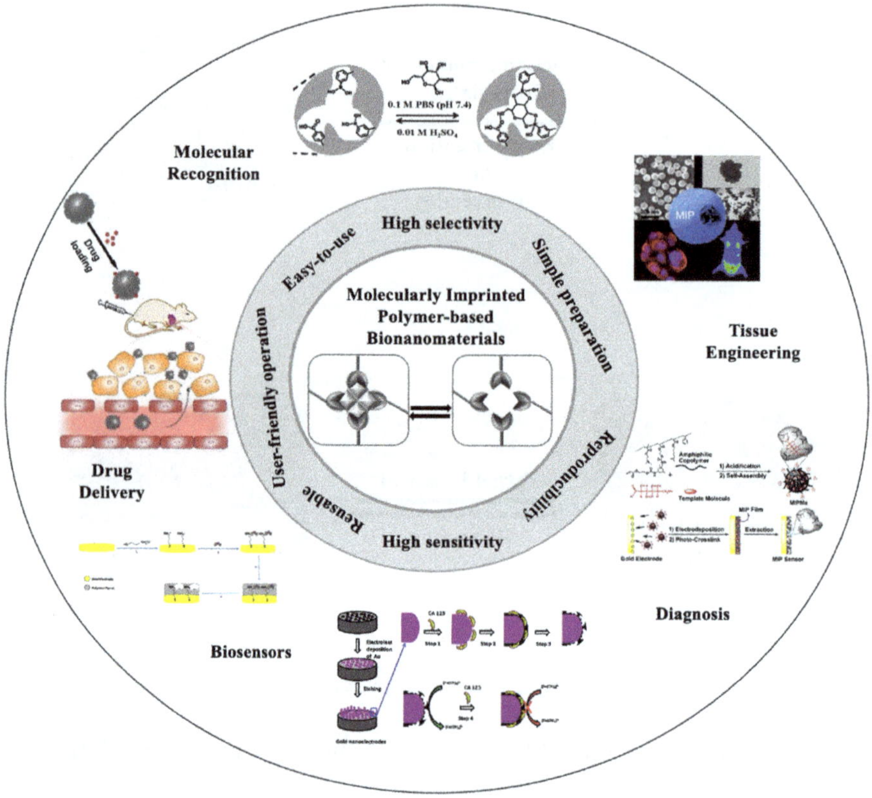

Figure 9.4. General overview of the physical and chemical features, structure–property relationship, and extensive biomedical applications of MIP-based polymeric nanomaterials. Reprinted with permission from [122]. Copyright (2020) American Chemical Society.

9.3.1 Types of bionanomaterials

9.3.1.1 Metallic bionanomaterials

Iron oxide nanoparticles, gadolinium-based nanoparticles, and gold nanoparticles are metallic bionanomaterials. Superparamagnetic and ultrasmall superparamagnetic iron oxides are two types of iron oxide nanoparticles that are named SPIOs (smaller size than 50 nm) and USPIOs (greater size than 50 nm), respectively. Generally, SPIOs are utilized as magnetic resonance imaging (MRI) contrast agents. Iron oxide nanoparticles, depending on the composition and size, can be developed and utilized for a variety of medical applications [43].

Gadolinium nanoparticles as metallic nanoparticles are synthesized using gadolinium acetylacetonate hydrate, gadolinium chloride hydrate, and gadolinium acetate hydrate from oxides (2–15 nm diameter). Naked gadolinium (Gd(III)) ions are very toxic, therefore, mostly multidentate ligands as chelates are used to coordinate with Gd(III) ions. The two coordinated for Gd(III) nanoparticles are 1,4,7,10-tetraazacyclododecane-1,4,7,10-tetraacetic acid and diethylene-triamine-penta-acetic acid. The complex of diethylene-triaminepenta-acetic acid and albumin is usually employed as a blood pool enhancing agent. These complexes can increase retention in the vascular compartment but are not widely used for medical purposes. Some disadvantages of these complexes are low elimination, inadequate stability, low water solubility [44].

Gold (Au) nanoparticles commonly are synthesized as nanocages, spherical particles, nanoshells, and nanorods. Unique optical properties of Au nanoparticles allow them to be made by easy synthesis techniques [45]. The high biocompatibility of Au nanoparticles indicates that they are convenient to use for biomedical applications. The ability to set the optical properties of Au nanoparticles such as scattering/near-infrared (IR) fluorescence and surface plasmon absorption can be achieved by controlling the shape, size, structure and composition of these nanoparticles. Au nanoparticles have been widely used for photothermal therapy, drug delivery, sensing applications, and cell tracking [46].

9.3.1.2 Nanofibers based bionanomaterials

Nanofibers such as cellulose make for attractive biomaterials with high surface/volume ratio, biocompatibility, tensile strength, low-density, low-cost, tensile strength, non-toxic, non-abrasive, biodegradable, and combustible properties. Cellulose is found as the amplest biopolymer in nature. Cellulose nanofibers can improve the mechanical properties of nanocomposite materials and as bionanomaterials. Cellulose nanofibers can be mostly obtained simply via bacteria as a non-plant resource, and/or wood, cotton as a plant resource, also polymerization procedures [47–50].

9.3.1.3 Carbon nanotube-based bionanomaterials

Nanotubes are rounded or arranged in graphite-like layers and synthesized with light elements (boron, nitrogen and their metal complexes). Nanotubes can form crystalline fibers, which can be very long compared to their diameter. These forms are small enough to settle in the lung, and their toxic effects can pose many risks, such as cancer [51]. Carbon nanotubes (CNTs) are given more attention than other nanotubes due to their biocompatible and environmentally friendly properties. There are two main types, single-walled and multi-walled CNTs. The electrical conductivity of CNTs with high electron mobility has been used to prepare electrochemical-based sensors from CNTs. The CNTs surfaces can be functionalized by placing appropriate hydroxyl or carboxyl groups on the surface [52]. The advantages of CNTs are that they are chemically stable and suitable for enabling combination with different materials and for the production of composite structures [53]. The surface of CNTs can be modified with molecularly imprinted technology [54].

9.3.1.4 Polymeric-based bionanomaterials

Besides some of the natural sources such as cellulose acetate, polyhydroxybutyrate (PHB), polyhydroxyalkanoate (PHA) etc, some synthetic sources can be used for the preparation of degradable polymeric green nanocomposite materials. Polyvinyl alcohol (PVA), aromatic polyesters and aliphatic polyesters are important synthetic sources that have recently been used for this purpose. Although these polymers are not renewable and degradable like natural polymers, they can be applied to obtain green nanocomposite materials [55]. Accordingly, these synthetic polymers are generally less preferred for use in biodegradable materials. In this chapter, some of these natural and synthetic polymers used in green nanocomposites material are given as particular examples from literature. Molecularly imprinted technology-based bionanomaterials have been widely used to prepare robust, stable, biocompatible and cheap materials for the minimization of organic pollution in the environment and wastewater [56].

9.3.1.5 Quantum dots-based bionanomaterials

Quantum dots (QDs) are nanometer-sized semiconductor crystals consisting of elements within the groups II to VI or III to V, which are called 'artificial atoms' because of their unique sizes [57, 58]. On the absorption of light, nanocrystals produce excitons and electron–hole recombination which leads to luminescence. QDs are often described as spheres, but they have a lattice structure similar to crystalline materials and bulk semiconductor materials. According to their size, they have thousands of atoms that can be found in each nanocrystal structure. They are suitable materials for molecular imprinting with a high surface area/volume ratio and suitable to use in biomedical applications [51, 59, 60].

9.4 MIP-based bionanomaterials for biomedical applications

The research for designing MIP-based nanomaterials has developed over the past decade in the field of biomedicine due to it being crucial to selectively quantify biomarkers or pathogens in clinical samples for the effective diagnosis and/or treatment of various diseases. Molecular imprinting has developed a unique method to apply in wide areas of biomedical application such as chromatographic stationary phases, designing sensor systems, separation of the proteins, antibody and enzyme mimics, bioimaging, and also drug delivery [14].

9.4.1 Biomimetic sensors

Sensors are devices which respond to a chemical physical stimulus by producing an electrical signal. Sensors are devices that utilize biological or chemical reactions for the detection of target analytes. Sensors couple a recognition element that interacts with the target analyte and a physical transducer that transforms the recognition interaction into a practical electrical signal. Transducer elements, including piezoelectric, optical, or electrochemical tools, generate frequency signals, light, or current, respectively [61]. The widespread use of MIP-based sensors has been published as for the sensing of various analytes such as proteins [62], enzymes [63], hormone [64], drugs [12], pesticides [65], metals [66], antibiotics [67] and pathogens [68]. The yield of biomimetic sensors must meet important criteria, such as stability, linearity, repeatability, high sensitivity, high selectivity, and reusability [69]. Biosensors capable of the accurate quantification and real-time monitoring of disease-related biomarkers including proteins, nucleotides, toxins, bacteria, and viruses have gained important interest and have provided an attractive research area for biomedical diagnosis [2]. In recent years, optic, piezoelectric and electrochemical biomimetic-based sensors have been studied for their capability in clinical biosensing, making biomedical diagnostics applications a quickly evolving topic. Molecularly imprinted-based bionanomaterials are an important material for biomarker detection.

The carbohydrate antigen 125 (CA-125) is a major biomarker in the detection of ovarian cancer [70]. Considering the high effect and mortality ratio of ovarian cancer, the detection of CA-125 as a biomarker has received attention in recent years. MIP-based electrochemical and optical biosensors were developed for ovarian cancer by Rebelo *et al.* In this study, CA-125 was chosen as the target protein. The MIPs were designed on the gold surface of the electrode. The electrochemical-based biosensor demonstrated good selectivity, and the limit of detection was calculated as 0.01 U·mL^{-1}. This study showed the 0.01 U·mL^{-1} and 500 U·mL^{-1} linear concentration range of the target. Moreover, this sensor also proved detection of CA-125 was also performed in artificial serum samples [71]. The synthesis steps are given in figure 9.5(a).

Viswanathan *et al* detected the epithelial ovarian cancer antigen-125 using a molecularly imprinted polymer-coated gold nanoelectrode sensor. They selected CA 125 as a protein biomarker. The preparation of the sensor scheme is displayed in figure 9.5(b). This electrode displayed good increases at the performed linear concentration range of 0.5 U·mL^{-1}–400 U·mL^{-1}. They reported that limit of detection was calculated as 0.5 U·mL^{-1} [72].

Another work for CA-125 detection was reported by Büyüktiryaki *et al.* They designed a rapid, and cheap sensor for the detection of CA-125. In this method, methacryloyl antipyrine europium (III) and methacryloyl antipyrine terbium (III) was utilized as novel metal-chelating monomers. The phosphoserine was utilized as a target molecule for CA-125 sensing. The limit of detection phosphoserine imprinted nanosensor was calculated as 0.49 U·mL^{-1} with perfect sensitivity and reusability [73].

To enhance the signal response of the MIP-based nanomaterials they have been constantly combined in the imprinting method. Pirzada *et al* recently developed a sensitive electrochemical-based sensor by using hybrid epitope imprinting. The hybrid epitope imprinting polymer was fabricated by electro-polymerization. The linear range was performed in concentration between from 25 pg·mL^{-1} to 4000 pg·mL^{-1} for the detection of neuron-specific enolase in human serum [74].

Early breast cancer detection and diagnosis are very important in terms of patient follow-up and/or treatment guidance. Pacheco *et al* reported an MIP-based electrochemical sensor for monitoring breast cancer. The cancer antigen 15-3 (CA 15-3) is utilized as a breast cancer biomarker. A linear relationship between of CA 15-3 concentration was performed between 5 to 50 U mL^{-1} and the limit of detection was calculated as 1.5 U·mL^{-1}. It is reported that the MIP-based sensor provided rapid analysis in about 15 minutes. This sensor is inexpensive, easy to prepare, disposable and can be easily integrated into small portable point-of-care devices [75]. In addition, Patheco *et al* reported an MIP-based electrochemical sensor for the detection of HER2-ECD breast cancer biomarker. The linear concentration range was performed between 10 ng·mL^{-1} to 70 ng·mL^{-1} HER2-ECD. The limit of detection and limit of quantification was calculated as 1.6 ng·mL^{-1} and

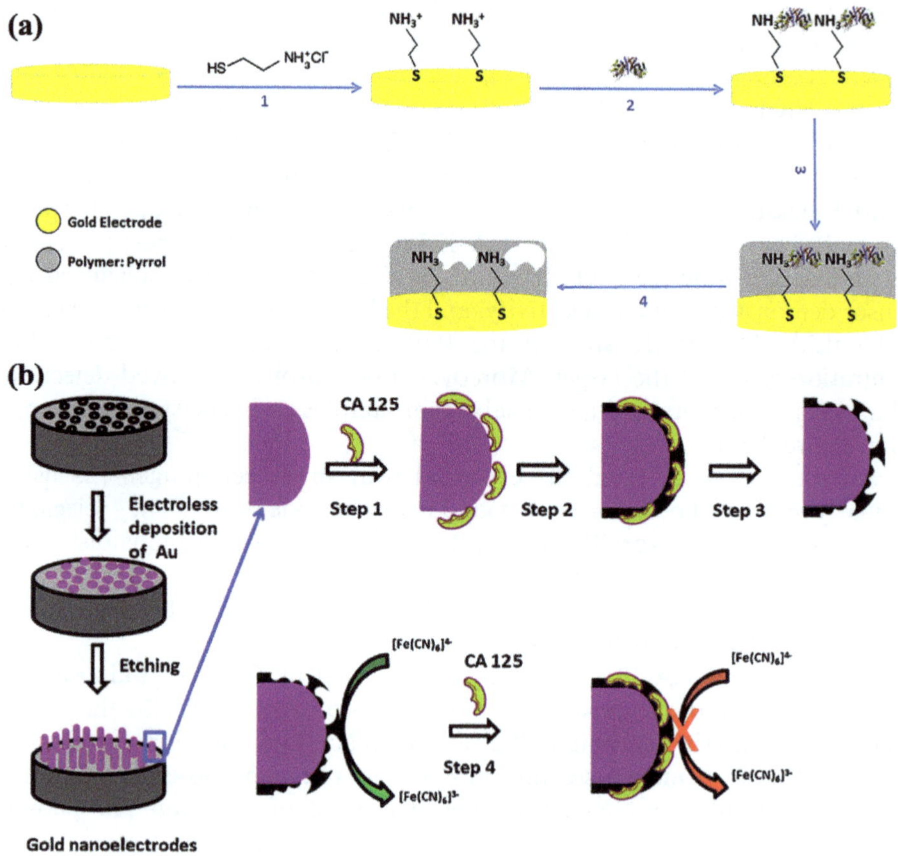

Figure 9.5. (a) Graphical representation of the different stages of MIP assembly (reprinted from [71], copyright (2019), with permission from Elsevier); (b) schematic representation of the protein imprinted nanosensor fabrication (reprinted from [72], copyright (2012), with permission from Elsevier).

5.2 ng·mL^{-1}, respectively. The MIP-based electrochemical sensor was found to be selective for HER2-ECD compared to other protein biomarkers [76]. Riberio *et al* detected the breast cancer biomarker CA 15-3 using MIP-based electrochemical sensor. The sensor showed a linear concentration response between 0.10 U·mL^{-1} to 100 U·mL^{-1} and the limit of detection was found to be below 0.10 U·mL^{-1}. The electrochemical sensor provided a novel approach for rapid, sensitive, and low-cost monitoring of CA 15-3 [77].

The utilization of implantable glucose sensors has been confined usually by their short term reliability in the human body. The occurrence of both chronic and acute inflammation in injured tissue can affect the function of the glucose sensor and shorten its lifetime [78, 79]. Wang *et al* developed a pH-sensitive MIP/hydrogel composite as a coating for implantable glucose sensors for the controlled release of dexamethasone-21 phosphate disodium (DXP) [80]. The MIP pH-sensitive nanospheres were successfully prepared via UV polymerization. The preparation of DXP-imprinted polymer is illustrated in figure 9.6.

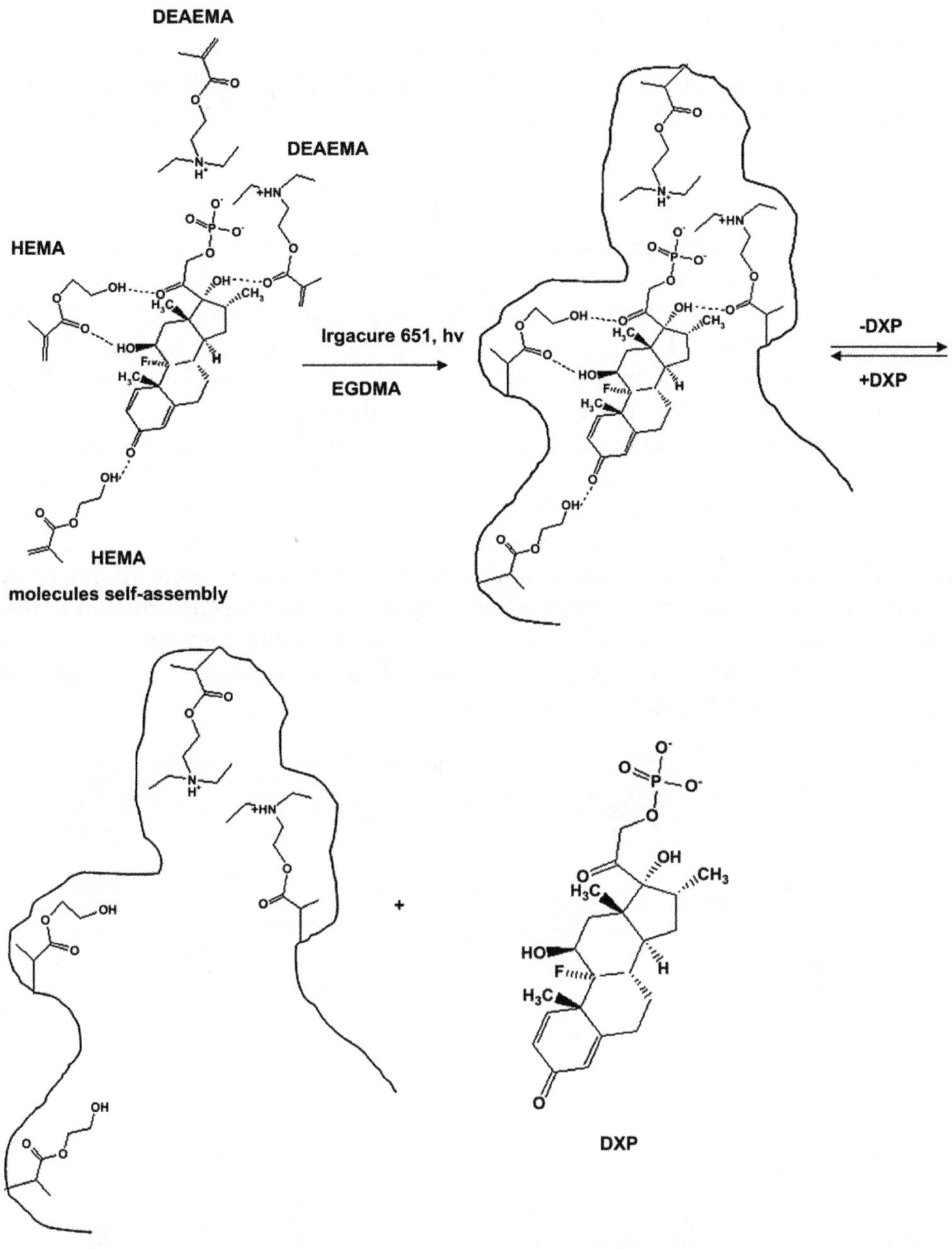

Figure 9.6. Scheme for the preparation of DXP-imprinted nanospheres. Reprinted from [80], copyright (2010), with permission from Elsevier.

Glucose is an energy source for cells and also comprises the main biomolecules in diabetes diagnosis [81]. Therefore, many research groups have prepared selective biosensors for detection and recognition of the glucose molecule in fluids of the body [82]. To determine glucose level they have utilized various methods such as fluorescent spectroscopy, colorimetry, optical, conductometry, and electrochemical [83]. Kim *et al* developed an MIP modified layer based non-enzymatic potentiometric sensor for the detection of glucose molecule [84]. The potentiometric sensor probe performed a broad linear range between 3.2×10^{-7} M to 1.0×10^{-3} M and the limit of detection was found to be 1.9×10^{-7} M. In the end, the non-enzymatic potentiometric-based sensor was used for the glucose detection. Figure 9.7(a) shows the fabrication of the MIP probe.

Another work, a novel glucose imprinted voltammetric sensor was prepared by Yang *et al* [85]. Firstly, they synthesized glucose imprinted micelles (MIPMs) from the self-assembly of a photo-cross-linkable amphiphilic copolymer in specific solution. The MIP-based voltammetric sensor design is depicted in figure 9.7(b). The glucose sensor exhibited a broad linear range from 0.2 mM to 8.0 mM. In addition, this MIP-based glucose sensor also displayed perfect stability and reversibility. In addition, Diouf *et al* developed a novel MIP-based non-enzymatic electrochemical sensor for the detection of glucose [86]. The MIP-based gold electrode was prepared by electropolymerized acrylamide/bis-acrylamide. The linear concentration range was performed between 0.5 $\mu g \cdot mL^{-1}$ and 50 $\mu g \cdot mL^{-1}$. They reported that the limit of detection and limit of quantification were found to be 0.59 $\mu g \cdot mL^{-1}$ and 1.9 $\mu g \cdot mL^{-1}$, respectively. Finally, glucose was determined in real saliva samples. This sensor has demonstrated a cheap, simple, and sensitive system for the detection of non-enzymatic glucose. The preparation of the glucose imprinted sensor is presented in figure 9.7(c).

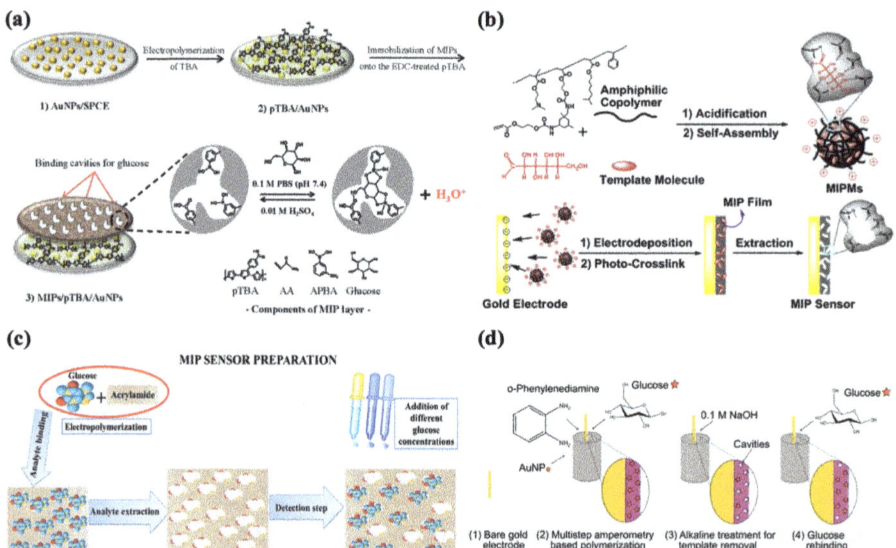

Figure 9.7. (a) Schematic representation of the fabrication of the MIP-based glucose sensor (reprinted from [84], copyright (2017), with permission from Elsevier); (b) schematic illustration of the MIP sensor fabrication (reprinted from [85], copyright (2011), with permission from Elsevier); (c) schematic representation of the Au-SPE/MIP procedures (reprinted from [86], copyright (2019), with permission from Elsevier); (d) manufacturing steps of AuNP decorated MIPs using o-PD as functional monomer and glucose as template molecules (reprinted from [87], copyright (2020), with permission from Elsevier).

Sehit *et al* reported a novel glucose imprinted non-enzymatic electrochemical sensor based on AuNPs (gold nanoparticles) and MIPs. The linear response of this glucose sensor ranged from 1.25 nM to 2.56 μM in human serum. The design of a sensitive and selective AuNPs/MIP-based electrochemical sensor is given in figure 9.7(d). The stability of this sensor was reported up to 95% during a storage period of 40 days [87]. Alexander *et al* developed a glucose imprinted electrochemical sensor [88]. The detection concentration linear range of this glucose sensor system was performed from 0.01 μM to 0.08 μM with a response time of ~2 min. A low limit of detection of 0.1 nM was achieved.

9.4.2 Drug delivery

Drug delivery systems (DDS) display many significant advances in using drug delivery via new optimized technology. The rate of drug-releasing plays an important role in the safety and efficacy of DDS. Also, the other significant factors in DDS are the delivery rate of the therapeutic dose, placing it in the appropriate place to reduce dosing frequency, reduce the side effects of the drug, and increase patient compliance [89–92]. Three approaches have been improved to control the drug release ratio:

i. Programming the ratio of the drug delivery: the diffusion of the drug has to follow a certain rate program;
ii. Modulating the activation of the drug delivery: the delivery of the drug needs to be activated by some chemical, physical processes;
iii. Regulating the feedback of the drug delivery: the release rate of the drug is organized via the concentration of a starting factor.

The combination of sensor systems with DDS has imitated the identification role of membrane receptors, enzymes, and antibodies in vital organisms for the reorganization of chemical reactions and for repair of the homeostatic equilibrium. Efficient bionanomaterials can be obtained using the unique properties of molecularly imprinted technology, for example, the ability of molecular imprinting to recognize specific bioactive molecules, and the absorption capacity [93–95]. There are some appearance characteristics that should be noticed in MIP-based DDS, as follows.

9.4.2.1 Rigidity or flexibility of the DDS structure

The stability of the cavities in the imprinted structure plays a significant role in these systems. The structure of MIP-based bionanomaterials should be strong without the template and protect the conformation of cavities. Also, the flexibility of the cavities should be planned as well as to release/rebinding the drug. These properties are an important factor in a sensor using diagnostic applications. Here, non-covalent based molecular imprinted technology prefers to prepare fast equilibrium kinetics [96, 97]. Another property of DDS has depended on the cross-linker. The hydrophobicity of the bionanomaterials can be increased by increasing the levels of the cross-linker agent, therefore, the conformation of the structure of the materials is stable during synthesis. But the high levels of cross-linker agent increase the strength of the materials, thus adapting of the materials to tissues will be difficult.

9.4.2.2 Chemical stability of the DDS structure

In drug delivery systems MIPs should be sufficiently stable to withstand chemical attack and mechanical stress. Bionanomaterials are contacted with biological fluids entering the body. Therefore, the chemical stability of MIP-based DDS should be controlled against different pH and mixed composition. Ethylene glycol dimethacrylate as an ideal cross-linker has obtained stable bionanomaterials in a broad range of pH and temperatures. A broad range of cross-linkers has been shown to be utilized as DDS. MIP in water is developed using hydrogels cross-linkers [98].

The significant weakness of hydrogen-bonding and electrostatic interactions in the water medium has revealed numerous difficulties such as decreasing the selectivity and binding and affinity of the target to the ligand in the MIP process. On the other hand, metal coordination and hydrophobic interactions show high interaction between functional monomer and target molecule in the water medium. Based on these explanations, solvent and materials composition play important roles in the success of decent imprinting [99, 100].

Several MIP-based DDS were recently developed for the controlled and sustained delivery of anti-inflammatory, antibiotic, and anticancer medicines in the literature. To date, many studies were focused on smart drug delivery based on MIP against the difficulties in this area. Smart delivery of the drug depends on small changes in pH, temperature, electric field, ionic strength, incident light or solvent composition [101].

In a study, Suksuwan *et al* used fluorescently active 2,6-bis(acrylamido)pyridine and *N,N′* methylene-bis-acrylamide to develop thermoresponsive R-thalidomide imprinted nanoparticles utilizing a physical and covalent approach. They reported 100 nm the size of the prepared nanoparticle. They showed that the high effectiveness of the drug for attacking multidrug-resistant cells was obtained via a physical approach [102].

Hemmati *et al* developed an MIP-based magnetic nanocomposite with graphene oxide. They used Rivastigmine as a template molecule. Rivastigmine is a carbamate type of an acetylcholine esterase inhibitor. They showed the Langmuir isotherm model and pseudo-first-order model with 71.41 mg/g capacity. They calculated and reported 1.98 selectivity factor compared to NIP materials. The high biocompatibility of bionanomaterials was demonstrated via cytotoxicity experiments. The 84.4% cell viability was obtained at 1.0 mg mL^{-1} loaded drug concentration [103].

In another study, Zhang *et al* prepared double responsive MIP-based mesoporous silica nanoparticles by using doxorubicin as a template drug. They can load 10.5 ± 0.2 wt% of doxorubicin over the bionanomaterials. They reported a 70% ± 8% loading efficiency value. They utilized pH and glutathione double responsive effects to the release of doxorubicin and showed high release due to the synergistic separation. Doxorubicin can inhibit TCA8113 cells growth. They reported low cytotoxicity in releasing experiments [104].

In another study, frontal polymerization was used for prepared gatifloxacin imprinted hydrogel by Wang *et al.* They used *N,N′*-methylenebisacrylamide and

N-isopropylacrylamide acrylic acid in hydrogels structure. They controlled releasing of gatifloxacin from the gatifloxacin imprinted hydrogel by temperature and pH [105]. L-DOPA has been utilized as a prodrug for Parkinson's disease treatment. L-DOPA is unstable when added to aqueous solutions and/or exposed to light, therefore, it can be degraded.

In the study, L-DOPA imprinted b-cyclodextrin was developed to be obtained as a nanocarrier for the release L-DOPA. The prepared MIP-based nanosponges delivered L-DOPA in the acidic condition. L-DOPA degraded at neutral condition but the authors showed the stability of L-DOPA in the acidic condition [106].

Bakhshizadeh *et al* reported a novel study to prepare a Mitox-antrone imprinted nanoparticles for drug delivery. They used poly(methacrylicacid-co-polycaprolactone diacrylate) and 4-vinyl pyridine as functional monomer. They used TiO_2 as core and MIP as a shell. They showed that the poly(methacrylicacid-co-polycaprolactone diacrylate)-based MIP demonstrated high binding capacity [107].

Kurczewska *et al* used DDS to obtain antibacterial wound dressing. To this aim, they utilized vancomycin drug encapsulated in alginate matrix. They reported decreasing vancomycin release from 87% to 47% for the alginate-MIP as compared to without the alginate. They reported non-Fickian transport diffusion. Also, the swelling controlled mechanism of this material was shown successfully [108].

Gu and their coworkers used DDS and nanotechnology combination to obtain a new strategy for use in cancer treatments to prevent the disadvantages of chemotherapy such as causing severe side effects and damaging healthy tissues. They improved a selective chemotherapeutic using MIP-based nanoparticles as a smart carrier. This group used 5′-Deoxy-5-fluorocytidine as a prodrug and sialic acid as a marker for tumor targeting. Drug imprinted nanoparticles accumulated at the tumor site and were then released (figure 9.8). They demonstrated new access to the development of smart release nanoplatforms [109].

There are various applications of MIP-based drug delivery according to their therapeutic administration routes such as intravenous routes, topical skin and transdermal routes, ocular routes and oral therapeutic applications. To improve drug bioavailability and avoid drug degradation, molecular imprinted polymers have also been conducted intravenously in *in vitro* analysis [110]. In a study, an effective nanomaterial was developed by using novel fluorescent multi-core shell structured biodegradable molecular imprinted magnetic nanoparticle, for sustained, targeted and controlled delivery of 5-fluorouracil as a drug. Asadi and coworkers synthesized nanoparticles using a mini-emulsion polymerization. Figure 9.9(a) shows the technique of this polymerization. They reported that the delivery of 5-fluorouracil was found to rely upon pH and also showed drug delivery within two hours in simulated gastric fluid. However, they reported a sustained release of 5-fluorouracil for up to 120 hours in plasma simulated fluid. They carried out an *in vivo* assay in a rat model, by injecting MIP solution intravenously and applied MIP-based drug nano-carriers into the liver as guided by an external magnetic field. They proved an effective nanocarrier system for cancer treatment [111].

Qin *et al* developed MIP-stabilized fluorescent zeolitic imidazolate tumor-sensitive biodegradable nanoparticles for drug delivery and targeted imaging. Targeting the

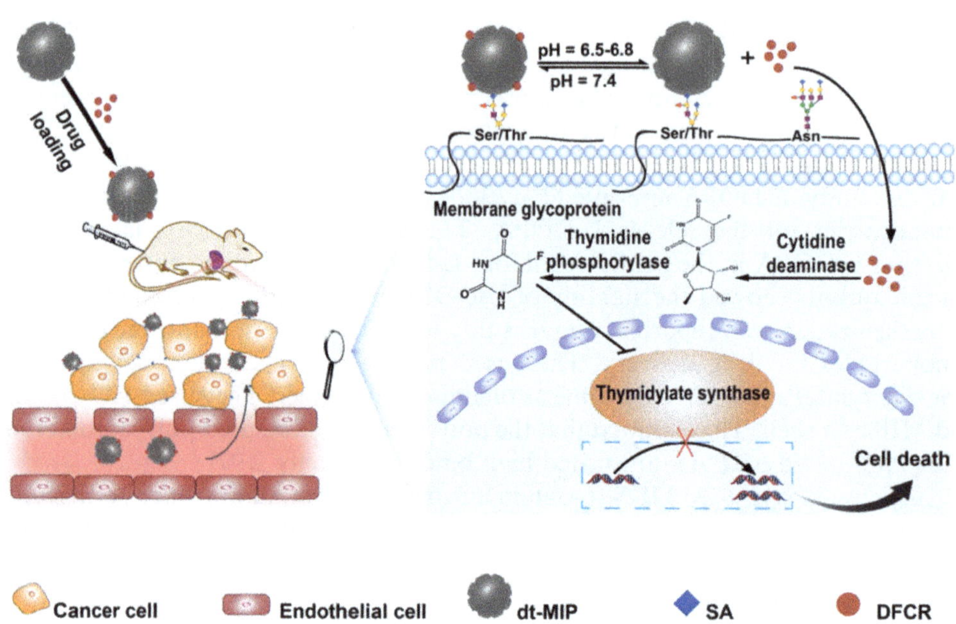

Figure 9.8. Schematic of the drug transport and action mechanism in a dual-templated MIP-based smart prodrug delivery system [109], copyright (2020) John Wiley & Sons.

enrichment of nanocarriers plays an important role in the effective anti-cancer drug delivery. Therefore, they utilized MIP-based fluorescent nanoparticles loaded with doxorubicin to synthesize tumor-sensitive biodegradable nanoparticles. The epitope of CD59 cell membrane glycoprotein was used as a target molecule. They used *N*,*N*′-diacrylylcystamine and dimethylamino ethyl methacrylate as the cross-linker and main monomer, respectively (figure 9.9(b)) [112]. Table 9.1 summarizes these bionanomaterials and their roles in drug delivery systems.

9.4.3 Cell imaging

There are considerations when developing the applications of MIPs *in vitro* and *in vivo*. Firstly, binding properties and physicochemical properties should be tested. MIPs should have properties such as hemocompatibility, cell biocompatibility, and inflammatory response in their *in vivo* applications [122]. Demir *et al* recently prepared MIPs templated with glucuronic acid (GlcA), an epitope of hyaluronan, which were applied for bio-labeling and bio-imaging of intracellular and extracellular hyaluronan on human skin tissues and cells. In this research were prepared the dye rhodamine or semiconductor quantum dots (QDs) with conventional fluorescent labels. They prepared N-doped CDs by using hydrothermal synthesis with starch as a carbon source and L-tryptophan used as a nitrogen atom provider (figure 9.10(a)). The targeting and imaging of hyaluronan on immobilized human cervical cancer cells is demonstrated by using CD MIP-core-shell nanocomposites. In this research was utilized human keratinocytes as noncancerous reference cells and indeed, less staining was observed by the CD-MIP. Unlike QDs, CDs show

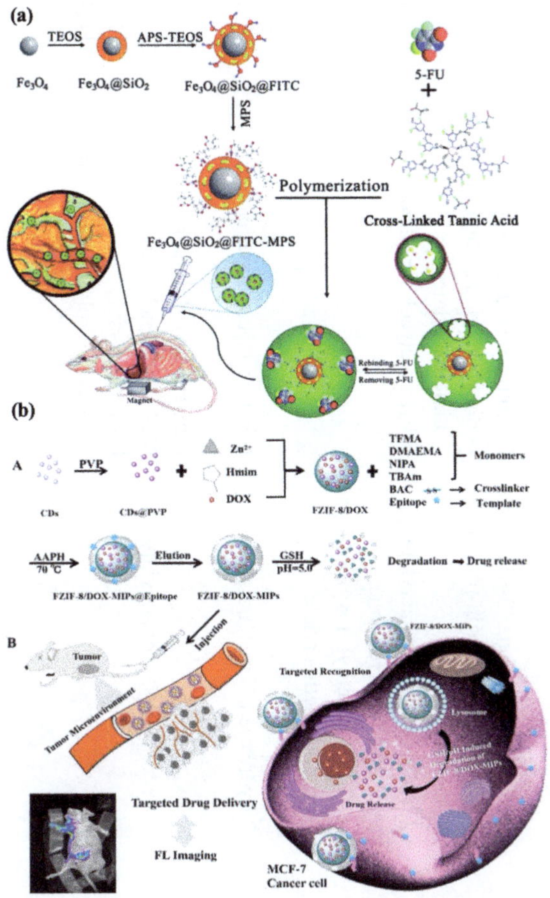

Figure 9.9. (a) The procedure followed for preparation and characterization of magnetic molecularly imprinted polymer nanoparticles as a 5-FU carrier (TEOS: tetraethyl orthosilicate, APS: 3-aminopropyl trimethoxysilane, FITC: fluorescein isothiocyanate, 5-FU: 5-fluorouracil, MPS: methacryloxypropyl trimethoxysilane) (reprinted from [111], copyright (2016), with permission of RSC); (b) synthesis of MIP-based nanoparticles and schematic illustration of targeted imaging and GSH/pH-responsive drug delivery of MIP-based nanoparticles (reprinted with permission from [112], copyright (2020) American Chemical Society).

more stable luminescence without blinking. In addition, CDs do not contain heavy metals and are more compatible than QDs [123]. In addition, Rangel *et al* utilized D-glucuronic acid (GlcA), an epitope of hyaluronic acid [124]. Hyaluronic acid, a glycosaminoglycan, has many important roles in human health and disease. It is also one of the main biomarkers of certain cancers. For this reason, detection of hyaluronic acid is important at an early stage. However, intracellular hyaluronic acid could be masked by other hyaluronic acid binding macromolecules, making its visualization a problem. Their perfect sensitivity, water compatibility, and small size, enabled the fluorescent-based molecularly imprinted nanogels to visualize hyaluronic acid, as evidenced by confocal fluorescence micrographs (figure 9.10(b)).

Table 9.1. Release of different targets with MIP-based bionanomaterials.

Template	Functional agent	Monomer	Cross-linker	Ref.
Ketotifen fumarate	Acrylic acid, Acrylamide, N-vinyl-2-pyrrolidone	2-hydroxyethyl methacrylate	Ethylene glycol dimethacrylate	[113]
Hydroxypropyl Methylcellulose	*N*,*N*-dimethylacrylamide, Acrylic acid	Betacon Macromere, 3-tris (trimethylsiloxy)silil-propyl methacrylate	Poly(ethylene glycol) (200) dimethacrylate, Ethylene glycol dimethacrylate	[114]
Ciprofloxacin	Acrylic acid	2-hydroxyethyl methacrylate, Polyvinylpyrrolidone, 3-tris(trimethylsiloxy)silil-propyl methacrylate	Ethylene glycol dimethacrylate	[115]
Timolol maleate	*N*-acetylated chitosan, Methacrylic acid	2-hydroxyethyl methacrylate	Ethylene glycol dimethacrylate	[116]
5-fluorouracil	Methacrylic acid	–	Ethylene glycol dimethacrylate	[117]
5-fluorouracil	Acrylic acid	2-hydroxyethyl methacrylate	*N*,*N*-methylenebisacrylamide	[117]
Insulin	Methacrylic acid	–	Ethylene glycol	[118]
Naltrexone	Acrylic acid, Methacrylic acid	–	Ethylene glycol dimethacrylate	[119]
Conformational epitope of HER2 and doxorubicin	Dopamine	–	–	[120]
Doxorubicin	3-(trimethoxysilyl)propyl methacrylate	*N*-isopropylacrylamide	Ethylene glycol dimethacrylate	[121]

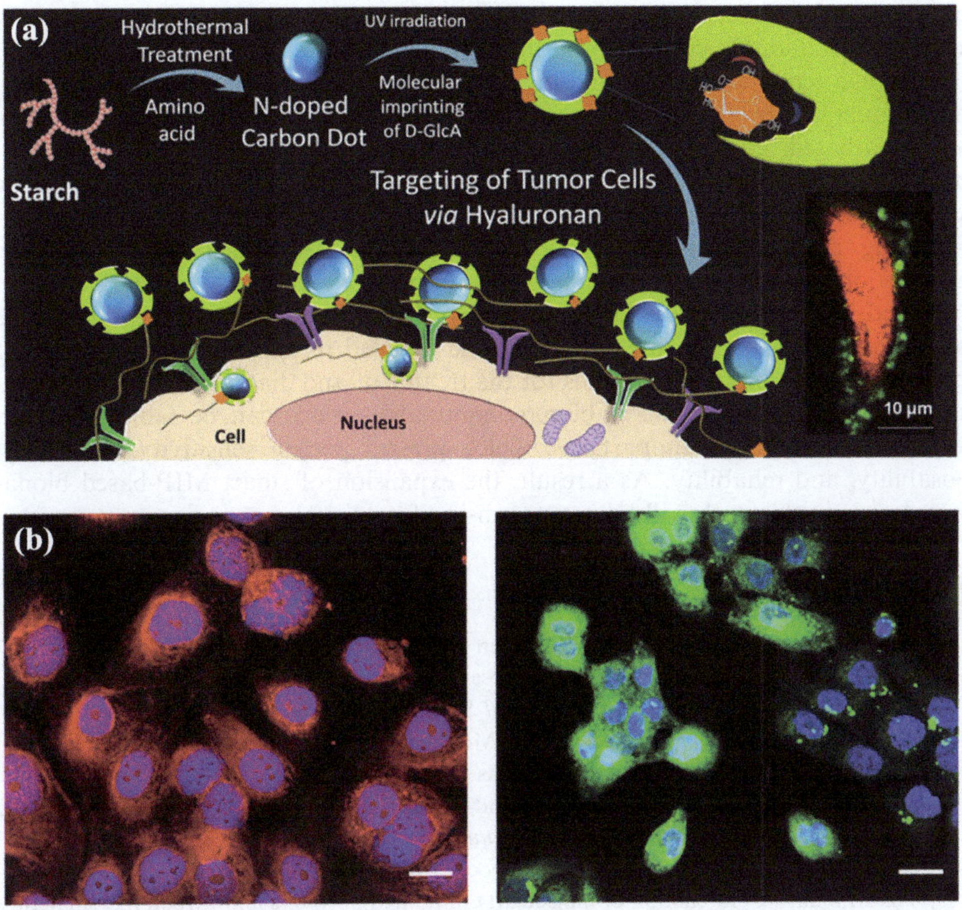

Figure 9.10. (a) CDs-MIP for cancer cell imaging (reprinted from [123], copyright (2018) American Chemical Society); (b) confocal images of fixed human keratinocytes showing extracellular, intracellular and nuclear labeling by MIPGlcA-NPs (red) (left) and by HABP/streptavidin FITC (green) (right), nuclear counterstaining with Hoechst (blue), scale bar: 20 μm ([124], copyright (2019), with permission of Springer).

9.5 Conclusions and future trends

With the discovery of MIPs in 1993, much research has been done on the applications of biocompatible, non-toxic, and eco-friendly nanomaterials. MIPs are cross-linked polymeric materials synthesized in the presence of a target analyte that serves as a mold for the creation of target-complementary recognition sites. Molecular imprinting technique provides a broad range of easy to imprint different biomolecules with size, three-dimensional structure, chemical, and physical features. The MIP-based bionanomaterials offer inexpensive, quick, easy-to-use, highly sensitive, and selective sensing approaches, especially for theranostics, diagnosis, and screening applications. Recently, in the MIPs area, a broad range of application areas have been presented, such as medical, pharmaceutical, food control, homeland security, and environmental As a result, polymeric bionanomaterials capable of recognizing the target molecule are obtained. These bionanomaterials are rapidly and easily produced in contrast to antibodies and are more stable in hard conditions such as high temperature, low and high pH, or the presence of organic solvents. In this chapter, we presented an overview of key recent advances in molecularly imprinted-based bionanomaterials and their biomedical applications, as well as of the direct utilization of the MIP-based bionanomaterials in biomimetic sensors drug delivery, tissue engineering, and cell imaging. These approaches make them promising materials for nanomedicine applications. A critical analysis of the information presented in examples illustrating the synthesis of MIPs is also presented. For example, when synthesizing MIPs against small peptides, it is essential to select the suitable epitope on the targeted receptor protein. Simple and novel MIP-based bionanomaterials for the treatment and diagnosis of a biomedical are described. The MIP-based bionanomaterials' surface can be fabricated with polymer thin film or nanoparticles, which present perfect sensitivity, selectivity, reusability, and reliability. As a result, the expansion of smart MIP-based bionanomaterials in this path will have a promising future.

References

[1] Yılmaz F, Saylan Y, Akgönüllü S, Çimen D, Derazshamshir A and Bereli N *et al* 2017 Surface plasmon resonance based nanosensors for detection of triazinic pesticides in agricultural foods *New Pesticides and Soil Sensors* (New York: Academic) pp 679–718

[2] Xu J, Miao H, Wang J and Pan G 2020 Molecularly imprinted synthetic antibodies: from chemical design to biomedical applications *Small* **16** 1–21

[3] Vlatakis G, Andersson L I, Müller R and Mosbach K 1993 Drug assay using antibody mimics made by molecular imprinting *Nature* **361** 645–7

[4] Haupt K 2010 Biomaterials: plastic antibodies *Nat. Mater.* **9** 612–4

[5] Ansari S 2017 Combination of molecularly imprinted polymers and carbon nanomaterials as a versatile biosensing tool in sample analysis: Recent applications and challenges *TrAC – Trends Anal. Chem.* **93** 134–51

[6] Ansari S and Karimi M 2017 Recent progress, challenges and trends in trace determination of drug analysis using molecularly imprinted solid-phase microextraction technology *Talanta* **164** 612–25

[7] Dai H, Xiao D, He H, Li H, Yuan D and Zhang C 2015 Synthesis and analytical applications of molecularly imprinted polymers on the surface of carbon nanotubes: a review *Microchim Acta* **182** 893–908

[8] Yáñez-Sedeño P, Campuzano S and Pingarrón J M 2017 Electrochemical sensors based on magnetic molecularly imprinted polymers: a review *Anal. Chim. Acta* **960** 1–17

[9] Ansari S and Karimi M 2017 Recent configurations and progressive uses of magnetic molecularly imprinted polymers for drug analysis *Talanta* **167** 470–85

[10] Ansari S 2017 Application of magnetic molecularly imprinted polymer as a versatile and highly selective tool in food and environmental analysis: Recent developments and trends *TrAC – Trends Anal. Chem.* **90** 89–106

[11] Belbruno J J 2019 Molecularly imprinted polymers *Chem. Rev.* **119** 94–119

[12] Akgönüllü S, Battal D, Yalcin M S, Yavuz H and Denizli A 2019 Rapid and sensitive detection of synthetic cannabinoids JWH-018, JWH-073 and their metabolites using

molecularly imprinted polymer-coated QCM nanosensor in artificial saliva *Microchem. J.* **153** 104454

[13] Battal D, Akgönüllü S, Yalcin M S, Yavuz H and Denizli A 2018 Molecularly imprinted polymer based quartz crystal microbalance sensor system for sensitive and label-free detection of synthetic cannabinoids in urine *Biosens. Bioelectron.* **111** 10–17

[14] Saylan Y, Akgönüllü S, Yavuz H, Ünal S and Denizli A 2019 Molecularly imprinted polymer based sensors for medical applications *Sensors (Switzerland)* **19** 1279

[15] Say R, Keçili R, Denizli A and Ersöz A 2016 Biomimetic imprinted polymers: theory, design methods, and catalytic applications *Molecularly Imprinted Polymers: Principles, Syntheses, and Applications* 2016 (Amsterdam: Elsevier) pp 103–20

[16] Czulak J, Guerreiro A, Metran K, Canfarotta F, Goddard A and Cowan R H *et al* 2016 Formation of target-specific binding sites in enzymes: Solid-phase molecular imprinting of HRP *Nanoscale* **8** 11060–6

[17] Xia Y, Zhao F and Zeng B 2020 A molecularly imprinted copolymer based electrochemical sensor for the highly sensitive detection of L-Tryptophan *Talanta* **206** 120245

[18] Saylan Y and Denizli A 2018 Molecular fingerprints of hemoglobin on a nanofilm chip *Sensors (Switzerland)* **18** 3016

[19] Babamiri B, Salimi A and Hallaj R 2018 A molecularly imprinted electrochemiluminescence sensor for ultrasensitive HIV-1 gene detection using EuS nanocrystals as luminophore *Biosens. Bioelectron.* **117** 332–9

[20] Dabrowski M, Zimińska A, Kalecki J, Cieplak M, Lisowski W and Maksym R *et al* 2019 Facile fabrication of surface-imprinted macroporous films for chemosensing of human chorionic gonadotropin hormone *ACS Appl. Mater. Interf.* **11** 9265–76

[21] D'Aurelio R, Chianella I, Goode J A and Tothill I E 2020 Molecularly imprinted nanoparticles based sensor for cocaine *Detection. Biosensors* **10** 22

[22] Saylan Y, Erdem Ö, Cihangir N and Denizli A 2019 Detecting fingerprints of waterborne bacteria on a sensor *Chemosensors* **7** 33

[23] Klangprapan S, Choke-arpornchai B, Lieberzeit P A and Choowongkomon K 2020 Sensing the classical swine fever virus with molecularly imprinted polymer on quartz crystal microbalance *Heliyon* **6** e04137

[24] Amatatongchai M, Sroysee W, Sodkrathok P, Kesangam N, Chairam S and Jarujamrus P 2019 Novel three-Dimensional molecularly imprinted polymer-coated carbon nanotubes (3D-CNTs@MIP) for selective detection of profenofos in food *Anal. Chim. Acta* **1076** 64–72

[25] Akgönüllü S, Yavuz H and Denizli A 2020 SPR nanosensor based on molecularly imprinted polymer film with gold nanoparticles for sensitive detection of aflatoxin B1 *Talanta* **219** 121219

[26] Bakhshpour M and Denizli A 2020 Highly sensitive detection of Cd(II) ions using ion-imprinted surface plasmon resonance sensors *Microchem. J.* **159** 105572

[27] Ayankojo A G, Reut J, Ciocan V, Öpik A and Syritski V 2020 Molecularly imprinted polymer-based sensor for electrochemical detection of erythromycin *Talanta* **209** 120502

[28] Eersels K, Lieberzeit P and Wagner P 2016 A review on synthetic receptors for bioparticle detection created by surface-imprinting techniques – from principles to applications *ACS Sensors* **1** 1171–87

[29] Zahedi P, Ziaee M, Abdouss M, Farazin A and Mizaikoff B 2016 Biomacromolecule template-based molecularly imprinted polymers with an emphasis on their synthesis strategies: a review *Polym. Adv. Technol.* **27** 1124–42

[30] Qin L, He X W, Yuan X, Li W Y and Zhang Y K 2011 Molecularly imprinted beads with double thermosensitive gates for selective recognition of proteins *Anal. Bioanal. Chem.* **399** 3375–85
[31] Ertürk G and Mattiasson B 2017 Molecular imprinting techniques used for the preparation of biosensors *Sensors (Switzerland)* **17** 1–17
[32] Mujahid A, Iqbal N and Afzal A 2013 Bioimprinting strategies: From soft lithography to biomimetic sensors and beyond *Biotechnol. Adv.* **31** 1435–47
[33] Lieberzeit P A, Gazda-Miarecka S, Halikias K, Schirk C, Kauling J and Dickert F L 2005 Imprinting as a versatile platform for sensitive materials – Nanopatterning of the polymer bulk and surfaces *Sens. Actuators B Chem.* **111–112** 259–63
[34] Whitcombe M J, Chianella I, Larcombe L, Piletsky S A, Noble J and Porter R *et al* 2011 The rational development of molecularly imprinted polymer-based sensors for protein detection *Chem. Soc. Rev.* **40** 1547–71
[35] Hillberg A L and Tabrizian M 2008 Biomolecule imprinting: Developments in mimicking dynamic natural recognition systems *Itbm-Rbm* **29** 89–104
[36] López-Puertollano D, Cowen T, García-Cruz Á, Piletska E, Abad-Somovilla A and Abad-Fuentes A *et al* 2019 Study of epitope imprinting for small templates: preparation of nanoMIPs for ochratoxin A *Chem. Nano Mat.* **5** 651–7
[37] Singh M, Gupta N and Raghuwanshi R 2017 Epitope imprinting approach to monitor diseases *J. Mol. Genet. Med.* **11** 1000270
[38] Rachkov A and Minour N 2000 Recognition of oxytocin and oxytocin-related peptides in aqueous media using a molecularly imprinted polymer synthesized by the epitope approach *J. Chromatog.* A **889** 111–8
[39] Nishino H, Huang C S and Shea K J 2006 Selective protein capture by epitope imprinting *Angew. Chem. Int. Ed. Engl.* **45** 2392–6
[40] Yang K *et al* 2019 Epitope imprinting technology: progress, applications, and perspectives toward artificial antibodies *Adv. Mater.* **31** 1902048
[41] Lehner R, Wang X, Marsch S and Hunziker P 2013 Intelligent nanomaterials for medicine: Carrier platforms and targeting strategies in the context of clinical application *Nanomed.: Nanotechnol., Biol. Med.* **9** 742–57
[42] Sitharaman B (ed) 2011 Nanobiomaterials Handbook 1st edn (Boca Raton, FL: CRC Press)
[43] Neuwelt E A, Hamilton B E, Varallyay C G, Rooney W R, Edelman R D and Jacobs P M *et al* 2009 Ultrasmall superparamagnetic iron oxides (USPIOs): A future alternative magnetic resonance (MR) contrast agent for patients at risk for nephrogenic systemic fibrosis (NSF)? *Kidney Int.* **75** 465–74
[44] Chang C and Mao D 2007 Thermal dehydration kinetics of a rare earth hydroxide, Gd $(OH)_3$ *Int. J. Chem. Kinet.* **39** 75–81
[45] Huang X and El-Sayed M A 2010 Gold nanoparticles: Optical properties and implementations in cancer diagnosis and photothermal therapy *J. Adv. Res.* **1** 13–28
[46] Lee K S and El-Sayed M A 2005 Dependence of the enhanced optical scattering efficiency relative to that of absorption for gold metal nanorods on aspect ratio, size, end-cap shape, and medium refractive index *J. Phys. Chem.* B **109** 20331–8
[47] Bakhshpour M, Tamahkar E, Andaç M and Denizli A 2017 Surface imprinted bacterial cellulose nanofibers for hemoglobin purification *Coll. Surf. B Biointerf.* **158** 453–9

[48] Bakhshpour M, Tamahkar E, Andaç M and Denizli A 2017 Affinity binding of proteins to the modified bacterial cellulose nanofibers *J. Chromatogr. B: Anal. Technol. Biomed. Life Sci.* **1052** 121–27
[49] Saylan Y, Tamahkar E and Denizli A 2017 Recognition of lysozyme using surface imprinted bacterial cellulose nanofibers *J. Biomater. Sci. Polym. Ed.* **28** 1950–65
[50] Göktürk I, Tamahkar E, Yılmaz F and Denizli A 2018 Protein depletion with bacterial cellulose nanofibers *J. Chromatogr. B Anal. Technol. Biomed. Life Sci.* **1099** 1–9
[51] Lim S Y, Shen W and Gao Z 2015 Carbon quantum dots and their applications *Chem. Soc. Rev.* **44** 362–81
[52] Karousis N, Tagmatarchis N and Tasis D 2010 Current progress on the chemical modification of carbon nanotubes *Chem. Rev.* **110** 5366–97
[53] Sinha N and Yeow J T W 2005 Carbon nanotubes for biomedical applications *IEEE Trans. Nanobiosci.* **4** 180–95
[54] Robertson J 2004 Realistic application of CNTs *Mater. Today* **7** 46–52
[55] Ren T, Wang G, Cao C, Yuan W, Song Y and Su J 2010 Electrospun poly(L-Lactide-co-ε-caprolactone)/polyethylene oxide/hydroxyapaite nanofibrous membrane for guided bone regeneration *J. Nanomater.* **8**
[56] Swetha M, Sahithi K, Moorthi A, Srinivasan N, Ramasamy K and Selvamurugan N 2010 Biocomposites containing natural polymers and hydroxyapatite for bone tissue engineering *Int. J. Biol. Macromol.* **47** 1–4
[57] Bailey R E, Smith A M and Nie S 2004 Quantum dots in biology and medicine *Physica E* **25** 1–12
[58] O'Farrell N, Houlton A and Horrocks B R 2006 Silicon nanoparticles: Applications in cell biology and medicine *Int. J. Nanomed.* **1** 451–72
[59] Maxwell T, Nogueira Campos M G, Smith S, Doomra M, Thwin Z and Santra S 2019 Quantum dots *Nanoparticles for Biomedical Applications: Fundamental Concepts, Biological Interactions and Clinical Applications* (Amsterdam: Elsevier) pp 243–65
[60] Wagner A M, Knipe J M, Orive G and Peppas N A 2019 Quantum dots in biomedical applications *Acta Biomaterialia* **94** 44–63
[61] García-Martinez G, Bustabad E A, Perrot H, Gabrielli C, Bucur B and Lazerges M *et al* 2011 Development of a mass sensitive quartz crystal microbalance (QCM)-based DNA biosensor using a 50 MHz electronic oscillator circuit *Sensors* **11** 7656–64
[62] Bakhshpour M, Ozgur E, Bereli N and Denizli A 2017 Microcontact imprinted quartz crystal microbalance nanosensor for protein C recognition *Coll. Surf. B Biointerf.* **151** 264–70
[63] Sener G, Ozgur E, Yilmaz E, Uzun L, Say R and Denizli A 2010 Quartz crystal microbalance based nanosensor for lysozyme detection with lysozyme imprinted nanoparticles *Biosens. Bioelectron.* **26** 815–21
[64] Lu C H, Zhang Y, Tang S F, Bin F Z, Yang H H and Chen X *et al* 2012 Sensing HIV related protein using epitope imprinted hydrophilic polymer coated quartz crystal microbalance *Biosens. Bioelectron.* **31** 439–44
[65] Gao N, Dong J, Liu M, Ning B, Cheng C and Guo C *et al* 2012 Development of molecularly imprinted polymer films used for detection of profenofos based on a quartz crystal microbalance sensor *Analyst* **137** 1252–58
[66] Yang Z P and Zhang C J 2009 Designing of MIP-based QCM sensor for the determination of Cu(II) ions in solution *Sens. Actuators B Chem.* **142** 210–15

[67] Ayankojo A G, Reut J, Boroznjak R, Öpik A and Syritski V 2018 Molecularly imprinted poly(meta-phenylenediamine) based QCM sensor for detecting Amoxicillin *Sens. Actuators B Chem.* **258** 766–74

[68] Spieker E and Lieberzeit P A 2016 Molecular imprinting studies for developing QCM-sensors for bacillus cereus *Procedia Eng.* **168** 561–4

[69] Bhalla N, Jolly P, Formisano N and Estrela P 2016 Introduction to biosensors *Essays Biochem.* **60** 1–8

[70] Sha R and Badhulika S 2020 Recent advancements in fabrication of nanomaterial based biosensors for diagnosis of ovarian cancer: a comprehensive review *Microchim. Acta* **187** 181

[71] Rebelo T S C R, Costa R, Brandão A T S C, Silva A F, Sales M G F and Pereira C M 2019 Molecularly imprinted polymer SPE sensor for analysis of CA-125 on serum *Anal Chim. Acta* **1082** 126–35

[72] Viswanathan S, Rani C, Ribeiro S and Delerue-Matos C 2012 Molecular imprinted nanoelectrodes for ultra sensitive detection of ovarian cancer marker *Biosens. Bioelectron.* **33** 179–83

[73] Büyüktiryaki S, Say R, Denizli A and Ersöz A 2017 Phosphoserine imprinted nanosensor for detection of Cancer Antigen 125 *Talanta* **167** 172–80

[74] Pirzada M, Sehit E and Altintas Z 2020 Cancer biomarker detection in human serum samples using nanoparticle decorated epitope-mediated hybrid MIP *Biosens. Bioelectron.* **166** 112464

[75] Pacheco J G, Silva M S V, Freitas M, Nouws H P A and Delerue-Matos C 2018 Molecularly imprinted electrochemical sensor for the point-of-care detection of a breast cancer biomarker (CA 15-3) *Sens. Actuators B Chem.* **256** 905–12

[76] Pacheco J G, Rebelo P, Freitas M, Nouws H P A and Delerue-Matos C 2018 Breast cancer biomarker (HER2-ECD) detection using a molecularly imprinted electrochemical sensor *Sens. Actuators B: Chem.* **273** 1008–14

[77] Ribeiro J A, Pereira C M, Silva A F and Sales M G F 2018 Disposable electrochemical detection of breast cancer tumour marker CA 15-3 using poly(Toluidine Blue) as imprinted polymer receptor *Biosens. Bioelectron.* **109** 246–54

[78] Patil S D, Papadmitrakopoulos F and Burgess D J 2007 Concurrent delivery of dexamethasone and VEGF for localized inflammation control and angiogenesis *J. Cont. Rel.* **117** 68–79

[79] Hickey T, Kreutzer D, Burgess D J and Moussy F 2002 Dexamethasone/PLGA microspheres for continuous delivery of an anti-inflammatory drug for implantable medical devices *Biomaterials* **23** 1649–56

[80] Wang C, Javadi A, Ghaffari M and Gong S 2010 A pH-sensitive molecularly imprinted nanospheres/hydrogel composite as a coating for implantable biosensors *Biomaterials* **31** 4944–51

[81] Wu H, Tian Q, Zheng W, Jiang Y, Xu J and Li X *et al* 2019 Non-enzymatic glucose sensor based on molecularly imprinted polymer: a theoretical, strategy fabrication and application *J Sol. State Electrochem.* 1379–88

[82] Bandodkar A J and Wang J 2014 Non-invasive wearable electrochemical sensors: A review *Trends Biotechnol.* **32** 363–71

[83] Wu Q, Wang L, Yu H, Wang J and Chen Z 2011 Organization of glucose-responsive systems and their properties *Chem. Rev.* **111** 7855–75

[84] Kim D M, Moon J M, Lee W C, Yoon J H, Choi C S and Shim Y B 2017 A potentiometric non-enzymatic glucose sensor using a molecularly imprinted layer bonded on a conducting polymer *Biosens. Bioelectron.* **91** 276–83

[85] Yang Y, Yi C, Luo J, Liu R, Liu J and Jiang J *et al* 2011 Glucose sensors based on electrodeposition of molecularly imprinted polymeric micelles: A novel strategy for MIP sensors *Biosens. Bioelectron.* **26** 2607–12

[86] Diouf A, Bouchikhi B and El Bari N 2019 A nonenzymatic electrochemical glucose sensor based on molecularly imprinted polymer and its application in measuring saliva glucose *Mater. Sci. Eng.* C **98** 1196–209

[87] Sehit E, Drzazgowska J, Buchenau D, Yesildag C, Lensen M and Altintas Z 2020 Ultrasensitive nonenzymatic electrochemical glucose sensor based on gold nanoparticles and molecularly imprinted polymers *Biosens. Bioelectron.* **165** 112432

[88] Alexander S, Baraneedharan P, Balasubrahmanyan S and Ramaprabhu S 2017 Highly sensitive and selective non enzymatic electrochemical glucose sensors based on graphene oxide-molecular imprinted polymer *Mater. Sci. Eng.* C **78** 124–9

[89] Liechty W B, Kryscio D R, Slaughter B V and Peppas N A 2010 Polymers for drug delivery systems *Annu. Rev. Chem. Biomol. Eng.* **1** 149–73

[90] Tiwari G, Tiwari R, Bannerjee S, Bhati L, Pandey S and Pandey P *et al* 2012 Drug delivery systems: An updated review *Int. J. Pharm. Investig.* **2** 2–11

[91] Tekade R K 2020 In Advances in pharmaceutical product development and research *Drug Delivery Systems* (New York: Academic)

[92] Kumari A, Yadav S K and Yadav S C 2010 Biodegradable polymeric nanoparticles based drug delivery systems *Coll. Surf. B Biointerf.* **75** 1–18

[93] Bakhshpour M, Idil N, Perçin I and Denizli A 2019 Biomedical applications of polymeric cryogels *Appl. Sci. (Switzerland)* **9** 553

[94] Tamahkar E, Bakhshpour M and Denizli A 2019 Molecularly imprinted composite bacterial cellulose nanofibers for antibiotic release *J. Biomater. Sci. Polym. Ed.* **30** 450–61

[95] Bakhshpour M, Yavuz H and Denizli A 2018 Controlled release of mitomycin C from PHEMAH–Cu(II) cryogel membranes *Artif. Cells, Nanomed. Biotechnol.* **46** 946–54

[96] Sung J C, Pulliam B L and Edwards D A 2007 Nanoparticles for drug delivery to the lungs *Trends Biotechnol.* **25** 563–70

[97] Pillai O and Panchagnula R 2001 Polymers in drug delivery *Curr. Opin. Chem. Biol.* **5** 447–51

[98] Csaba N, Garcia-Fuentes M and Alonso M J 2006 The performance of nanocarriers for transmucosal drug delivery *Exp. Op. Drug Deliv.* **3** 463–78

[99] Challa R, Ahuja A and Ali J *et al* 2005 Cyclodextrins in drug delivery: An updated review *AAPS PharmSciTech* **6** E329–57

[100] Wanakule P and Roy K 2012 Drug delivery *Tissue Engineering: Principles and Practices* ed J P Fisher, A G Mikos, J D Bronzino and D R Peterson (Boca Raton, FL: CRC Press)

[101] Alvarez-Lorenzo C and Concheiro A 2004 Molecularly imprinted polymers for drug delivery *J. Chromatogr. B: Anal. Technol. Biomed. Life Sci.* **804** 231–45

[102] Suksuwan A, Lomlim L, Rungrotmongkol T, Nakpheng T, Dickert F L and Suedee R 2015 The composite nanomaterials containing (R)-thalidomide-molecularly imprinted polymers as a recognition system for enantioselective-controlled release and targeted drug delivery *J. Appl. Polym. Sci.* **132** 1–21

[103] Hemmati K, Sahraei R and Ghaemy M 2016 Synthesis and characterization of a novel magnetic molecularly imprinted polymer with incorporated graphene oxide for drug delivery *Polymer* **101** 257–68

[104] Zhang K, Guan X, Qiu Y, Wang D, Zhang X and Zhang H 2016 A pH/glutathione double responsive drug delivery system using molecular imprint technique for drug loading *Appl. Surf. Sci.* **389** 1208–13

[105] Wang X L, Yao H F, Li X Y, Wang X, Huang Y P and Liu Z S 2016 pH/temperature-sensitive hydrogel-based molecularly imprinted polymers (hydroMIPs) for drug delivery by frontal polymerization *RSC Adv.* **6** 94038–47

[106] Trotta F, Caldera F, Cavalli R, Soster M, Riedo C and Biasizzo M *et al* 2016 Molecularly imprinted cyclodextrin nanosponges for the controlled delivery of L-DOPA: perspectives for the treatment of Parkinson's disease *Expert Opin. Drug Deliv.* **13** 1671–80

[107] Bakhshizadeh M, Sazgarnia A, Seifi M, Hadizadeh F, Rajabzadeh G and Mohajeri S A 2017 TiO_2-based mitoxantrone imprinted poly (methacrylic acid-co-polycaprolctone diacrylate) nanoparticles as a drug delivery system *Curr. Pharm. Des.* **23** 2685–94

[108] Kurczewska J, Cegłowski M, Pecyna P, Ratajczak M, Gajęcka M and Schroeder G 2017 Molecularly imprinted polymer as drug delivery carrier in alginate dressing *Mater. Lett.* **201** 46–9

[109] Gu Z, Dong Y, Xu S, Wang L and Liu Z 2020 Molecularly imprinted polymer-based smart prodrug delivery system for specific targeting, prolonged retention and tumor microenvironment-triggered release *Angew. Chemie. Int. Ed.* 1–6

[110] Zaidi S A 2016 Latest trends in molecular imprinted polymer based drug delivery systems *RSC Adv.* **6** 88807–19

[111] Asadi E, Abdouss M, Leblanc R M, Ezzati N, Wilson J N and Azodi-Deilami S 2016 *In vitro/in vivo* study of novel anti-cancer, biodegradable cross-linked tannic acid for fabrication of 5-fluorouracil-targeting drug delivery nano-device based on a molecular imprinted polymer *RSC Adv.* **6** 37308–18

[112] Qin Y T, Feng Y S, Ma Y J, He X W, Li W Y and Zhang Y K 2020 Tumor-sensitive biodegradable nanoparticles of molecularly imprinted polymer-stabilized fluorescent zeolitic imidazolate framework-8 for targeted imaging and drug delivery *ACS Appl. Mater. Interf.* **12** 24585–98

[113] Tieppo A, White C J, Paine A C, Voyles M L, McBride M K and Byrne M E 2012 Sustained *in vivo* release from imprinted therapeutic contact lenses *J. Contr. Rel.* **157** 391–7

[114] White C J, McBride M K, Pate K M, Tieppo A and Byrne M E 2011 Extended release of high molecular weight hydroxypropyl methylcellulose from molecularly imprinted, extended wear silicone hydrogel contact lenses *Biomaterials* **32** 5698–705

[115] Hui A, Willcox M and Jones L 2014 In vitro and *in vivo* evaluation of novel ciprofloxacin-releasing silicone hydrogel contact lenses *Investig. Ophthalmol. Vis. Sci.* **55** 4896–904

[116] Kim H J, Zhang K, Moore L and Ho D 2014 Diamond nanogel-embedded contact lenses mediate lysozyme-dependent therapeutic release *ACS Nano* **8** 2998–3005

[117] Singh B and Chauhan N 2008 Preliminary evaluation of molecular imprinting of 5-fluorouracil within hydrogels for use as drug delivery systems *Acta Biomater.* **4** 1244–54

[118] Li S, Tiwari A, Ge Y and Fei D 2010 A pH-responsive, low crosslinked, molecularly imprinted insulin delivery system *Adv. Mater. Lett.* **1** 4–10

[119] Rostamizadeh K, Vahedpour M and Bozorgi S 2012 Synthesis, characterization and evaluation of computationally designed nanoparticles of molecular imprinted polymers as drug delivery systems *Int. J. Pharm.* **424** 67–75

[120] Hashemi-Moghaddam H, Zavareh S, Karimpour S and Madanchi H 2017 Evaluation of molecularly imprinted polymer based on HER2 epitope for targeted drug delivery in ovarian cancer mouse model *React. Funct. Polym.* **121** 82–90

[121] Kaamyabi S, Habibi D and Amini M M 2016 Preparation and characterization of the pH and thermosensitive magnetic molecular imprinted nanoparticle polymer for the cancer drug delivery *Bioorganic Med. Chem. Lett.* **26** 2349–54

[122] Haupt K, Medina Rangel P X and Bui B T S 2020 Molecularly imprinted polymers: Antibody mimics for bioimaging and therapy *Chem. Rev.* **120** 9554–82

[123] Demir B, Lemberger M M, Panagiotopoulou M, Medina Rangel P X, Timur S and Hirsch T *et al* 2018 Tracking hyaluronan: molecularly imprinted polymer coated carbon dots for cancer cell targeting and imaging *ACS Appl. Mater. Interf.* **10** 3305–13

[124] Medina Rangel P X, Laclef S, Xu J, Panagiotopoulou M, Kovensky J and Tse Sum Bui B *et al* 2019 Solid-phase synthesis of molecularly imprinted polymer nanolabels: Affinity tools for cellular bioimaging of glycans *Sci. Rep.* **9** 1–9

Chapter 10

Bionanomaterials for green bionanotechnology

Charles Oluwaseun Adetunji, Olugbemi T Olaniyan, Osikemekha Anthony Anani, Abel Inobeme, Kingsley Eghonghon Ukhurebor, Ruth Ebunoluwa Bodunrinde, Juliana Bunmi Adetunji, Kshitij RB Singh, Vanya Nayak, Wadzani Dauda Palnam and Ravindra Pratap Singh

Bionanomaterials are widely applied for green bionanotechnology, most especially in the biomedical sector and their application can be linked to several factors, namely interconnected porous network, biodegradability, nontoxic by-products, and immune biocompatibility. These bionanomaterials are applied for tissue regeneration and *in* and *ex situ* tissue engineering for regeneration of tissue such as orthopedic implants, cardiovascular implants, dental implants, and their utilization as antimicrobial agents. Hence, this chapter provides detailed information on bionanomaterials utility for tissue implant and regeneration, treatment of diseases caused by microbes. Along with synthesis and characterization of bionanomaterials for biomedical application.

10.1 Introduction

The application of nanobiotechnology has transformed medical sciences such as physiology, microbiology, anatomy and pharmacology. Advancements in these fields have huge potential in transforming health care practices where physiologists help to elucidate the mechanisms and design of sub-cellular levels of nanodevice, drug delivery specificity and therapeutic efficacy, thereby minimizing side effects [1]. The role of bionanoparticles in various fields of human endeavor cannot be overemphasized due to their wide applications in catalysis, as sensors, film coatings, biological probes, diagnostic sensors and in medical fields. Their uses cover different areas of the medical field. The synthesis of nanoparticles and composites has found unique utilization in the biomedical area like tissue engineering, medical implanting, delivery of drugs and prosthetic components, detection of various biomolecules; hence they have affected the medical field remarkably. Bionanoparticles are useful in bioprinting usage due to their biodegradability and compatibility with biological

doi:10.1088/978-0-7503-3767-0ch10

systems. The design and synthesis of bionanomaterials and composites have been done to exhibit advanced functionalities such as photonic coatings, adhesive films or mimicking a unique biological parameter and function [2].

Also, much attention has been drawn by nano-based calcium phosphate such as tricalcium phosphate in bionanomaterials due to some of their properties such as exceptional sizes, high surface area with respect to volume ratio and high biocompatibility with natural bones. In a study, the formulated 3D nanobiocomposite scaffolds were based on calcium phosphate and carbonated hydroxyapatite. Findings from the *in vitro* analysis showed that the introduction of the bionanomaterial brought about an improvement of SaOS-2 cell proliferation and the alkaline phosphate activity. It was revealed from the investigation that scaffolds obtained from nanomaterials introduced a biomimetic medium suitable for the attachment of osteoblastic cells, which found immense relevance in the area of bone tissue technology [3]. Advances in the study of nanomaterials have also benefited the livestock industries as they helped in monitoring animal breeding patterns and health checkups by delivering genes and drugs to the desired cell or tissues [4].

This chapter intends to provide detailed information on various applications of bionanomaterials for green bionanotechnology in the biomedical domain, principally highlighting tissue implant and regeneration, treatment of various microbial diseases caused by bacterial, viruses and fungi. Detailed emphasis is also laid on various synthesis and characterization methods of bionanomaterials for biomedical application, highlighting biosynthesis methods.

10.2 Synthesis of bionanomaterials for biomedical application

There are different methods available for the synthesis of bionanomaterials. Some of the methods available for the synthesis of bionanoparticles are discussed below.

10.2.1 Biosynthetic method

Various approaches to synthesize nanoparticles have now focused on the biological routes as they are relatively easy to fabricate, cost-effective, green and environmentally friendly. These biosynthesis methods have unique advantages: introducing less toxic materials, low-temperature requirement and fast reaction rate [5]. The chemical approach possesses various limitations like excess use of toxic chemicals and high temperature and energy usage, which makes the synthesized nanoparticles non-biocompatible and hazardous for the environment. However, these problems can be solved using a green approach, known as the biosynthesis method and can be completed through the Tollen methods, polyoxometalates methods, and irradiation methods. The biological route utilizes various parts of plants and algae, microorganisms like bacteria, fungi, yeast, and other biological ways, including nutrient mediums like egg yolk, starch, honey, pectin, etc. These biosynthesized nanomaterials have shown a potential role in controlling various diseases with minimum side effects. Figure 10.1 shows various biological routes used in the biosynthesis of nanomaterials. Many reviews and articles have focused on biological methods to synthesize nanomaterials. The most commonly synthesized nanomaterials are from noble metals such as cadmium sulfide, platinum,

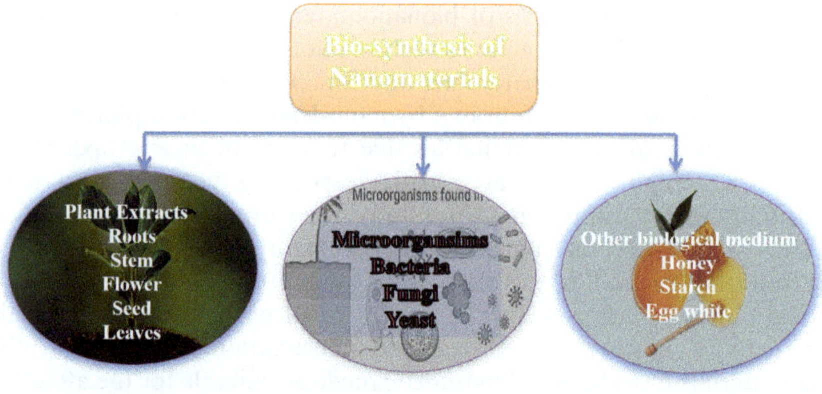

Figure 10.1. Various biological routes used in the biosynthesis of nanomaterials.

gold, cerium magnesium, barium, titanate, amongst others [6–8]. Biosynthesis of nanomaterials is now widely recommended as building blocks of the upcoming generations in controlling and diagnosing various diseases.

10.2.2 Hydrolysis method

Unlike other nanomaterials, bionanomaterials are readily prepared from animal and plant sources with properties showing high similarity with perfect crystal. Some of the preparation methods include acid hydrolysis, which aids in removing the lower order components to help in the conversion of the higher crystalline region that does not dissolve in water into a stable suspension through mechanical shearing [9]. Typical biodegradable and renewable molecules like chitin, cellulose and starch occur naturally and can be prepared by various approaches, including hydrolysis in acidic medium both naturally and in the laboratory. The nanoparticles of synthetic origin are usually synthesized using different physical and chemical processes that involve various reducing agents; some are mild in their reducing properties while others are strong. Examples are sodium citrate and sodium borohydrides. These reducing agents are, however, not environmentally friendly due to their corrosive effects on the ecosystem. Numerous researchers have used the method of hydrolysis and dialysis to prepare nanocellulose whiskers from different starting materials such as biomass and farm wastes [10].

Favier *et al* [11] extracted nanocellulose crystal from *Microcosmus* spp. The tunic of the animal is 1 cm thick. They were able to prepare nano-cellulose whiskers using simple hydrolysis and dialysis steps, and the observed length of the nanoparticles ranged from 100 nm to several micrometers while the order of the width was 10–20 nm. In a related study, Bondeson and Oksman [12] synthesized nanocellulose whisker using spruce microcrystalline cellulose by utilizing dialysis and hydrolysis to extract the nanowhiskers. Grunert and Winter [13] produced nanocrystals using hydrolysis of microfibril nanocrystals.

Similarly, Tokoh *et al* [14] prepared nanocrystals through sulfuric acid hydrolysis. The blending of the graphene oxide (GO) was done with polylactic acid and thermoplastic polyurethane (TPU) using a solvent-based mixing process. They successfully produced nanocomposites using FDM and showed their biocompatibility. Findings from the study revealed that there is the possibility of improving mechanical properties with a rise in the GO content. Aside from this, there was also a significant increase in the thermal parameters due to GO fillers' introduction. Results from *in vitro* studies showed that the nanocomposites have a high degree of compatibility with the biological system [13].

10.2.3 Bioreduction method

The bioreduction method is one of the techniques for the synthesis of bionanomaterials, as plants have many natural compounds like saponins, alkaloids, tannins, flavonoids, steroids, and other nutritional compounds obtained from different plant parts like flowers, leaves, stems, roots shoots, barks, and seeds. Extracts of plants are safe and, therefore, can be used as a potential precursor for nanomaterial synthesis. The plant extracts contain various secondary metabolites, which are utilized as stabilizing and reducing agents in the bioreduction reaction. The reduction process is induced by the presence of phenolic compounds, reducing sugars, enzymes and proteins. This synthetic process is regulated by factors such as the concentration of the reaction medium, pH of the system, and the starting materials [6].

10.2.4 Hydrothermal method

The hydrothermal approach is one of the best for preparing nanoparticles such as titanium oxide, which has wide application in the medical field. The reaction is carried out at a lower temperature when compared to other methods. Manipulation of various parameters such as heating duration and temperature aid in varying the particle sizes, composition and morphology of the nanoparticles. This method makes it possible to synthesis nanoparticles of size ranges within 6–10 nm [15]. There are some other green approaches that are also highly simplified and suitable for the synthesis of photoactive bionanoparticles.

In the hydrothermal method, an oxidizing and reducing agent is used in an aqueous medium. The microwave-assisted process also exists, which is also hydrothermal and used to prepare titanium oxide using titanium chloride. Some other studies have compared the preparation using the traditional hydrothermal approach and the microwave-assisted [16]. Fuchigami *et al* [17] synthesized Fe–Pt nanoparticles using the hydrothermal method by treating Fe–Pt silica composites resulting in the formation of nanoparticle shells of Fe–PT. They then investigated the potencies of magnetic porous nanoparticles for the targeted delivery of drugs in lung and gastric cancer treatment within cell lines. The anti-cancer drug (doxorubicin) was then filled into the hollow space.

10.2.5 Microfluidization method

Microfluidization is a method suitable for the preparation of nanofibrils of cellulose and their micro-fibrils and is completed at a consistent shear rate. It involves the pumping of the fluid slurry through a chamber that is z shaped, which is used to achieve an elevated shear force [18].

10.3 Characterization of bionanomaterials

Characterization of the synthesized bionanomaterial includes the regulation of structural, magnetic, electric, optical, and mechanical properties, which highly determine their applications. The characterization of nanomaterials is mainly divided into four types: structural, optical, electrical, and magnetic. Structural characterization involves the detection of morphology and arrangement of atoms, and the optical characterization includes detection of light absorption and light emission characteristics and how it affects the characters of the synthesized nanomaterials, the characterization is done using various methods such as coupled plasma spectrometry (ICP), Fourier transforms infrared spectroscopy (FTIR), ultraviolet–visible spectroscopy (UV), energy-dispersive x-ray spectroscopy (EDS) and photo-electron spectroscopy (XPS). Figure 10.2 shows various techniques that are used to characterize the synthesized nanomaterials.

10.3.1 UV–visible spectroscopic

This technique is one of the useful tools in the characterization of bionanomaterials. Initial characterization of the silver nanoparticle is mostly done using this method. This is suitable for detecting and monitoring the reduction process, for example, of silver ions to silver metals, which occur at a particular wavelength (e.g., 400 to 1200 nm for silver) [19].

10.3.2 X-ray diffraction

X-ray diffraction (XRD) is non-destructive and widely used to obtain details on the crystallographic structure and chemical compositions of materials. In their work, Mathew *et al* [20] used this technique to characterize chitosan and chitin crystal nanoparticles. Angellier *et al* [21], in their study, characterized solid nanocomposite

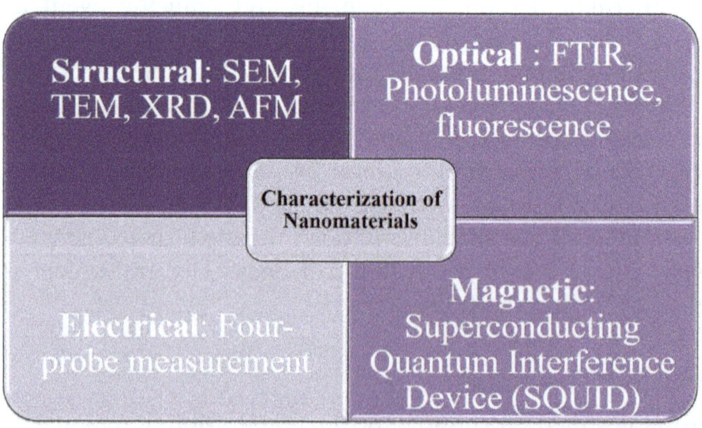

Figure 10.2. Various techniques used in the characterization of synthesized nanomaterials.

obtained from natural rubber latex and nanocrystals of starch using scanning electron microscopy, x-ray diffraction analysis and toluene absorption experiments.

10.3.3 Atomic force microscopy

This is a useful instrumental technique for the detection of sizes of nanoparticles. In this process, the fractured surface of films is observed at a temperature of liquid nitrogen. This technique makes it possible to deduce information on the presence of voids, aggregates, homogeneity, and the whisker's orientation. Force microscopy of nanoparticles could be used alternatively for electron microscopy with good resolution [22]. In x-ray diffraction, the extract is mixed first with the silver salt solution and the gradual conversion in the silver nanoparticles is allowed to take place. The resulting mixture is then centrifuged and then filtered, and the nanoparticles obtained subjected to analysis using x-ray diffraction techniques.

10.3.4 Fourier transformed infrared spectroscopy (FTIR)

Fourier transform infrared spectroscopy (FTIR) is highly utilized to study the infrared spectrum of absorption, emission, and photoconductivity of nanoparticles [23]. In FTIR, the nanoparticle powder prepared is subjected to measurements using the FTIR machine in the presence of potassium bromide pellets on a reflectance mode. Some other samples are usually employed as control during the measurement.

10.3.5 Transmission electron microscopy

This is useful in the characterization of bionanoparticles, as well as to detect the morphology and sizes of the synthesized nanoparticles. Preparation of samples for TEM analysis is done using 1 ml of the mixture, which contains the synthesized nanoparticle followed by dilution and sonication in an ultrasonic bath. Drops are then placed on a copper grid. Grunert *et al* [13], in their work, documented the size of the extracted cellulose from bacteria using the images from TEM. Different studies have reported the use of TEM for this purpose.

10.3.6 Potentiometric analysis

This is based on the variation in the redox potentials of the elementary metals during the conversion of the ions into metals and is usually done over a period of time using the combination of calomel and platinum electrodes [24]. In another study, Sanpui *et al* [25] synthesized silver nanoparticle chitosan for nanocarrier function and investigated the cytotoxic potential on cancer cells in the colon. This study was done using the colon cancer cell lines. The low content of silver nanoparticle chitosan carrier was prepared in phosphate buffer solution and incubated for 24 hours. Guo *et al* [26], in their study, synthesized polyvinylpyrrolidone containing silver nanoparticle coating of varying sizes through the use of the electrochemical method and this was then applied for assessing the cytotoxic activity of the silver nanoparticles on acute myeloid leukemia of the bone marrow. The nanoparticles' effect on the clinical isolates and cell lines was assessed using six different cell lines. Bone marrows from affected patients as well as healthy donors were also investigated. The effect of the synthesized nanoparticles on DNA damage, cell apoptosis, generation of ROS and viability was assessed.

One of the widely applied nanomaterials in biological systems is titanium oxide, which is also photoactive in nature. It exists in various forms, either amorphous or crystalline. There are different routes available to prepare titanium oxide and related bionanoparticles, which are sensitive to light. As reported by Fan *et al* [27], some of these methods include gas phase method, combustion, emulsion polymerization, hydrothermal method, and alcohol thermal approach. Various studies are carried out on the synthesis of bionanocomposites by reinforcing and blending bionanomaterials in different polymeric matrices [28]. Chitin whiskers with a higher aspect ratio are useful in reinforcing filler in the synthesis of polycaprolactone based nanocomposites. Parallel rod shapes have been documented as the geometry of chitin whiskers obtained from Riftia tubes with an aspect ratio of 1:20 [29].

10.4 Biomedical applications of bionanomaterials

Due to their small size and unique properties, nanomaterials have found their profound use in the biomedical domain. They are highly used to treat various kinds of diseases like cancer, neurodegenerative diseases, microbial infections, etc. They are highly used as nanocarriers in drug and gene delivery systems. They are also utilized in the generation of tissues, implants, and scaffolds. Not just in therapeutics, nanomaterials have found their potential role in the diagnosis of various diseases by detecting various biological components like DNA, RNA, proteins, antibodies, antigens, enzymes, etc. Thus, nanomaterials play a theranostic role in the biomedical domain, and many review articles and books have focused on the biomedical perspective of various nanomaterials [30, 31].

10.4.1 Tissue implant and regeneration

Neves *et al* [32] reported that patient-oriented solutions in personalized tissue engineering and regenerative medicine require cell-based therapies utilizing cell sources for easier induced pluripotent stem cells (iPSC cells) technologies or autologous set-ups. Thus, scaffold biomaterials or tissue-engineered bioproducts are customized to fit a patient's tissue in a defective state by adopting rapid prototyping technologies such as 3D printing. Similarly, Xavier *et al* [33] reported that nanobiotechnology utilizing nanobiomaterials for structural and mechanical bio-integration had become a powerful tool in different biomedical applications, particularly in drug delivery, tissue regeneration, and gene transfection, biosensor, and medical imaging. The authors revealed that reduced toxicity, high surface-to-volume ratio and improved cellular response are the major features of these nanobiomaterials, such as carbon-based, ceramic and metal nanoparticles. Many of the advanced synthetic nanoparticles such as bioglass, hydroxyapatite, zirconia, silver and titanium nanoparticles are utilized for dental restoration due to high biocompatibility and unique bioactive characteristics. The authors suggested that in the nearest future, developmental physiology, tissue engineering plus cell and molecular biology will play an active role in the field of dental regeneration due to the regenerative capacity of dental tissues, ameloblasts, dentin, and cementum, which are absent in adult dental tissue and also with limited regenerative potentials. These dental issues can be enhanced utilizing nanobiomaterials or nanoscale materials through physiological mechanisms involving signals for the development of morphological characters, scaffolds for mimicking an extracellular matrix and stem cells to respond to morphogenesis, growth factors such as BMP, Shh, FGFs, plus Wnt signaling, thereby forming composites, fibers and injectable materials.

Chen *et al* [34] reported that tissue engineering techniques had grown significantly in the past few decades even though different limitations have been witnessed due to the conventional method's restrictions to certain fields of study. Many advanced techniques have been developed to overcome these limitations, such as cell culture harvested from intact sheets without applying proteolytic enzymes (dispase or trypsin). Cell sheets are generally known to possess channels, extracellular matrix, growth factors, cell surface proteins, receptors, and nexin. Studies have identified some nanobiomaterials applications with the cell sheet combined with scaffolds for tissue reconstruction and repairs through superposition and implantation. Some other techniques involve pretreated hypoxia, mesenchymal sheet cell combined growth factors and gene transfer or iPSC-derived cell sheets, ESC for repairs and regenerative medicine. Sidhu *et al* [35] revealed that organ transplant through tissue engineering application had grown significantly utilizing different techniques and approaches such as scaffolding, advanced 3D printing technology, bio-fabrication with inkjet bioprinters, laser-assisted and extrusion-based bioprinting using an extracellular matrix. The authors showed that the use of extracellular matrix as bio-ink has higher limits, particularly to non-vascularized organs. Thus advancement in biotechnology has brought about the development of decellularized extracellular matrix. Bhat and Kumar [36] showed that nanobiomaterials are currently being utilized to restore and repair tissue engineering and regenerative medicine. The characteristics or features of the nanobiomaterials enable them to be the right choice for several tissue-specific applications. These include nanobiomaterials such as immune biocompatibility, biodegradability, nontoxic by-products, and interconnected porous network. Today, many nanobiomaterials are developed into tissue regeneration products, such as orthopedic implants, cardiovascular implants, and dental implants.

Abdulghani and Mitchell [37] reported that *in* and *ex situ* tissue engineering for regeneration of tissue has developed significantly in approach with some unexplored strands of regenerative medicine such as designing of scaffolds for implants, solvent-casting, particulate-leaching, sol–gel, phase-separation, 4D printing of 3D object, electrospinning and predictive modeling. The authors reported that biopolymers, bioceramics and other natural materials could be utilized to synthesize nanobiomaterials in bone generation therapy through predictive modeling strategies. Mostafavi *et al* [38] reported that recently, conductive nanomaterials in tissue regeneration such as neural, cardiovascular, muscle and bone have come to the forefront. The authors noted that the application of electroconductive nanobiomaterials enhances cell to cell crosstalk such as cell growth, proliferation, migration, plus differentiation. Pogorielov *et al* [39] reported that technological advancement has led to increased tissue engineering development for regeneration and repair of damaged tissue or organ. The authors highlighted that biomolecules and polymers like collagen, chitosan and chitin can be improved upon to increase the mechanical properties with the application of nano-based materials. Tao *et al* [40] reported that increased versatility in scaffold designs is seen when tissue engineering is combined with nanobiotechnology to promote proliferation, cell adhesion and differentiation in vascular (endodontics), periodontal, bone tissue regeneration, plus temporomandibular joint. The authors revealed that to promote periodontal tissue regeneration, scaffold materials, like polylactic acid, polyamide, collagen, poly (lactic-co-glycolic acid), chitosan, and polycaprolactone, can be combined with nanohydroxyapatite facilitating revascularization of periapical tissue and pulp regeneration. Polymeric nanofibers, nanofibrous-type, nanocomposite-based scaffolds are utilized for tissue growth, adhesion, cell differentiation, plus the synthesis of the cartilaginous extracellular matrix. Also, nanomodified mineral-like graphene, trioxide aggregate is currently being tested for biofabrication of scaffolds.

Banigo *et al* [41] reported that many techniques and nanobioproducts are generally utilized for tissue engineering, such as biomolecules, nanoparticles, biomaterials, cells, medical data, informatics, predictive modeling, differentiation factors, 3D tissue growth, bioreactors, enzymes, cell expansion, biophysical, biochemical, biomechanical, biocompatibility and biodegradability procedures plus signaling. Many biomaterials are utilized to manufacture orthopedic implants due to their chemical nature like biodegradability, strength, being chemical inert, nontoxic by-products, low elasticity, and resistance to corrosion, stability to biological tissues. Shi *et al* [42] showed that polymeric materials are currently being utilized for bone regeneration through different techniques involving bioactive surface modification with nanobiomaterials to modify its structural, physicochemical, biophysical, geometric structure, surface chemistry, plus biological properties. Ansari [43] reported that orthopedic technologies and biomaterials of superior properties like advanced computational modeling, nanoparticles, biomaterial-based three-dimensional (3D) cell-printing substitutes, cell-based products, nonfibrous substitutes, biomimetic fibrous, stem cells, bioactive porous polymer/inorganic composites had shown tremendous characteristics and potential in the development of synthetic substitutes for tissue regeneration. Different strategies have been developed utilizing advanced technologies such as bone graft replacements, optimized 3D structure, implantable scaffolds and biomaterials like polypeptides, enzymes, signaling factors, and small biomolecules.

Lowe *et al* [44] reported that tissue engineering involves the physiological mechanisms of combining different biomaterials to address regenerative and repair tissues in the body. For instance, nanohydroxyapatite can contribute to the physiological behavior of any biomaterial, such as biocompatibility, bonding chemistry, surface-area-to-volume ratio, interfacial chemistry, mechanical strength, bioresorbability, micropore architectures, rate of degradation, pore size, pore interconnectivity, topographical parameters, porosity, pore morphology plus substrate functionality. The authors highlighted different techniques and approaches that biomedical scientists should utilize to help design and optimize biomolecules in tissue regeneration, such as advanced qualitative and quantitative studies, advanced computational modeling, cell culture, and animal model experiments. Idumah [45] reported that tissue engineering involves fabrication and physiological replacements of damaged tissue through bioactive biomolecules. Nair *et al* [46] revealed that a natural extracellular matrix is known to act as a 3D structure with biochemical and mechanical cues to control and support cell functions and organization through macro- and micro-fabrication techniques. Engel *et al* [47] revealed that biological functionality could be enhanced utilizing nanobiomaterials during regenerative medicine techniques by producing sufficient signals stimulating cells towards physiological behavior in triggering the regeneration process. Rodríguez-Vázquez *et al* [48] reported that tissue engineering could serve as a therapeutic strategy utilizing functional biomaterials such as nanobiomaterials to develop scaffoldings to repair damaged organs or tissue in regenerative medicine. Frey *et al* [49] reported that there are three physiological components such as cells, growth factors and scaffolds or cell-based therapies, immunomodulation, and gene therapy using stem plus progenitor cells in tissue engineering. The authors noted that basic sciences like nanotechnology, bioinformatics, biomechanics, material science, physiology, polymer chemistry had witnessed increased research output concerning the promotion of functionalized organogenesis. Physiological approaches concerning stem cell populations, neurogenic niches, growth factors, immune modulation, bioreactor technology, transcription factors and regulators, scaffold production, cell expansion, reprogramming, transplantation additives have transformed the application of nanobiomaterials in tissue engineering.

Pina *et al* [50] reported exciting technologies and approaches in basic medical sciences for tissue engineering and regenerative medicine, like solvent casting, particulate-leaching, phase separation, and freeze-drying electrospinning, rapid prototyping in combination with nanobiotechnology, that have transformed and promoted cell adhesion, new bone growth and proliferation. The authors noted that nanocomposites, such as collagen, silk fibroin, gelatin, chitosan, hyaluronic acid, alginate, gellan gum, and derivatives as natural polymeric matrices, HAp plus β-TCP as bioactive fillers, are biomaterials with excellent characteristics for tissue regeneration. Mao and Mooney [21] reported that several nanomaterials have been utilized for medical therapy, such as orthopedics applications, wound healing, immune modulation, controlling cell behavior and repairing tissue. Salata [51] and España-Sánchez *et al* [52] revealed that tissue engineering requires physiological platforms for specific characteristics like morphology, surface chemistry, and interconnectivity to facilitate cell adhesion and cellular migration, the supply of nutrients, removal of waste molecules, plus proliferation. Hill *et al* [53] revealed that reconstructive bone surgeries and joint replacement are now increasing globally. They noted that poor healing and integration is a major problem that could only be tackled by basic scientists like physiologists, microbiologists, tissue engineering, regenerative medicine and anatomists through a multidisciplinary approach. Through advancement in technology, nanobiomaterials are now being utilized for the fabrication of devices, tissues and drug delivery systems at the nanoscale with higher biocompatibility, biodegradability and zero immune rejection. Cutting-edge technologies are also adopted to provide replacing, regenerating, and imaging tissues to address any pathological conditions associated with body tissues or organs. Nanofabrication of bone tissues through advanced fabrication techniques such as multi-material bioprinting, high-resolution printing techniques, and novel bio-inks combined with big-data science, proteomics, genomics, algorithms utilizing modeling and hydrogels are the current technologies. In personalized medicine, patient data could be utilized for tissue engineering using iPSCs tailored to an individual. The authors noted that chiral amino acids' addition to calcium carbonate influences crystal handedness and morphology, which are currently adopted in nanomedicine to develop nontoxic nanobiomaterials.

Kapat *et al* [54] reported that non-centrosymmetric crystalline biomaterial displays piezoelectric properties. Thus piezoelectric nano-biomaterials are currently being investigated as highly attractive biomolecules for therapeutic applications, drug delivery, along tissue regeneration in regenerative medicine. Many piezoelectric materials are now being fabricated for tissue engineering, such as nano-piezoceramics, piezopolymers, barium titanate, polyvinylidene fluoride, zinc oxide. The physiological mechanisms of these piezoelectric materials for tissue regeneration involve subjecting a cell to electric stimulation, leading to phenotypic and genetic alterations, thereby accelerating tissue regeneration processes. The authors noted that advancements in piezoelectric nano-biomaterials have led to regenerating cartilage, nerves, tendons, skin, muscle and ligaments. Other applications include therapeutics, actuation, sensing, reconstruction, cochlear implants, osteochondral and T/L grafts, synthetic skin, nano-transducers and nerve conduits. Piezoelectric nano-biomaterials are piezopolymers such as PVDF, PLLA, P(VDFTrFE), PHBV, and piezoceramics such as BN and BT, ZnO, HA, BFO. Boisseau and Loubaton [55] reported that artificial molecular assemblies, nanodevices, plus biomolecules exhibit biocompatible materials that facilitate cell therapy through growth, biodistribution, strong protection and drug delivery system. Nanodevices are also utilized for *in vivo* diagnostics like swallowable imaging drug for smart measurement of blood, glucose, biomarkers, and enzymes, proteins in different disease conditions such as diabetes, HIV/AIDS and cancer. Neel *et al* [56] reported that tissue engineering could transform the practice of dentistry and reconstruction surgery utilizing bionanomaterials and bioproducts of many periodontal diseases. The authors noted that a thorough understanding of genetics, stem cell embryology, plus cell and molecular biology is needed to manufacture and characterize many biomolecules.

10.4.2 Utilization of nanoparticles in the therapy of antimicrobial infections

The emergence of nanotechnology has played a remarkable role in curtailing several challenges linked with various antibacterial, antifungal, and antiviral drugs in the therapy of disease caused by microorganisms [57]. On this note, several groups of nanoparticles have been assessed for use to improve various medical uses while reducing the side effects during the therapy of maladies [58]. The mechanisms of action of the nanoparticles involve an increase in the drug's solubility, enhancement of the overall bioavailability, increase in the duration of circulation, focusing on the affected sites, and ease in overcoming of biological obstacles and efficient modulation of the release profile of drugs. Also, there are increasing documented proofs that there are promising potentials for reducing developed resistances and even a possible reversal through the application of techniques based nanomaterials, which involves the alteration of the route of delivery of the drugs, promotion of drug intake at the intracellular level, alternating of pathogen and drug interaction, and the conferring of anti-biofilm occurrence [59].

Anti-toxin-safe microorganisms have developed into a genuine danger to the wellbeing of humans. Among them, pathogenic microorganisms, such as *Staphylococcus* sp. and *Streptococcus* sp. were held accountable for different genuine illnesses [60]. Contaminations from bacteria and the sicknesses caused could prompt the death of an affected individual at the stage of infection. Xiong *et al* [61] utilized integrated Cu nanoparticles as a preservative and reducing agent. Tomar and Garg [62] reported that Au nanoparticles are now being used antimicrobially in distinguishing malignant cell growth. Fellahi *et al* [63] noticed during their work the antibacterial activity of Ag nanoparticles and Cu nanoparticles against *Escherichia coli.* Research uncovered that CuO nanoparticles demonstrated high antimicrobial potency against various bacterial strains, like *S. typhimurium, Proteus vulgaris, E. coli, E. faecalis* and *S. aureus*. They discovered that *E. faecalis* and *E. coli* introduced the most extreme susceptibility to CuO nanoparticles, while *Klebsiella pneumonia* was not affected [64]. Leung *et al* [65] reported that MgO nanoparticles appeared to have a great antimicrobial impact on microorganisms.

Although nanomaterials' mechanism against viral infections is still unclear, various nanomaterials have found their potential use in combating viral diseases. Antiviral medications should have the option to pervade through principle body obstructions to arrive at significant infection sites and are especially significant for AIDS treatment since significant human immunodeficiency infections (HIV) supplies are available in the bone marrow and fat tissue [66]. The improvement of nanocarriers for antiviral medications has just ended up being effective in dodging or limiting antiviral medications' most significant restrictions, especially through their small sizes. The principle attributes of each nanoparticle will impact the instruments associated with drug conveyance [67]. However, sometimes, these medications are insufficient, or they can cause basic results [68]. Medication opposition has additionally been accounted for. Hence, new compelling treatments are required. Over the most recent ten years, nanoparticles have arisen as a significant apparatus to battle infections [69]. Silver nanoparticles (AgNPs) were seen to exhibit antiviral action in the study of [70]. SARS-CoV-2 infection is the latest pandemic around the world. Social moderation systems and vague medication treatments have been actualized [71].

The scope and landscape of biotechnology and pharmaceutical sectors have been enhanced and broadened with the advent of nanotechnology in medicine. There are more than a hundred nanodrugs currently licensed for clinical use in various areas such as bioimaging, implantation of biomaterials and delivery of drugs. Nanomaterials' properties have made them potential antimicrobial agents in contrast to conventional antimicrobial agents [72]. Nanomedicine's potential in tackling various kinds of infectious disease caused by microorganisms has also been well documented [73]. Some nanomaterials used against bacteria and fungus are elaborated below.

10.4.2.1 For the treatment of bacterial diseases

The extracellular vesicles of bacteria are another unique kind of bacteria based nanoparticles. They are also known as the outer membrane vesicles (OMVs) with a bilayer spherical shape containing various nucleic acids and proteins. They have been assessed for potential application in biomimicry and as vehicles for drug delivery. The therapeutic use of extracellular vesicles derived from microbiota has also been examined [74]. Also, various compounds are present in these vesicles that have the potential to affect different pathways within the host. Aside from this, OMVs have been employed to formulate several useful nanomaterials that have coated bacterial membrane that is remarkable in nano-vaccination and bacteriocidal effects. The production of OMVs is by membrane budding or blebbing followed by isolations for different uses [75]. A remarkable effort has been put into the use of bionanomaterials in microbial diagnosis. In a related study on the medical use of nanoparticles in treating bacterial diseases, Lowery *et al* formulated a T2 (T2MR) based platform for diagnosis, capable of detecting rapidly several species of bacteria, including *Candida* species that are present in a blood sample. A significant change in the T2MR signals was observed due to the hybridization of an oligonucleotide using amplified DNA of Candida. The fabrication of magneto DNA nanoparticles for targeting the RNA of bacteria was done by Park *et al*, making microbes profiling in various samples easier. With the incorporation of the tiny NMR component to read out the signals, this assay can simultaneously detect and phenotype varying bacteria groups simultaneously [76].

There are numerous toxins produced by fungi and bacteria, which are grouped as exotoxins and endotoxins responsible for causing different infections in plants and animals. Findings from studies have shown the potencies of nanoparticles in biodetoxification through the neutralization of toxins. A typical example documented is the synthetically obtained nanoparticle based on various copolymers such as *N*-tert-butyl acrylamide and acrylic acid, which can detect and neutralize various toxicities of peptide toxin (melittin) through the electrostatic and hydrophobic mechanism of interaction [77]. Das *et al* [78] developed a nanoplatform capable of selectively neutralizing toxins due to cholera around the epithelial cells through nanoparticles monosialotetrahexosylganglioside coating on its surface and it was observed to be effective in attenuating the secretory responses of *V. cholera* in the models considered. Due to the minimal biodegradability of some acryl compounds in a physiological environment, there is a need to assess and ensure safety in *in vivo* applications. The current use of lipid-based membrane developed more recently, which helps the neutralization of toxins efficiently.

Similarly, Henry *et al* [79] formulated liposomes made of sphingomyelin based on the known compositions of the plasma membrane, which include sphingolipids, cholesterol and glycerophospholipid. This new formulation provides easy removal of toxins across the membrane. The use of these artificial liposomes also enhances the efficient sequencing of a wide range of toxins produced by varieties of bacteria, including streptococcal and staphylococcal pathogens. The use of liposomes capable of absorbing exotoxins intravenously also results in a significant rescuing of the studied mice from *S. pneumonia*. Also, *in vivo* efficacy of liposomes can be improved through combination with antibiotic treatment, as illustrated in using a model antibiotic known as vancomycin. As a result of the presence of toxins receptors, there is a spontaneous reaction of natural lipoproteins with different toxins that are membrane-active, bringing about the abrogation of the lytic effects [80].

In a study by Fang *et al* [77], it was reported that nanostructures that are cell membrane functionalized could act as decoys that neutralize toxins. Apart from the area of diagnosis of infections due to bacteria, bionanomaterials have also been employed to determine the metabolic activities of bacteria. In a related study, Perez and co-workers designed two SPION-based assays to assess bacterial susceptibility to antibiotics present in blood using magnetic relaxation. The two main antibiotic resistance mechanisms that prevent toxicity due to the high contents of antimicrobial drugs are increased drug efflux and uptake reduction. An extra barrier against uptake is provided by the outer membrane of bacteria such as *E. coli* and *P. aeruginosa*, which are Gram-negative, resulting in lower susceptibility to some hydrophobic antibiotics. It has been reported by Singh *et al* [81] that a number of vehicles for the delivery of nanoparticles tend to compromise these mechanisms of resistance. The fusogenic liposome that is made up of lipids can fuse very fast with the microorganism's cell membrane, resulting in the release of a high dose of the drug into the cytoplasm, which could lead to saturation of the pumps of trans-membrane [82]. Various nanomaterials and conjugated nanomaterials have shown their antibacterial activity against bacteria, but still there is a lot of room left to explore antibacterial efficiency of nanomaterials.

10.4.2.2 For the treatment of fungal diseases

Synthesis of the nanoparticles has been done using various fungal and bacteria components to realize the focused treatment of fungal and bacterial diseases easily. For effective entrance into the targeted cells, identifying the various interactive mechanisms within biomolecules on the fungi and bacteria membrane is the first stage. A typical example was the use of chitosan obtained from the cell wall of *C. neoformans* in the formulations of nanomaterials bringing about a drug delivery mechanism that is *Neoformans* targeting [83]. Fungi have recently developed strains with high resistance to several drugs, both conventional and modern synthetic. On this basis, nanomaterials can also be utilized to overcome various drug resistance mechanisms such as rise in the efflux of drugs from microbial cells, fall in absorption, the formation of biofilm and intracellular. There is high accuracy in delivering drugs in the right doses to the site of infections using nanoparticles with a marked reduction in adverse reactions [84]. There are few known antifungal agents as well as problems associated with the development of resistance and toxicity. There is, therefore, a pressing need for an alternative. The nanoparticle is useful in this dimension in conveying antifungal drugs, reducing toxicity, and ensuring effective targeting. Nanomaterials were first employed for antifungal therapy in the 1990s with the formulation of Amphotericin B. There are different antifungal drug delivery systems, such as dendrimers, polymeric nanomaterials, and liposomes, with each system having its advantages and disadvantages. It brings about a rise in the antifungal potentials, including bioavailability of drugs, decrease in overall toxicity, thus enhancing innovative therapeutic approaches [85].

One of the groups of the most difficult disease to be controlled globally is the Mycoses. Invasive mycoses could be predisposed to some conditions, for example, neoplasia, chronic diseases and immunosuppression. The most common diseases caused by fungi are vaginal and oral candidiasis. These mycoses at the superficial level usually affect 25% to 30% of the human population [86]. Few studies exist on the antifungal potential aided by dendrimers. The solubility of clotrimazole and its impact against fungi, especially of the species, was improved by polyamidoamine dendrimers [87]. Janiszewska *et al* [88], in their work, reported that the antifungal potential of dendrimeric lipopeptides results in morphological alterations in the fungal cells as well as inhibition of enzymatic activities.

Not much study has been done on the antifungal potential for other delivery systems, for example, CNTs and silica nanotubes. CNTs have been well explored globally for other applications. In a related study, Benincasa *et al* [89] reported that AmB conjugated with CNTs was useful against isolates of *Candida* sp. using scanning electron microscopy; the potency against fungi and bacteria was shown. The results revealed that the cells of microorganisms were trapped and wrapped by the CNTs' networks. Antifungal potentials against *Aspergillus oryzae, Fusarium oxysporum* and *Aspergillus niger* have been reported in nanosheets of graphene oxide. Cui *et al* [90], in their study, reported graphene oxide as a unique two-dimensional nanomaterial that could be employed as health biomedicines with remarkable antifungal potential. Hussein *et al* reported the antimicrobial potential of nanoparticles packed with ampicillin forming a nanocomposite that brought about a reduction in the activity of *C. albicans* [91]. Niemirowicz *et al* [92] documented the inhibiting potential of nanoparticles on the growth of *C. albicans.* The growth was inhibited in samples from blood, cerebrospinal fluid, and human plasma. Gold nanoparticle (AuNPs) can subvert the cell layer of the microorganism via direct cooperation with proteins and lipids. Rózalska *et al* [93] considered the potency of AgNPs against *C. albicans* and *C. parapsilosis*, and then discovered that the nanoparticles were potent at reduced concentration with a zone of inhibition ranging from (1.56–6.25 $\mu g\ mL^{-1}$), indicating no cytotoxic effects. The individuals from the variety of *Aspergillus* infection are depicted as pioneering microorganisms fit for inciting hypersensitive responses to fundamental diseases in people, and nanoparticles were found to be effective against *Aspergillus* sp. [94].

10.4.3 Use of nanotechnology in biosensors

Broza and Haick [95] reported that rapid and recent development in the field of nanobiotechnology had expanded the frontiers of medical sciences in the utilization of sensors and other biosensor techniques for the analysis of many disease conditions and biomolecules in the environment and human body, which are capable of altering metabolic pathways. The biosensor is defined as a device containing a physicochemical detector, which enables detection of the desired analyte with the help of a biological component [96]. These biosensors can detect fluctuations in biomarkers and molecules through bio-tracking in many diseases such as cancer, diabetes, obesity and hypertension. The authors noted that the physiological measurement of many biomolecules such as uric acid, dopamine, glucose, peptides, DNAs, proteins, enzymes, antigens, and hormones in disease conditions is an important aspect of therapeutic management associated diseases. Fluctuations or depletions in many of these biomolecules are correlated with abnormal physiological regulations such as diabetes, Parkinson's, Alzheimer's, renal disease and Lesch–Nyhan syndrome, and metabolic syndrome hypertension, cardiovascular disease, gout, oxidative stress, and multiple sclerosis. The authors noted that carbonaceus nanomaterials serve as a novel biomaterial that could be utilized to manufacture and design portable, cost-effective, rapid and fast response nanobiosensor devices. The characteristics of carbon nanoparticles, nanodiamonds, carbon nanohorns, nanodots such as tunable electrical, photoluminescence properties, nanoscale size, high photostability, chemical inertness, biocompatibility have prompted the interest of many biomedical scientists in the adoption and construction of these chemical vapor sensors or biosensors that can detect biomolecules and biomarkers from serum, urine, and tears.

Studies have indicated that non-invasive sampling techniques have gained more popularity in the medical practice to diagnose diseases [97]. These biosensors are designed to detect either single target or multiple biomarkers simultaneously. Many diseases are interrelated in terms of biomarkers. Thus, in the design of biomarkers based biosensors, the analytical performance plus the kinetics should be allowed for comparison, high sensitivity, stable and selective to differentiate different biomarkers, and link to a particular dysfunction. Senf *et al* [97] reported that disease prevention is based on early detection and accurate diagnosis of diseases using biomarkers from body fluids such as saliva, blood, sweat, and urine. Yezdani *et al* [98] revealed that nanoelectronic biosensors are rapidly gaining attention in medical applications for disease detection, diagnosis, screening and treatment. The huge potential in DNA sequencing using nanopores, drug delivery systems, and single-virus detection has greatly impacted the medical sciences such as physiology and biophysics, bioengineering, molecular biology, immunology, medicine, pharmacy, etc. In cancer physiology, nanobiomaterials are utilized for cancer detection and therapy and other neurodegenerative diseases such as Alzheimer's, Parkinson's and epilepsy. The characteristic physiological feathers like high surface area, nanoscale effects, biocompatibility, charge, agglomeration and solubility of the nanobiomaterials in the human body makes them suitable for medical applications such as gene and drug delivery, diagnostic biosensors, biomedical imaging, analytical, therapeutic and detection purposes plus procedures, like targeting diabetes, cancer, and infertility, improving material–cell interactions, drug delivery, scaffolds for tissue regeneration, innovative approaches in the fight against incurable diseases. Today, nanoparticles' physiological applications include cancer imaging techniques, delivery transporters, genomics science, artificial intelligence and robotics, computational modeling, stem cell physiology and pharmaceuticals through nanosystems, nanodevices, nanoimplants, nanodrugs. Medical scientists are currently utilizing nanobiotechnology to detect, diagnose, and treat cancer, diabetes, gout, neurodegenerative diseases, cardiovascular diseases, and reproductive dysfunctions.

Nasimi and Haidari [99] reported that drugs are now being encapsulated in nanoparticles for effective delivery systems, reduced side effects, and dosage. The authors also noted that nanotechnology is currently utilized to diagnose and detect diseases such as atherosclerosis, diabetes, cancer, and other cardiovascular dysfunction. The characteristic physiological features of nanoparticles like specificity, biodegradability, nontoxicity, and bio-availability enable them to be a highly attractive platform for many medical and biological applications such as biomolecular recognition and biosensing bioimaging and therapeutic delivery. In medical sciences, medical imaging has advanced tremendously as a tool for diagnosing many diseases. These techniques involve *in vivo* and *in vitro* analysis, which includes optical imaging (OI), ultrasound imaging (USI), magnetic resonance imaging (MRI), and positron emission tomography (PET) for many biological samples. Nasimi and Haidari [99] also noted that nanobiosensors such as nanotubes, cantilevers, nanowires, and atomic force microscopy are being utilized to detect and diagnose several diseases with their sensitivity, specificity, and accuracy. These biosensors have encapsulated nanoparticles for specific chemokines, tumor cells, antibodies, and biomarkers to rapidly detect diseases.

Noah and Ndangili [100] revealed that timely detection, rapid diagnosis utilizing smart data analysis, informatics analysis and bionanotechnology is key for the detection and screening of analytes, biomolecules, enzymes, biomarkers, and antibodies such as nucleic acids, sugars, proteins, whole cells, circulating tumor cells, extracellular vesicles cytogenetic parameters, small metabolites and cytokinetic parameters in disease conditions to start early treatment protocol. For bioanalytical performance, the authors suggested that biosensors for electrochemical enzymatic measurements are critical components as point-of-care tools for personalized health care management. Today, diabetes monitoring utilizing graphene-based glucose biosensor using chitosan and graphene is becoming more popular among medical scientists. Nanobiotechnology is currently utilized to diagnose and detect infectious diseases such as malaria, dengue fever, viral hepatitis, cholera, avian influenza, severe respiratory syndrome, lassa fever, and COVID-19. Bionanosensors have very high sensitivity, accuracy, specificity, robustness, are inexpensive and user friendly technology promoting the rapid prevention and prompt treatment of diverse infectious diseases. These biosensors utilize portable magnetic barcode assay systems for different biological molecules such as antibodies, biomarkers, enzymes, metabolites and antigens from urine, saliva, tears, and blood to detect infections diseases. For instance, detection of β-hematin utilizing biosensors in the serum of patients has been correlated to malaria parasite infections, the nanoplasmonic-based sensor for the detection of HIV from immobilized antibodies like HIV-1 capsid antigen p24 in human serum, anti-cardiac troponin 1 for cardiovascular diseases, and anti-cyclic

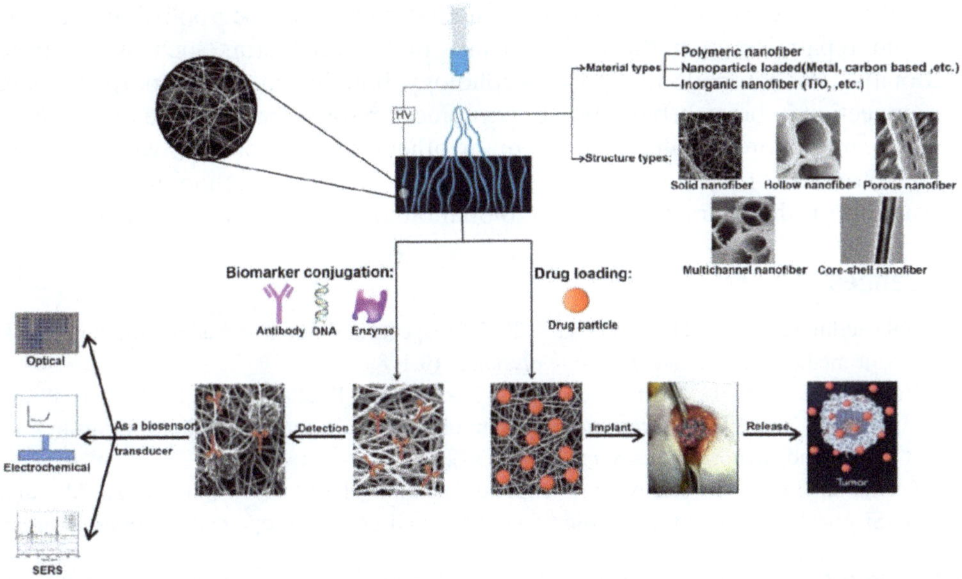

Figure 10.3. Various fabricated forms of nanofibres and their potential applications in diagnosing and treating various types of cancers. Reproduced with permission from [104].

citrullinated peptide for rheumatoid arthritis, immunosensor detection of soluble egg antigen for the detection of bilharzia, schistosome infection [101].

Salata [102] and Buzea *et al* [103] reported that many biomaterials display desirable characteristics relevant to many industrial applications. They noted that nanomaterial manufacturing and industries increase the exposure of many individuals to nanotoxicity. Thus relevant stakeholders should develop laws and policies for safety management of every aspect of nanotechnology. Asghari *et al* [104] reported that environmental stress causing several diseases, particularly cancer, has caused a significant increase in the development of cost-effective biosensors for early detection and diagnosis of disease progression. Figure 10.3 depicts various fabricated forms of nanofibres and their potential applications in diagnosing and treating various types of cancers [104]. There have been identified several important biomaterials for bioengineering applications such as electrospun nanofibers, and polymeric materials for the manufacturing of paper-based microfluidic biosensors. Further, it was also revealed that many nanobiomaterials such as gold nanoparticles, quantum dots, magnetic nanoparticles, gold nanowires, and CNTs could be developed into biosensors for the detection of biomarkers, proteins, DNA fragments, antibody fragments, RNA fragments, enzymes, antigens, and cytokines in cancer detection with great precision, accuracy plus sensitivity.

10.5 Conclusion

This chapter has provided detailed information on utilizing bionanomaterials with the wider application of green bionanotechnology, especially in the biomedical sector. It was discovered that some bionanomaterials could be applied as regenerative and repair issues in the body because of several factors such as substrate functionality, biocompatibility, pore morphology, bonding chemistry, porosity, pore interconnectivity, bioresorbability, topographical parameters, surface-area-to-volume ratio, micropore architectures and many others. The comprehensive application of bionanomaterial as an antimicrobial agent was also highlighted. Relevant information on the characterization of bionanomaterial was also highlighted.

References

[1] Fakruddin Md, Zakir H and Hafsa A 2012 Prospects and applications of nanobiotechnology: a medical perspective *J. Nanobiotechnol.* **10** 1–8

[2] Valo H, Peltonen L, Vehviläinen S, Karjalainen M, Kostiainen R, Laaksonen T and Hirvonen J 2015 Electrospray encapsulation of hydrophilic and hydrophobic drugs in poly (L-lactic acid) nanoparticles *Small Mol.* **5** 1791–8

[3] Olakanmi E O 2013 Selective laser sintering/melting (SLS/SLM) of pure Al, Al–Mg, and Al–Si powders: Effect of processing conditions and powder properties *J. Mater. Process. Technol.* **213** 1387–405

[4] Singh R P and Singh K R B 2021 Nanobiotechnology in animal production and health ed S Mondal and R L Singh *Advances in. Animal Genomics* (Amsterdam: Elsevier) pp 185–98

[5] Nguyen P T N, Salim C, Kurniawan W and Hinode H 2014 A non-hydrolytic sol–gel synthesis of reduced graphene oxide/TiO_2 microsphere photocatalysts *Catal. Today* **230** 166–73

[6] Siavash I, Hassan K, Seyed V and Mirmohammadi B Z 2014 Green and sustainable synthesis of nanomaterials *Synth. Silver Nanopart.: Chem., Phys. Biol. Meth. Res. Pharmaceut. Sci.* **9** 385–406

[7] Singh K R, Nayak V, Sarkar T and Singh R P 2020 Cerium oxide nanoparticles: properties, biosynthesis and biomedical application *RSC Adv.* **10** 27194–214

[8] Fernandes M, Singh K R, Sarkar T, Singh P and Singh R P 2020 Recent applications of magnesium oxide (MgO) nanoparticles in various domains *Adv. Mater. Lett.* **11** 20081543

[9] Rossi M, Cubadda F, Dini L, Terranova M L, Aureli F, Sorbo A and Passeri D 2014 Scientific basis of nanotechnology, implications for the food sector and future trend *Trends Food Sci. Technol.* **40** 127–48

[10] Torres F G, Troncoso O P, Pisani A, Gatto F and Bardi G 2019 Natural polysaccharide nanomaterials: an overview of their immunological properties *Int. J. Mol. Sci.* **20** 5092

[11] Favier V, Chanzy H and Cavaille J Y 1996 Polymer nanocomposites reinforced by cellulose whiskers *V. J. Macromol.* **28** 6365–7

[12] Bondeson D and Oksman K 2007 Polylactic acid/cellulose whisker nanocomposites modified by polyvinyl alcohol *J. Compos. Part* A **38** 2486–92

[13] Grunert M and Winter W T 2002 Nanocomposites of cellulose acetate butyrate reinforced with cellulose nanocrystals *J. Polym. Environ.* **10** 27–30

[14] Tokoh C, Takabe K, Fujita M and Saiki H 1998 Cellulose synthesized by acetobacter xylinum in the presence of acetyl glucomannan *J. Cellulose* **5** 249–61

[15] Khan I, Saeed K and Khan I 2019 Nanoparticles: Properties, applications and toxicities *Arabian J. Chem.* **12** 908–31

[16] Gan Y X, Jayatissa A H, Yu Z, Chen X and Li M 2020 Hydrothermal synthesis of nanomaterials *J. Nanomater.* **2020** 8917013

[17] Fuchigami T, Kawamura R, Kitamoto Y, Nakagawa M and Namiki Y 2012 *Biomaterials* **33** 1682

[18] Kluge J, Muhrer G and Mazzotti M 2019 High pressure homogenization of pharmaceutical solids *J. Supercrit. Fluids* **66** 380–8

[19] Zhang X, Liu Z, Shen W and Gurunathan S 2016 Silver nanoparticles: synthesis, characterization, properties, applications, and therapeutic approaches *Int. J. Mol. Sci.* **17** 1534

[20] Mathew A P, Laborie M P G and Oksman K 2009 Cross-linked chitosan/chitin crystal nanocomposites with improved permeation selectivity and pH stability *J. Biomacromol.* **10** 1627–32

[21] Mao A S and Mooney D J 2009 Regenerative medicine: Current therapies and future directions *PNAS* **112** 14452–97

[22] Abadias G 2018 Review article: Stress in thin films and coatings: Current status, challenges, and prospects *J. Vac. Sci. Technol.* A **36** 020801

[23] Sindhu R, Binod P and Pandey A 2015 Microbial poly-3-hydroxybutyrate and related copolymers *Industrial Biorefineries and White Biotechnology* (Amsterdam: Elsevier) pp 575–605

[24] Sahayaraj K 2012 Bionanomaterials: Synthesis and Applications *Proc. of the First National Seminar on New Materials Research and Nanotechnology (NSNMRN 2012) ((12–14 Sept. 2012, Govt. Arts College, Ooty. TamiiNadu))*

[25] Sanpui P, Chattopadhyay A and Ghosh S S 2011 Induction of Apoptosis in Cancer Cells at Low Silver Nanoparticle Concentrations using Chitosan Nanocarrier *ACS Appl. Mater. Interfaces* **3** 218–28

[26] Guo D L *et al* 2013 Anti-leukemia activity of PVP-coated silver nanoparticles via generation of reactive oxygen species and release of silver ions *Biomaterials* **34** 7884–94

[27] Fan W, Lai Q, Zhang Q and Wang Y 2011 Nanocomposites of TiO_2 and reduced graphene oxide as efficient photocatalysts for hydrogen evolution *J. Phys. Chem.* C **115** 10694–701

[28] Uddin A J, Araki J, Fujie M, Sembo S and Gotoh Y 2012 Interfacial interaction and mechanical properties of chitin whisker-poly(vinyl alcohol) gel-spun nanocomposite fibers *Polym. Int.* **61** 1010–15

[29] Kumirska J, Czerwicka M, Kaczyński Z, Bychowska A, Brzozowski K and Stepnowski J 2010 Application of spectroscopic methods for structural analysis of chitin and chitosan *Mar. Drugs* **8** 1567–636

[30] Nayak V, Singh K R, Singh A K and Singh R P 2021 Potentialities of selenium nanoparticles in biomedical science *New J. Chem.* **45** 2849–78

[31] Singh R P and Singh K R B 2021 Introduction to composite naterials *Composite Materials* 1st edn (Boca Raton, FL: CRC Press) pp 1–28

[32] Neves L S, Rodrigues M T, Reis R L and Gomes M E 2016 Current approaches and future perspectives on strategies for the development of personalized tissue engineering therapies *Exp. Rev. Prec. Med. Drug Dev.* **1** 93–108

[33] Xavier J R, Desai P, Varanasi V G, Al-Hashimi I and Gaharwar A K 2015 Advanced nanomaterials: promises for improved dental tissue regeneration *Nanotechnology in Endodontics* (Cham: Springer) pp 5–22

[34] Chen G, Qi Y, Niu L, Tuoyu D, Jinwei Z, Tingting F and Weiqi Y 2015 Application of the cell sheet technique in tissue engineering (Review) *Biomed. Rep.* **3** 749–57

[35] Sidhu P, Kumar S, Kumar K, Vyas V, Vyas R, Dhillon P S and Kaur T 2020 Recent advances in tissue engineering and regenerative medicine *Biomed. J. Sci. Tech. Res.* **26** 19733–9

[36] Bhat S and Kumar A 2012 Biomaterials in regenerative medicine *J. Postgrad. Med. Edu. Res* **46** 81–9

[37] Abdulghani S and Mitchell G R 2019 Biomaterials for *in situ* tissue regeneration: a review *Biomolecules* **9** 1–24

[38] Mostafavi E, Medina-Cruz D K, Kalantari A T, Soltantabar P and Thomas J W 2020 Electroconductive nanobiomaterials for tissue engineering and regenerative medicine *Bioelectricity* **2** 2

[39] Pogorielov M, Oleshko O and Hapchenko A 2017 Tissue engineering: challenges and selected application *Adv. Tiss. Eng. Regener. Med.* **3** 330–4

[40] Tao O, Wu D T, Pham H M, Pandey N and Tran S D 2019 Nanomaterials in craniofacial tissue regeneration: a review *Appl. Sci.* **9** 1–13

[41] Banigo A T, Iwuji S C and Iheaturu N 2019 Application of biomaterials in tissue engineering: a review *J. Chem. Pharmaceut. Res* **11** 1–16

[42] Shi C, Yuan Z, Han F, Zhu C and Li B 2016 Polymeric biomaterials for bone regeneration *Ann. Joint* **1** 1–14

[43] Ansari M 2019 Bone tissue regeneration: biology, strategies and interface studies *Prog. Biomater.* **8** 223–37

[44] Lowe B, Hardy J G and Walsh L J 2020 Optimizing nanohydroxyapatite nanocomposites for bone tissue engineering *ACS Omega* **5** 1–9

[45] Idumah C I 2020 Progress in polymer nanocomposites for bone regeneration and engineering *Polym. Polym. Compos.* 1–19

[46] Nair L S, Bhattacharyya S and Laurencin C T 2006 Nanotechnology and tissue engineering: the scaffold based approach *Nanotechnologies for the Life Sciences* vol 9 (New York: Wiley)

[47] Engel E, Michiardi A, Navarro M, Damien L and Planell J A 2007 Nanotechnology in regenerative medicine: the materials side *Trends Biotechnol.* **26** 39–47

[48] Rodríguez-Vázquez M, Vega-Ruiz B, Ramos-Zúñiga R, Saldaña-Koppel D A and Quiñones-Olvera L F 2015 Chitosan and its potential use as a scaffold for tissue engineering in regenerative medicine *BioMed Res. Int.* **2015** 821279

[49] Frey B, Steffen M and Zeisberger S P H 2016 Tissue engineering and regenerative medicine —new initiatives for individual treatment offers *Transfus. Med. Hemother.* **1–24** 318–9

[50] Pina S, Oliveira J M and Reis R L 2014 Natural-based nanocomposites for bone tissue engineering and regenerative medicine: a review *Adv. Mater.* **2915** 1–27

[51] Salata O V 2004 Applications of nanoparticles in biology and medicine *J. Nanobiotechnol.* **2** 1–6

[52] España-Sánchez B L *et al* 2018 Trends in tissue regeneration: bio-banomaterials *Tissue Regeneration* (Rijeka: InTech) pp 218–28

[53] Hill M J *et al* 2019 Nanomaterials for bone tissue regeneration: updates and future perspectives *Nanomedicine* **14** 22

[54] Kapat K, Shubhra Q T H, Zhou M and Leeuwenburgh S 2020 Piezoelectric nano-biomaterials for biomedicine and tissue regeneration *Adv. Funct. Mater.* **30** 1909045

[55] Boisseau P and Loubaton B 2012 Nanoscience and nanotechnologies: hopes and concerns *C R Phys.* **12** 620–36

[56] Neel E A A, Chrzanowski W, Salih V M, Kim H-W and Knowles J C 2014 Tissue engineering in dentistry *J. Dentistry* **2** 915–28

[57] Milovanovic M, Arsenijevic A, Milovanovic J, Kanjevac T and Arsenijevic N 2017 Nanoparticles in antiviral therapy *Antimicrobial Nanoarchitectonics* ed A M Grumezescu (Amsterdam: Elsevier) 383–410

[58] Xiong M H, Bao Y, Yang X Z, Zhu Y H and Wang J 2014 Delivery of antibiotics with polymeric particles *Adv. Drug Deliv. Rev.* **78** 63–76

[59] Han C, Romero N, Fischer S, Dookran J, Berger A and Doiron A L 2017 Recent developments in the use of nanoparticles for treatment of biofilms *Nanotechnol. Rev.* **6** 383–404

[60] Olishevska S, Nickzad A and Déziel E 2019 *Bacillus* and *Paenibacillus* secreted polyketides and peptides involved in controlling human and plant pathogens *Appl. Microbiol. Biotechnol.* **103** 1189–215

[61] Xiong J, Wang Y, Xue Q and Wu X 2011 Synthesis of highly stable dispersions of nanosized copper particles using L-ascorbic acid *Green Chem.* **13** 900–4

[62] Tomar A and Garg G 2013 Short review on application of gold nanoparticles *Glob. J. Pharmacol* **7** 34–8

[63] Fellahi O, Sarma R, Das M, Saikia R, Marcon L and Coffinier Y 2013 The antimicrobial effect of silicon nanowires decorated with silver and copper nanoparticles *Nanotechnology* **24** 495101–12

[64] Ahamed M, Alhadlaq H A, Khan M A, Karuppiah P and Al-Dhabi N A 2014 Synthesis, characterization, and antimicrobial activity of copper oxide nanoparticles *J. Nanomater.* **2014** 637858

[65] Leung Y H, Ng A M, Xu X, Shen Z, Gethings L A and Wong M T *et al* 2014 Mechanisms of antibacterial activity of MgO: non-ROS mediated toxicity of MgO nanoparticles towards *Escherichia coli Small* **10** 1171–83

[66] Wallet C M *et al* 2019 Microglial cells: the main HIV-1 reservoir in the brain *Front. Cell. Infect. Microbiol.* **9** 362

[67] Cojocaru F D, Botezat D, Gardikiotis I, Uritu G, Dodi L, Trandafir C, Rezus E, Rezus B I, Tamba and Mihai C T 2020 Nanomaterials designed for antiviral drug delivery transport across biological barriers *Pharmaceutics* **12** 171

[68] Antipov E and Pokryshevskaya E 2019 The effects of adverse drug reactions on patients' satisfaction: evidence from publicly available data on Tamiflu (oseltamivir) *Int. J. Med. Inform.* **125** 30

[69] Rudramurthy G R and Swamy M K 2018 Potential applications of engineered nanoparticles in medicine and biology: an update *J. Biol. Inorg. Chem.* **23** 1185

[70] Morris D, Ansar M, Speshock J, Ivanciuc I, Qu Y, Casola A and Garofalo R 2019 Antiviral and immunomodulatory activity of silver nanoparticles in experimental RSV infection *Viruses* **11** 732

[71] Sallard E, Lescure F X, Yazdanpanah Y, Mentre F and Peiffer-Smadja N 2020 Type 1 interferons as a potential treatment against COVID-19 *Antivir. Res.* **178** 104791

[72] Hemeg H A 2017 Nanomaterials for alternative antibacterial therapy *Int. J. Nanomed.* **12** 8211–25

[73] Patra J K *et al* 2018 Nano based drug delivery systems: recent developments and future prospects *J. Nanobiotechnol.* **16** 71

[74] Guerrero-Mandujano A, Hernández-Cortez C, Ibarra J A and Castro-Escarpulli G 2017 The outer membrane vesicles: secretion system type zero: OMVs as type zero secretion system *Traffic* **18** 425–32

[75] Brown L, Wolf J M, Prados-Rosales R and Casadevall A 2015 Through the wall: extracellular vesicles in gram-positive bacteria, mycobacteria and fungi *Nat. Rev. Microbiol.* **13** 620–30

[76] Park K S *et al* 2016 A magneto-DNA nanoparticle system for the rapid and sensitive diagnosis of enteric fever *Sci. Rep.* **6** 32878

[77] Fang J H, Lee Y T, Chiang W H and Hu S H 2015 Magnetoresponsive virus-mimetic nanocapsules with dual heat-triggered sequential-infected multiple drug-delivery approach for combinatorial tumor therapy *Small* **11** 2417–28

[78] Das S, Angsantikul P, Le C, Bao D, Miyamoto Y and Gao W 2018 Neutralization of cholera toxin with nanoparticle decoys for treatment of cholera *PLOS Negl. Trop. D.* **12** e0006266

[79] Henry B D, Neill D R, Becker K A, Gore S, Bricio-Moreno L and Ziobro R 2015 Engineered liposomes sequester bacterial exotoxins and protect from severe invasive infections in mice *Nat. Biotechnol.* **33** 81–8

[80] Bozzuto G and Molinari A 2015 Liposomes as nanomedical devices *Int. J. Nanomed.* **10** 975–99

[81] Singh R, Smitha M S and Singh S P 2014 The role of nanotechnology in combating multi-drug resistant bacteria *J. Nanosci. Nanotechnol.* **14** 4745–56

[82] Gupta S and Kumar P 2012 Drug delivery using nanocarriers: Indian perspective *Proc. Natl. Acad. Sci., India, Sect. B Biol. Sci.* **82** 167–206

[83] Ali M A *et al* 2020 Advancements in plant and microbe-based synthesis of metallic nanoparticles and their antimicrobial activity against plant pathogens *Nanomaterials* **10** 1146

[84] Varier K M 2019 Nanoparticles: antimicrobial applications and its prospects *Advanced Nanostructured Materials for Environmental Remediation. Environmental Chemistry for a Sustainable World* vol 25 ed M Naushad, S Rajendran and F Gracia (Cham: Springer)

[85] Srinivasan A, Lopez-Ribot J L and Ramasubramanian K A 2014 Overcoming antifungal resistance *Drug Discov. Today Technol.* **11** 65–71

[86] Ramos-E-Silva M, Lima C M O, Schechtman R C, Trope B M and Carneiro S 2010 Superficial mycoses in immunodepressed patients (AIDS) *Clin. Dermatol.* **28** 217–25

[87] Winnicka K, Sosnowska K, Wieczorek P, Sacha P T and Tryniszewska E 2011 Poly (amidoamine) dendrimers increase antifungal activity of clotrimazole *Biol. Pharm. Bull.* **34** 1129–33

[88] Janiszewska J, Sowińska M, Rajnisz A, Solecka J, Łącka I, Milewski S and Urbańczyk-Lipkowska Z 2012 Novel dendrimeric lipopeptides with antifungal activity panel *Bioorg. Med. Chem.* **22** 1388–93

[89] Benincasa M, Pacor S, Wu W, Prato M, Bianco A and Gennaro R 2011 Antifungal activity of amphotericin B conjugated to carbon nanotubes *ACS Nano* **5** 199–208

[90] Cui J, Yang Y, Zheng M, Liu Y, Xiao Y, Lei B and Chen W 2014 Facile fabrication of graphene oxide loaded with silver nanoparticles as antifungal materials *Mater. Res. Express* **1** 045007

[91] Hussein-Al-Ali S, El Zowalaty M, Hussein M Z, Geilich B and Webster T 2014 Synthesis, characterization, and antimicrobial activity of an ampicillin-conjugated magnetic nano-antibiotic for medical applications *Int. J. Nanomed.* **9** 3801–14

[92] Niemirowicz K, Durnaś B, Tokajuk G, Piktel E, Michalak G, Gu X, Kułakowska A, Savage P B and Bucki R 2017 *Sci. Rep.* **7** 4610

[93] Różalska B, Sadowska B, Budzyńska A, Bernat P, Różalska S and Mukherjee A 2018 Biogenic nanosilver synthesized in *Metarhizium robertsii* waste mycelium extract—as a modulator of *Candida albicans* morphogenesis, membrane lipidome and biofilm *PLoS One* **13** e0194254

[94] Paulussen C, Hallsworth J E, Álvarez-Pérez S, Nierman W C, Hamill P G and Blain D 2017 Ecology of aspergillosis: insights into the pathogenic potency of *Aspergillus fumigatus* and some other *Aspergillus* species *Microb. Biotechnol.* **10** 296–322

[95] Broza Y Y and Haick H 2013 Nanomaterial-based sensors for detection of disease by volatile organic compounds *Nanomedicine* **8** 785–806

[96] Singh R P 2016 Nanobiosensors: potentiality towards bioanalysis *J. Bioanal. Biomed.* **8** e143

[97] Senf B, Woon-Hong Y and Jong-Hoon K 2020 Recent advances in portable biosensors for biomarker detection in body fluids *Biosensors* **10** 1–23

[98] Yezdani U, Khan M, Kushwah N, Verma A and Khan F 2018 Application of nanotechnology in diagnosis and treatment of various diseases and its future advances in medicine *World J. Pharm. Pharmaceut. Sci. SJIF* **7** 1611–33

[99] Nasimi P and Haidari M 2013 Medical use of nanoparticles: drug delivery and diagnosis diseases *Int. J. Green Nanotechnol* **1** 1–5

[100] Noah N and Ndangili P 2019 Current trends of nanobiosensors for point-of-care diagnostics *Hindawi J. Anal. Meth. Chem.* **2019** 2179718

[101] Qasim M, Lim D J, Park H and Na D 2014 Nanotechnology for diagnosis and treatment of infectious diseases *J. Nanosci. Nanotechnol.* **14** 7374–87

[102] Salata O V 2004 Applications of nanoparticles in biology and medicine *J. Nanobiotechnol.* **2** 1–6

[103] Buzea C, Pacheco I I and Robbie K 2007 Nanomaterials and nanoparticles: sources and toxicity *Biointerphases* **2** MR17–71

Angellie H, Molina-Boisseau S, Lebrun L and Dufresne A 2005 Processing and structural properties of waxy maize starch nanocrystals reinforced natural rubber *J. Macromol.* **38** 3783–92

[104] Asghari S, Rezaei Z and Mahmoudifard M 2020 Electrospun nanofibers: a promising horizon toward detection and treatment of cancer *Analyst* **145** 2854–72

Lightning Source UK Ltd.
Milton Keynes UK
UKHW021424140821
388797UK00003B/72

9 780750 337656